George A. Patterson

RESPIRATORY PHYSIOLOGY

RESPIRATORY PHYSIOLOGY

N. BALFOUR SLONIM, M.D., Ph.D.
Director, Cardiopulmonary Diagnostic Laboratory,
Denver, Colorado

LYLE H. HAMILTON, Ph.D.
Principal Scientist, Wood VA Center;
Professor of Physiology and Director, Clinical Physiology Section
The Medical College of Wisconsin,
Milwaukee, Wisconsin

SECOND EDITION

With 77 illustrations

SAINT LOUIS
The C. V. Mosby Company

1971

SECOND EDITION

Second printing

Previous edition copyrighted 1967

Printed in the United States of America

Standard Book Number 8016-4666-9

Library of Congress Catalog Card Number 76-172884

Distributed in Great Britain by Henry Kimpton, London

PREFACE

The major objective of this monograph is to present clearly and concisely the physiology of respiration. We have stressed fundamental principles and also indicated the applications of the basic science to the clinical practice of medicine. We have further attempted to identify and to propound the pressing problems of the field and to distinguish established fact from unproved speculation. We hope the reader will sense our fascination with this vital subject. We aim to pique his curiosity for the unanswered questions of respiratory physiology.

The present material is the product of experience gained in both teaching physiology and practicing medicine. This book is designed primarily for the medical student, but it should also prove useful to the physician, the physiologist, and the environmental scientist. Paramedical personnel, such as nurses, anesthetists, and inhalation therapists, will find some sections of interest.

Almost all the illustrations have been drawn especially for this monograph. The illustrative material includes electron micrographs of healthy human lung. In addition to the standard material, the text contains material on the respiratory aspects of pH homeostasis (Chapter 10), the respiratory physiology of the newborn (Chapter 13), respiratory responses to unusual environments and special atmospheres (Chapter 14), and the clinical evaluation of pulmonary function (Chapter 15). The Appendix includes a table of symbols and abbreviations for respiratory physiology and a set of equations for use in respiratory calculations. A glossary of key terms follows the Appendix.

We are keenly aware that mathematics is the language of science and therefore of physiology, lending itself to objective, precisely quantitative, and unambiguous expression. In this regard we have aimed for a realistic balance, to avoid the delusion of mathematical precision on the one hand and the misfortune of unnecessary complication on the other.

We are sorry to have had to omit, for the sake of brevity, the names of many contributors to the field of respiratory physiology, as well as the specific references to their published works. However, we believe that the inclusion of such a large and constantly increasing volume of detail would defeat the objective of this monograph. We have attempted to reach a compromise by listing selected references for further study in a section at the end of the book.

Our sincere appreciation goes to numerous reviewers whose frank criticism has been invaluable in the revision, and the improvement, of our text. We also acknowledge with pleasure the capable and dedicated assistance of N. Karen Estridge, Alison C. Brown, Catherine A. Walther, and Judith G. Broaddrick in the preparation of our manuscript and of Carole A. Russell for the many new illustrations in this second edition.

N. BALFOUR SLONIM
LYLE H. HAMILTON

CONTENTS

INTRODUCTION

ON PHYSIOLOGY

We define physiology broadly as the science of processes and function of living biologic systems. Its roots are in anatomy, biochemistry, and biophysics, and its spreading branches bear the blossoms and fruit of clinical medicine. The physiologist studies sensors, intercommunicating neurohumoral pathways, effectors, feedback control systems, and the differentiating and integrating intermediation of the central nervous system. All physiologic explanations involve the elements of cell function and biologic control mechanisms that, in turn, reduce to sequences of physicochemical events. The application of feedback control theory to physiology is a step toward thinking in terms of dynamic processes.

There are two stages of conceptualization in the evolution of a science—early static description and entity thinking and a later stage of thinking in terms of dynamic process and function. As knowledge accumulates and the unity of science is discovered, the classic artificial boundaries between the departmentalized disciplines basic to physiology blur and then disappear. Having served their original purpose, these carefully defended borders now appear less and less meaningful. On analysis today, physiologic processes resolve inevitably into the more basic biologic sciences of biochemistry, biophysics, and anatomy—the science of structure. In this resolution process pharmacologic tools are often used as molecular dissecting needles with which to unravel physiologic processes. At molecular level the apparent dichotomy disappears as structure and function fuse into a single identity. Synthetically, physiologic processes are the manifestation of highly organized molecular processes; analytically, physiologic processes resolve inevitably into biochemical and biophysical events.

Of basic importance to physiology are the concepts of internal environment, homeostasis, and steady state. Many different feedback control systems operate to assure the fitness of the internal environment, or milieu interieur, and the constancy of its regulated quantities throughout a wide range of environmental conditions. When an environmental influence perturbs a biologic system, appropriate counterreactions begin. Homeostasis is a consequence of successful counterreactions, both physiologic and behavioral, to environmental influences; it is thus the tendency to maintain a condition of relative constancy, or stability, of the internal environment of the organism through a series of interacting physiologic processes. It is this mean physiologic state that maintains the organism as a viable entity distinct from its external environment. The essence of physiology is regulation.

Thermodynamically, a living biologic system is an open system in a steady state. Such a system is to a large extent self-regulatory. If a stimulus is applied to it, it reacts to reestablish the steady state or, if the stimulus continues to act, it assumes a different steady state. The whole organism, its organs, its cells, and the reaction systems within the cells are all open systems.

Physiologically, a steady state is a balanced condition of responsive adjustment to any particular environmental condition, influence, or stress. In health every environmental change that displaces a biologic system from its mean steady state evokes appropriate countermeasures. Since the dynamic adjustments operating to reestablish a steady state involve many physiologic processes that proceed at different rates, one must define the relevant physiologic parameters for a given condition and it is more precise to speak of a *nearly* steady state. On close examination a steady state is seen to contain many transient processes for which time is important in terms of fractions of a second.

An unsteady state is characterized by changing physiologic parameters in the course of transition from one nearly steady state to another. Unsteady states may result from breathing unusual gas mixtures, hyperventilation, hypoventilation, breathholding, exercise, anesthesia, drugs, increasing apparatus dead space, and changes in posture or cardiac output. These causes may occur singly or in combination.

The present forms of terrestrial life have evolved upon this rotating, revolving earth out of millions of generations of ancestry. It is not surprising, then, that all living organisms undergo continuous variations, or fluctuations, as does the geophysical environment with which they continuously interact. We are now in the process of discovering and describing the manifestations of this fundamental biologic phenomenon.

Some fluctuations contain no regularly recurring patterns of change with time and are termed *aperiodic*. In contrast, some relatively regular patterns of change repeat at nearly constant intervals; phenomena that recur with such regularity are termed *periodic*, or rhythmic, and can be analyzed in terms of amplitude, frequency, and phase. Some biorhythmic variations are linked to natural fluctuations of the geophysical environment such as the cycles of light and temperature, the ebb and flow of the ocean tides, and the annual rotation of the seasons. A host of periodic phenomena in animals and plants follow these periodic environmental changes. Many such oscillations have periods of approximately 24 hours and, accordingly, are termed *circadian* rhythms.

Biorhythmicity is also manifest as a variation of susceptibility to a variety of stressors, such as drug overdose, endotoxins, and high-intensity noise. Susceptibility is a function of the circadian system phase at the time the stress is applied. Indeed, experiments can be designed so that circadian system phase makes the difference between survival and death.

Biologic rhythms of large amplitude can be a source of considerable error in estimating mean values and normal ranges. Unfortunately, sampling at a fixed clock hour is not a sufficient precaution to control circadian rhythms as a source of variation in experimental studies.

Circadian rhythms persist even in coma and for several months after elimination of the most obvious time cues. However, during prolonged isolation the circadian system as a whole becomes desynchronized from the 24-hour clock (external circadian desynchronization).

Can a circadian rhythm, as some evidence suggests, desynchronize from other physiologic rhythms of the same organ system? What is the etiologic, diagnostic, and therapeutic significance of abnormalities of amplitude, period, or phase of physiologic rhythms? Certainly, we must consider the significance of physiologic rhythms in both health and disease.

ON TELEOLOGY

Teleology is a belief that natural phenomena are determined by an overall design or ultimate purpose in nature. As such, it is an aspect of the classic vitalism-versus-mechanism controversy. Because much of physiology appears to "make sense" we are tempted to think in terms of need and purpose. When scientists ask "Why?" they generally mean "How does it happen?" rather than "What is its purpose?" They avoid *teleology*, or *purpose*, as an explanation for natural events. Indeed, not every physiologic occurrence serves a useful purpose. Lack of purpose, however, does not imply lack of cause.

Goose pimples (cutis anserina) may, at one time, have kept furry animals warm, but this erection of skin papillae does nothing for modern man. It is likewise unrewarding to spend time worrying "What are hiccups for?" They are not "for" anything. There are wrong questions as well as wrong answers.

The word "function" is used by some to mean "purpose." If one asks, "What is the function of a yawn?" he is apparently assuming that because people yawn, yawning must serve some useful purpose. Yawning may be useful, but this is not guaranteed by the fact that people yawn.

If we think in terms of need and purpose, then we must conclude that the body makes mistakes. Scar tissue can impair function as well as localize infection; immune mechanisms can kill as well as protect. Books have been written about the "stupidity" as well as the "wisdom" of the body.

The remarkable adaptation of many molecules, processes, and mechanisms to the conditions of life is to be understood in terms of environment, mutations, biologic survival value, and natural selection. The natural selection of effective feedback control systems is the real reason that biologic phenomena appear to be purposeful. This appearance is also the chief argument for teleology. Thus, although teleology is an attractive projection of the mind, in this book we will ask "How?" rather than "Why?"

ON TEACHING RESPIRATORY PHYSIOLOGY

The process of respiration is different in lower animals from that in mammals. In microscopic forms, such as protozoa, gas exchange involves only simple diffusion; a respiratory system does not exist. In insects, where the respiratory system is independent of the circulatory system, gases diffuse freely through a tracheal system that terminates in tracheoles in the deeper tissues. Coelenterates, fish, amphibia, and reptiles differ with respect to the coordination of their "ventilatory" and circulatory systems for the function of respiration. Birds have a unique ventilatory system in which a undirectional flow of gas through the lungs is assisted by air sacs that fill and empty through the action of adjacent skeletal muscles.

The functions of respiration, circulation, electrolyte and water balance, metabolism, and body temperature are so interlocked that alterations of one evoke responsive adjustments in the others to establish a new dynamic steady state. When any such changes occur, respiration adjusts rapidly to metabolic demand, assuring the tissues an adequate supply of O_2 and removing excess CO_2.

Respiratory gas exchange produces arterial from mixed venous blood and is the essence of pulmonary function. The regulation of gas exchange to meet the changing *demands of the body* is the essence of respiratory physiology.

In health the mammalian cardiorespiratory system supplies O_2 to the metabolizing tissues of the body and removes excess CO_2 from them, maintaining optimal pressures of these two respiratory gases in the cells. This vital function is accomplished by the coordinated operation of two fluid pump systems—a blood circulatory system and a gas exchange system. The thorax is a variable displacement, variable frequency, air pump that moves air back and forth through the airways by active expansion followed by passive elastic recoil, thus presenting large volumes of inspired gas to large volumes of mixed venous blood. This air pump is devoid of valves and operates by creating a subatmospheric pressure. The right ventricle is a variable displacement, variable frequency, blood pump that drives the cardiac output in one direction through thin-walled capillaries in the alveoli of the lung. This blood pump has valves and operates by creating a positive pressure. Ventilation is phasic, or intermittent, whereas lung perfusion is essentially continuous if pulsatile. In spite of the rather unlikely combination of flows, gas exchange is both efficient and well controlled. Inspired wetted gas moves into contact with moist warm respiratory surfaces convoluted within the lung. Here blood flow matches gas flow.

Respiration in air-breathing animals involves a set of coordinated, regulated physiologic processes. To appreciate the integrated function of the whole set we must first understand the function of each component process. We will thus dissect the respiratory system into its component processes for presentation and study. However, as we will show, the functioning whole is somewhat greater than the sum of the functions of its separated parts because new functions are derived from the coordinated interaction of various components. The components that comprise the respiratory system include pulmonary ventilation, pulmonary circulation, ventilation/perfusion distribution, diffusion, transport of gases, and regulation of respiration.

Pulmonary ventilation. Ventilation is the process by which air is moved into the lungs toward the alveoli where gas exchange takes place. The muscles of respiration produce the intrathoracic pressure changes that move air into and out of the lung.

Pulmonary circulation. The pulmonary circulation supplies mixed venous blood to the pulmonary capillaries at the rate required for delivery of CO_2 and uptake of O_2 in the gas exchange region of the lung. Since the rate of pulmonary blood flow is normally determined by, and essentially equal to, cardiac output, it is under circulatory control. Thus pulmonary circulation is as vital to respiratory physiology as is pulmonary ventilation.

Ventilation/perfusion distribution. Respiratory gas exchange requires adequate rates of ventilation and perfusion (pulmonary capillary blood flow) and requires that these two flows be delivered to adjacent areas to minimize the diffusion impediment. If all ventilation went to the right lung and all circulation went to the left lung, respiratory gas exchange would not occur. Although the distribution of neither ventilation nor perfusion is ideal, mechanisms exist to minimize regional variation of ventilation/perfusion ratios. In the consideration of ventilation/perfusion problems we cannot separate respiratory function from circulatory function.

Diffusion. Gases move by diffusion from regions of high pressure to regions of low pressure through membranes that separate alveolar gas from blood in the pulmonary capillaries. Equalization of gas pressure is achieved more quickly when the capacity for diffusion is large.

Transport of gases. Respiratory processes supply O_2 to the cells and remove the CO_2 produced by metabolism. Efficient transport and delivery of O_2 and CO_2 depends upon the remarkably well-adapted properties of hemoglobin, the physical chemistry of blood, and the precise regulation of the systemic arterial circulation that perfuses the body tissues to maintain optimal respiratory gas tensions.

Regulation of respiration. The central nervous system coordinates and regulates both ventilation and perfusion and, to some degree, their distribution in the lung. This function, together with adjustment of the systemic circulation, controls blood-gas transport and delivery. Respiration changes efficiently to meet the demands of gas exchange throughout the wide range of conditions to which the body is exposed. Although we study each of the foregoing component processes separately, we must remember that efficient pulmonary gas exchange and circulatory transport and delivery are the result of coordination and regulation of all of the foregoing processes.

ON LEARNING RESPIRATORY PHYSIOLOGY

The medical student must learn and the physician must know respiratory physiology for proper diagnosis and effective treatment of bronchopulmonary disease. With the advent of potent and effective therapeutic modalities—the result of advances in pharmacology and medicine—the physician, now more than ever before, has an obligation to understand the physiology of the body systems with which he deals. In the past, therapeutic impotence often made diagnosis academic so that comprehension of pathologic physiology was less a practical necessity. Today, however, it is necessary to know the meaning of alterations in blood-gas tensions, to understand the causes of change in expired gas composition, and to appreciate the factors affecting gas diffusion in the lung so that we can distinguish problems of ventilation/perfusion distribution from problems of diffusing capacity. Today it is useful to understand that spirometric measurements of flow rates and lung volume measurements can differentiate airways obstruction from loss of lung elasticity. A knowledge of pathologic physiology is basic to the precise diagnosis of the cyanotic patient and further essential for selection of proper treatment. A good grasp of the material contained in this text is essential to the physician in facing the questions, problems, and decisions of clinical medicine.

Each time we are introduced to a new field we must learn a new vocabulary to communicate precisely with others in the field. As we learn mathematics, it is first necessary to become familiar with the symbols for addition, subtraction, multiplication, and division; then with those for exponents and logarithms; and later with those for the operations of differentiation and integration. Physics and chemistry require a new vocabulary and a new set of symbols for valences, atomic weights, isotopes, etc. It is not surprising, therefore, that there is a special terminology with definitions, abbreviations, and symbols for respiratory physiology. This terminology is generally consistent with that of chemistry, physics, and mathematics. The student must learn this basic vocabulary to comprehend this book as well as the literature of physiology. The table of Symbols and Abbreviations for Respiratory Physiology in the Appendix presents the system. We will define them again where they first appear in the text.

HISTORIC REVIEW

Respiratory physiology has developed enormously since Hippocrates (460-377 B.C.) first suggested that the main purpose of breathing is to cool the heart. Galen (A.D. 130-201) came close to understanding the circulation but continued to believe, as Hippocrates, that breathing serves to cool the heart. His most significant teachings in respiratory physiology dealt with diaphragmatic contraction and chest wall movement.

For centuries no important progress in the understanding of respiratory physiology was made. Then, anatomists of the early Renaissance, such as Leonardo da Vinci (1452-1519), set the stage for further progress. Michael Servetus (1511-1553) understood that blood passes from the pulmonary artery through the lungs into the pulmonary vein and that during this passage it becomes crimson. A short time thereafter it was realized that the passage of blood through the lungs is accompanied by the uptake of something from air.

William Harvey (1578-1657) established the relationship of the circulation to the lungs in his classic publication, *De Motu Cordis,* which appeared in 1628. Robert Boyle (1627-1691) observed that small animals die promptly in an evacuated chamber, a fact that led him to deduce that air contains a vital ingredient. The next important steps were made by Joseph Priestley (1733-1804), who discovered oxygen, and Antoine Laurent Lavoisier (1743-1794), who overthrew the phlogiston theory and saw the basic chemical identity of respiration with combustion in the disappearance of O_2 and the appearance of CO_2.

Joseph Black (1728-1799) made an important contribution to the chemistry of respiration through his studies of CO_2. Black discovered that when limestone or chalk are heated, a gas evolves and that the same volume of gas effervesces when these substances are treated with strong acid. He named this gas "fixed air." He also found that when limewater is exposed to air, a white precipitate of chalk is formed, suggesting that "fixed air" is a natural component of the atmosphere. Again, using limewater as a test, he proved that "fixed air" is produced when charcoal burns, in the fermentation of beer, and during the process of respiration. He confirmed the latter in Glasgow in 1764. In an air duct in the ceiling of a church where 1,500 people congregated for a religious service for a period of 10 hours, he dripped a solution of limewater over rags, producing a quantity of crystalline lime ($CaCO_3$). He knew that this gas would extinguish both flame and life.

In 1754 Black published his M.D. dissertation entitled "Experiments on Magnesia Alba, Quicklime, and Some Other Alkaline Substances." Although from a chemical point of view Black did not characterize "fixed air" completely, he is generally given credit for the discovery of CO_2.

Heinrich Gustav Magnus (1802-1870) made the first quantitative analyses of arterial and venous blood for O_2 and CO_2. John Hutchinson (1811-1861) devised the spirometer, measured the vital capacity in both health and disease, and described the other subdivisions of the lung volume. Lothar Meyer (1830-1895) showed that the oxygenation of blood is dependent upon atmospheric pressure. Paul Bert (1833-1886) first demonstrated that a reduced inspired O_2 tension (hypoxia) is a cause of hyperventilation, as well as the cause of signs and symptoms of altitude sickness. His work, *La Pression Barométrique: Recherches de Physiologie Experimentale,* appeared in 1878.

John Scott Haldane (1860-1936), John Gillies Priestley (1880-1941), and Yandell Henderson (1873-1944) showed the importance of blood CO_2 tension, both as a normal stimulus to respiration and as a factor in the maintenance of respiratory homeostasis. Joseph Barcroft (1872-1947) made important contributions to our understanding of blood-gas transport, oxyhemoglobin dissociation curves, and the physiologic effects of altitude. He strongly supported the fact, then in dispute, that pulmonary alveolocapillary gas exchange involves only the simple process of diffusion.

Since the turn of the century, the field of respiratory physiology has grown almost exponentially. The rising flood of contributions challenges teacher and student alike to study, evaluate, and assimilate a wealth of new data, ideas, and conceptual models. The inexorable evolution of physiology brings with it a number of problems. These include the dissemination and presentation of information, the proper role of computer technology, the emphasis due molecular biology as opposed to classic system biology, productivity as opposed to creativity, and the optimal balance of resources to be invested in basic as opposed to applied physiology. What is the future of the science of physiology? As we wrestle with these questions and problems it is encouraging to know that science is the first common enterprise of mankind.

CHAPTER 1 Respiration and metabolism

RESPIRATION AND VENTILATION

The biochemist and the physiologist use the term *respiration* differently. When the biochemist says respiration, he refers to the intracellular processes of hydrogen transport involving cytochromes and other enzymes. The physiologist uses the term to mean those processes by which air is breathed, O_2 is extracted from it by the blood and delivered to the tissues, and CO_2 is delivered from blood to lungs and then breathed out. This latter definition gives the context in which the term respiration will be used in this book.

The primary function of respiration is thus a gas exchange, in which the mixed venous blood is arterialized by O_2 uptake and in which the CO_2 resulting from body metabolism is discharged. This exchange takes place at such a rate that the arterial blood O_2 pressure, CO_2 pressure, and pH remain within narrow limits throughout a wide range of physiologic conditions. The three fundamental respiratory processes involved in gas exchange are ventilation, diffusion, and circulation.

Four processes actively change respired gas—O_2 loss, CO_2 gain, saturation with water vapor, and temperature adjustment to 37° C. Unless the respiratory exchange ratio (R_E) is 1.0, the nitrogen concentration is *passively* increased or decreased. The respired gas washes intermittently into and out of the lungs in a discontinuous, but essentially exponential, process.*

*This is only one example of the many exponential processes in biology.

The lung presents a special situation with regard to its circulation and tensions of O_2 and CO_2. It is unique in the fact that without circulation its oxygen tension (P_{O_2}) is greater and its carbon dioxide tension (P_{CO_2}) is less than are those of any other organ. Further, it is an organ that depends upon wet gas as an air supply, has endogenous stores of substrate for nutrition, and lives for hours to days after excision from an experimental animal; hours are required to observe the metabolic effects of pulmonary artery ligation.

BASAL METABOLIC RATE

Metabolism includes all the simultaneously occurring *anabolic* (synthetic) and *catabolic* (degradative) biochemical processes in the animal body. The sum total of these processes is termed the *metabolic rate* and is expressed in terms of energy change per unit time. Metabolic rate thus includes a multitude of intermediary reactions. When there is no synthesis of either body substance (as during growth or repair) or products (such as milk or eggs), metabolic rate equals catabolic rate, as there is no *net* anabolism. If the body performs no outside work and does not change the total energy content of its reservoir of high-energy phosphate bonds, then catabolic rate equals the rate of heat production. The estimation of this rate by measurement of chemical changes in the body is termed *indirect calorimetry*.

Metabolic rate has been carefully studied. *Basal metabolic rate* (BMR) is the standard for comparison and is measured with the subject at rest and fasting, but not asleep. The term *basal* is arbitrary because during sleep, metabolic rate falls. The dimensions of metabolic rate are heat production units per unit time. However, the rate of O_2 consumption is more easily measured. Assuming 4.7 to 4.8* Kcal/L of O_2 consumed permits conversion of the steady state basal O_2 consumption to heat production units per unit time. In clinical practice this conversion is sidestepped by expressing BMR in terms of percent of predicted, or normal, rather than in absolute units.

Oxygen consumption varies with species, size, sex, age, hormonal factors, diet, temperature, activity, and season. The rate of O_2 consumption varies from tissue to tissue within the same organism and correlates appreciably with energy production. The rate of O_2 consumption by tissues or organisms is subject to both neural and hormonal influence and may adapt during exposure to changing environmental conditions. The bulk of O_2 is consumed by the mitochondria.

Metabolic rate is subject to many influences and regulatory mechanisms. Diverse factors such as cold acclimatization, body temperature, hormones, sedation, sleep, anesthesia, and certain chemical substances (e.g., dinitrophenol and salicylates) can exert significant effects. The basal metabolic rate of human residents of very cold regions or cold-acclimatized animals may be 15% to 30% higher than the BMR before acclimatization or that of the same species living in a temperate zone. A low level of oxidative metabolism, or aerobiosis, occurs during hibernation, hypothermia, and other states in which there is no lack of O_2 but, rather, a reduced requirement for it. The term *hypoxidation* has been proposed for these situations.

The rate at which different cells "live" varies enormously; and one of the factors responsible for this variation is activity. The metabolic rate of resting muscle is quite low, whereas exercising muscle displays an extremely high rate. Conversely, the "level of living" of brain cells apparently varies little with mental "exercise" or activity; indeed, if thinking has a metabolic cost, it has yet to be measured. The lowest metabolic rates are found during sleep and anesthesia. Digestion of food involves heat-producing metabolic conversions, termed the *specific dynamic action* of protein; one may feel warm after a large protein meal.

One important physiologic homeostatic mechanism involves the pituitary and thyroid glands. In response to tissue needs the hypothalamic paraventricular nuclei elaborate a neurohumoral factor, thyroxine releasing hormone (TRH), that moves via the hypophyseal-portal vascular system to the adenohypophysis. The adenohypophysis then releases thyrotropic hormone (TSH), which is carried by the general circulation to the thyroid gland. Thyrotropic hormone, in turn, acts upon the thyroid gland, effecting release of the thyroid hormone, which reaches the body tissues via the general circulation, increasing metabolic rate.

BMR is widely used for clinical assessment of thyroid function. The test is of value when properly done and carefully interpreted. However, many factors besides thyroid function can influence the metabolic rate. Further, the picture of hypothyroidism may result from fault at any step in the thyroid regulatory cycle. It is quite possible to have marked hypometabolism with normal thyroid function. It is also possible for a completely athyrotic patient to register a normal BMR.

*The precise value of this conversion factor varies somewhat with the respiratory quotient. In a fasting animal catabolizing mainly fat and protein, heat production per liter of O_2 varies only from 4.7 (fat) to 4.8 (protein) Kcal. For carbohydrate, such as starch, it would be 5.0 Kcal. For calculation of heat production in a fasting state, use 4.7 Kcal/L (STPD) of O_2 consumed, or 105 Kcal/mole of O_2.

Similarly, hypermetabolism does not necessarily mean hyperthyroidism.

The average young adult male consumes about 250 ml of O_2 per minute in a basal state. Women consume somewhat less, due to smaller size and a higher proportion of fat, which metabolizes at a considerably slower rate than lean tissue. Women live at an oxidative pace which is 5% to 10% slower than that of men. Oxygen consumption declines with age in both sexes as a result, partly, of replacement of lean tissue with fat.

BMR declines continuously after the first few years of life. The BMR of children depends upon size and body composition, but the rate per unit weight is higher than that of adults. Small children might be expected to be displaced along the log-log plot of metabolism toward small animals and to share with these a high metabolic rate per gram of tissue.

BODY VOLUME, SURFACE AREA, AND TEMPERATURE

The velocity of chemical reactions generally depends upon temperature—the higher the temperature the faster is the reaction. For some reactions the speed is doubled when the temperature is raised 10° C or halved if the temperature is lowered 10° C. The same law appears to hold for biologic systems. If such a temperature change occurred in a whole animal, its Q_{10} (the change in metabolic rate for a 10° C change in temperature) would be 2.0. Actually, many animals show a Q_{10} closer to 3.0, since their metabolic rate drops to one third of normal if the body temperature is lowered 10° C. Hibernating mammals are able to live on a small fraction of the fuel they would use if their temperature remained high.

The rate of diffusion of molecules through water is a factor that effectively limits the size of living cells and thus determines the maximum possible distance of a cell from its capillary blood supply; in this sense it determines the structure of tissue. Fick recognized the analogy between the process of diffusion and heat transfer by conduction and first put diffusion on a quantitative basis, adopting the equation of Fourier. Diffusion in an isotropic* medium assumes that the rate of transfer of the diffusing substance through a unit area of a section is proportional to the concentration gradient measured normal to the section. Krogh estimated that a spherical organism of 1 cm radius, which used 100 ml of O_2/kg/hr, would need an ambient O_2 pressure of 25 atmospheres, or 19,000 mm Hg, to supply O_2 to its center by diffusion. He also calculated that such an organism cannot have a radius greater than 0.5 mm if it is to live by diffusion alone in water which is almost in equilibrium with air at 1 atmosphere pressure.

Living cells produce heat as a by-product of the slow burning of food known as metabolism. This heat is liberated to the surroundings from the surface of the organism containing these cells. But if all cells produced the same amount of heat, large organisms would get hotter than small organisms because surface area does not increase at the pace of volume as organisms increase in size. For example, a cube that measures 1 cm on a side has a volume of 1 ml and a surface area of 6 cm^2, giving a volume:surface area ratio of 1/6; a cube 2 cm on a side has a volume of 8 ml and a surface area of 24 cm^2, giving a volume:surface area ratio of 1/3; a cube 3 cm on a side has a volume of 27 ml and a surface area of 54 cm^2, giving a ratio of 1/2. In general, animals produce metabolic heat in rough proportion to their surface areas and not their volumes. The most widely used method for estimating the body surface area of human beings is the formula of DuBois:

$$BSA = 71.84 \times H^{0.725} \times W^{0.425}$$

*An isotropic medium is one whose diffusion properties are the same in all directions.

where BSA is body surface area in square meters, H is body height in centimeters, and W is body weight in kilograms.

Two of the smallest groups of warm-blooded animals are shrews and hummingbirds. Both groups have low volume: surface area ratios, and both have very high metabolic rates. Animals belonging to the smallest species in each of these groups metabolize at rates so high that they generally cannot store enough fuel to last them overnight at these high rates. Each has a different solution to the problem. The shrew gets up periodically through the night to hunt for food; the hummingbird lowers its body temperature, thereby cutting the rate at which fuel is burned.

Whales and elephants produce far more heat than mice, but a gram of mouse tissue produces far more heat than a gram of elephant tissue. If one plots the logarithm of the heat produced per gram of tissue against the weight of the animal, all warm-blooded animals including shrews, mice, rats, cats, dogs, man, horses, elephants, and whales fall approximately on the same straight line. Thus, the catabolic rate of homeotherms, from mice to elephants, shows a high positive correlation with body weight, which is seen best in a log-log plot of the two variables. The law that describes this relationship between body size and metabolic rate for interspecies comparison is as follows:

$$B = 70 \times W^{3/4}$$

where B is basal metabolic rate in Kcal/day and W is body weight in kilograms.

OXYGEN CONSUMPTION AND CARBON DIOXIDE PRODUCTION

Oxygen uptake as opposed to consumption

A sprinter may run a 100-meter dash holding his breath. During this brief period he has essentially no O_2 *uptake*, although his O_2 *consumption* from lung and blood stores is high and his metabolic rate is still higher. A distance runner will consume less O_2 at the start than he will a few minutes later. During this transitional *unsteady state*, his O_2 consumption will not accurately reflect his metabolism. He gets a portion of his energy from anaerobic breakdown of glucose to lactic acid, but this *oxygen debt* will be paid off at the end of his run by hyperventilation, during which his O_2 consumption will exceed his metabolic rate. During a *steady state*, however, O_2 uptake is a measure of both O_2 consumption and metabolic rate.

Some O_2 diffuses through the skin into the blood. In a frog this is adequate to supply the metabolic requirement below a certain critical temperature. Not only are the frog's metabolism and, consequently, O_2 consumption decreased at a low temperature, but O_2 is more soluble in cold water than it is in warm, and hence is available in larger quantities. However, in dry-skinned man this *diadermic* breathing is apparently small enough to be neglected.

Carbon dioxide output as opposed to production

Every aerobic metabolizing cell consumes O_2 and produces CO_2. During a steady state, CO_2 output equals CO_2 production. However, the quantity of CO_2 stored in the body is large. Small changes in breathing can increase or decrease the level of CO_2 stores. When this occurs, the measured CO_2 output does not accurately reflect CO_2 production. Carbon dioxide is the most important acid end product of metabolism. The lungs excrete some 13,000 mEq/day of carbonic acid, whereas the kidney excretes less than 100 mEq/day of sulfates, phosphates, and other fixed acids. Since the CO_2 production of an average man is about 200 ml/min, the lungs eliminate about 300 L of CO_2 daily.

Respiratory exchange ratio as opposed to respiratory quotient

The metabolic respiratory quotient (R) is the molar ratio of CO_2 production to the corresponding O_2 consumption. During a steady state, this metabolic respiratory quotient can be calculated by dividing the CO_2 output by the O_2 uptake, because $R = R_s = R_E$. The value of R depends upon the kind of fuel being used by the metabolizing cells. If glucose is the only fuel, the following equations show that R = 1.00:

$$C_6H_{12}O_6 + 6\ O_2 \longrightarrow 6\ CO_2 + 6\ H_2O$$

$$R = \frac{CO_2 \text{ production}}{O_2 \text{ consumption}} = \frac{6\ CO_2}{6\ O_2} = 1.00$$

Fat contains relatively little O_2; thus more O_2 must be supplied to burn it. The metabolic respiratory quotient for fat, therefore, is low—about 0.70; the exact value depends upon the particular fat that is burned. Protein has a metabolic respiratory quotient of slightly less than 0.80.

Rarely, if ever, does the entire body burn only one kind of fuel. Rather, a mixture of all three foodstuffs is metabolized, giving rise to metabolic respiratory quotient (R) values of 0.80 to 0.85 at rest. Early in the course of exercise the proportion of carbohydrate burned increases; this is reflected in an increased value for R. After prolonged heavy exercise, high proportions of fat are burned and rather low R values (below 0.80) result.

Unsteady states preclude accurate measurement of R by the usual methods. Oxygen uptake does not reflect O_2 consumption if an O_2 debt is being incurred or paid off. Carbon dioxide output does not reflect CO_2 production if body CO_2 stores are undergoing change. In such unsteady states the ratio of CO_2 output to the O_2 uptake as determined by analysis of mixed expired gas is known as the respiratory exchange ratio (R_E). There are brief periods in which R_E climbs to values well over 1.0 (e.g., early hyperventilation) or falls to values below zero (e.g., sudden breathing of a gas mixture low in O_2 and high in CO_2, so that O_2 moves from blood to lungs and CO_2 moves from lungs to blood). However, if metabolic activity and level of breathing are constant, R_E approaches R_s, although it may be many minutes before it truly reflects R_s.

The metabolic respiratory quotient does not change during unsteady states except in the case of exercise, where it rises. The respiratory exchange ratio, R_E, therefore, usually reflects changes in the O_2 and CO_2 stores of the body. The CO_2 stores are large compared with the O_2 stores. The former are largely in the body tissues and change slowly, whereas the latter are nearly all in the blood and change quickly. During an unsteady state, therefore, changes in R_E simply reflect the rates of adjustment of CO_2 and O_2 stores.

EXERCISE AND METABOLISM

The waking hours of a person's day might be construed as being made up of three kinds of metabolism: basal, digestive, and exercise. If a young man whose basal O_2 consumption is 250 ml/min were basal for 24 hours, he would burn about 1,750 Kcal/day. Actually, he consumes almost twice that number of Kcal, or 3,000 to 3,500 Kcal/day. Most of this difference is due to varied levels of physical activity. Individuals employed in heavy work for many hours a day, particularly those working outside during cold weather, may consume two, three, or four times as much as the average young man on a 3,000 Kcal diet.

Certain forms of physical exercise such as running, grade walking, swimming, or cross-country skiing may tax the exerciser to his limit. This limit, unsteady state exercise in young men, has been measured in excess of 5 L (STPD) of oxygen uptake per minute, or in excess of twenty times basal. During spurts of maximal activity, this multiple must be presumed to be even higher, but since such spurts are highly unsteady states the associated metabolic rates are difficult to measure.

What is the energy cost of descending stairs or of going downhill? Subjects who walked up a downward-moving escalator at a rate necessary to remain in the same place and who then walked down on an upward-moving escalator at the same rate found that the energy over and above that necessary for quiet standing was one third as great in walking down as it was in walking up the escalator. The same ratio should hold in climbing and descending stairs or mountains. Of the total energy expended in raising and lowering one's self against gravity, about 75% is attributable to climbing and 25% to descending. Another study has shown that it is more economical to run upstairs than it is to walk up. The energy cost per unit time is greater in running upstairs, but the overall cost is less.

The physical work of the body may be classified into the various components of total metabolic rate as follows:

- Internal, or invisible, work
  - Basal metabolic rate
  - Body position maintenance, if not recumbent or otherwise supported
  - Body function, if in excess of basal
  - Internal resistance to motion
- External, or visible, work
  - Work against gravity
    - Effective, resulting in potential energy increase and measured as
      - Body weight × vertical ascent
    - Ineffective
  - Accelerations and decelerations of body parts

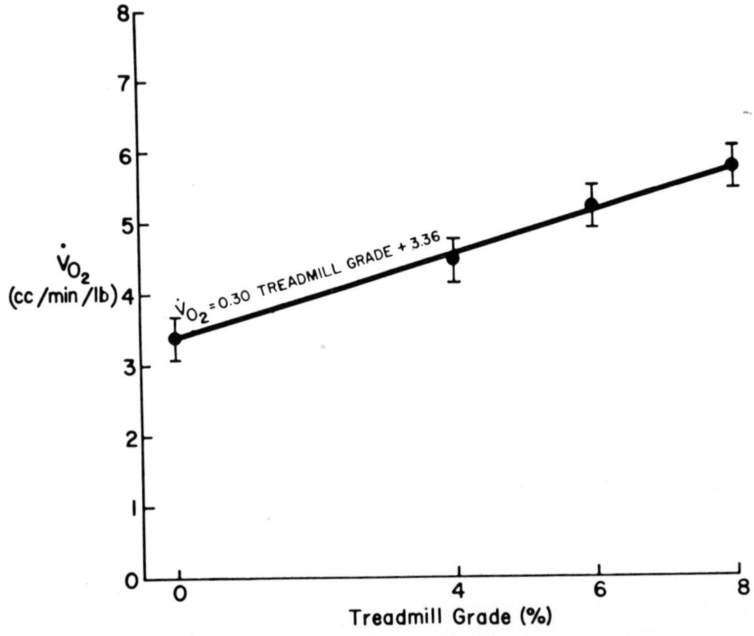

Fig. 1-1
Rate of oxygen uptake versus treadmill grade. Response to treadmill exercise in ten healthy untrained Denver-acclimatized (P_B = 623 ± 5.8 mm Hg) young men after breakfast ad libitum. Mean ± standard deviation. All measurements made from eighth to tenth minutes of treadmill exercise. Treadmill belt speed was 2 mph in all studies. Percent grade as used here is sine of angle of inclination of treadmill multiplied by 100, giving the ratio of vertical ascent to belt travel or distance walked. (From unpublished data of N. B. Slonim.)

Some investigators have argued, on theoretic grounds, that treadmill walking cannot simulate mountain or hill climbing, since the exercising subject does not actually lift his weight against gravity; it is possible, by bending the knees while walking on a treadmill, to keep the eyes on a level with a particular point on an adjacent wall. However, actual experience on a hill and on a treadmill at the same grade with the same subjects show that these two forms of activity are, essentially, equivalent. The percentage grade of a treadmill is usually expressed as the sine of the angle of inclination multiplied by 100; thus at any given speed for any given time the distance walked is the belt travel (Fig. 1-1 and Table 1).

Minute volume of breathing, O_2 uptake, and heart rate all vary quite linearly with metabolic rate throughout a wide central range of exercise levels. The mechanism coordinating these physiologic parameters with the metabolic level is still unknown. The pumping ability of the heart normally limits cardiac output, and therefore O_2 uptake, during exhausting exercise. *Peak O_2 uptake* may be defined as the highest value obtained for rate of O_2 uptake as determined by measurement and analysis of mixed expired gas collected during the sixth minute of exhausting exercise.

Table 1

Characteristics of ten healthy untrained Denver-acclimatized young men who were subjects of the study shown in Fig. 1-1

	Age (years)	Height (inches)	Weight (pounds)	Body surface area (square meters)
Mean	23.9	70.7	166	1.94
Standard deviation	3.2	1.6	17	0.10

Because this determination involves strenuous physical exertion, it is usually reserved for healthy, trained subjects. It is essential that a physician assure the health of subjects during this most strenuous exertion. A common termination or end-point with highly motivated subjects is abrupt collapse. Provision must be made to avoid injury in such event or in the event of syncope.

Various methods of determining peak O_2 uptake are used, and these differ with regard to exercise apparatus, duration of test, and approach to the limit. The treadmill, vertical ladder treadmill, and bicycle ergometer are all used as exercise apparatus. A common mistake is the failure to use a *low-resistance* breathing system in exercise studies; this point cannot be emphasized too strongly. The breathing system must be of uniform, high caliber from low-resistance respiratory valve all the way to the expired gas receiver.

The performance-limiting symptom of *healthy, trained* subjects is almost always weakness of the lower extremities. In no instance is dyspnea a performance-limiting factor. Syncope has been observed on rare occasion. Premature ventricular systoles are occasionally seen during exercise at heart rates in excess of 180 beats/min. Expiratory minute volume during exercise is customarily expressed at BTPS, but it is questionable whether either saturation or temperature equilibration is complete at high ventilatory rates. Because environmental conditions strongly affect exercise physiology and physical working capacity it is well to record such simple environmental factors as barometric pressure, ambient temperature, and relative humidity. An appreciable correlation has been found between peak O_2 uptake and body surface area (correlation coefficient $r = 0.70$). In a study of forty-one normal men, 25 to 45 years of age, an appreciable negative correlation was found between peak O_2 uptake and age.

LUNG METABOLISM AND LUNG FUNCTION

The metabolism of the lung supports a number of general as well as specific functions. The general functions include (1) performance of external work, including mechanical, osmotic, and electrical work, (2) the maintenance of gradients and unstable structures, and (3) the maintenance of lung temperature in its exposed situation. The specific functions include (1) maintenance and repair of structure, (2) smooth muscle contraction, including the normal tonus of bronchial smooth muscle, (3) ciliary activity, (4) phagocytic activity of alveolar macrophages, (5) synthesis of lipids such as pulmonary surfactant, (6) active transport, (7) nerve conduction, and (8) synthesis of macromolecules such as proteins, DNA, and RNA.

Biochemical processes supply energy for the various general and specific functions. In the lung, as elsewhere, anaerobic glycolysis is accomplished in the cellular cytoplasm, whereas the aerobic phase, which produces thirteen times as much energy, is carried out in the mitochondria. Ninety percent of the succinate oxidase in the lungs is found in the mitochondria.

The lung itself is estimated to account for about 10% of the total body O_2 consumption. Fetal lung tissue, in its intrauterine state of primary atelectasis, is characterized by a high metabolic rate and low blood flow. Energy is obtained chiefly from two sources—blood glucose, a source that is quite circulation dependent, and fatty acids, a source that is less circulation dependent. Thus the lung is less sensitive to occlusion of its blood supply than, for example, the brain, which is almost completely dependent upon glucose. Glucose deprivation has no significant short-term effect on the rate of O_2 consumption in the lung. The lung has a considerably more active hexose-monophosphate shunt than, for example, does liver. As in other tissues, adenosine triphosphate (ATP) is the major immediate source of energy in lung tissue. A Pasteur effect has been noted in rat lung slices, implying a competition for adenosine diphosphate (ADP).

Standard tissue slice as well as homogenate technics have been used to study the metabolism of lung tissue. It should be noted that tissue homogenation involves not only the loss of normal structural relationships but also inactivation and denaturation of biochemical substances, such as proteins. For example, it has been found that calcium ions inhibit certain reactions in lung homogenates, but not in lung slices.

With the discovery of surfactant, lung phospholipids have assumed importance for the mechanics of breathing. The lung appears particularly oriented to the biosynthesis of phospholipids from a number of substrates. Lipogenesis from acetate is an active process in the lung. A major substrate for oxidative metabolism in many body tissues is the lipid fraction of plasma, termed free fatty acids (FFA). This long-chain fatty acid fraction, bound to serum albumin, derives from adipose tissue storage depots. It is potentially an important source of readily available energy. Whereas liver incorporates a large fraction of FFA into triglyceride molecules, lung converts them predominantly to phospholipids; of this, 85% to 90% is found in the lecithin component.

Serotonin is converted to 5-HIAA by the lung, norepinephrine is rapidly metabolized, but histamine is apparently not metabolized by the lung. Amyl nitrite inhalation is said to accelerate pulmonary destruction of the circulating catecholamines, norepinephrine and epinephrine, thus preventing their angina-producing effect upon the myocardium. There is evidence that the lung removes from the circulation or destroys such chemical substances as prostaglandins, serotonin, bradykinin, and that it converts angiotensin I into angiotensin II.

Many substances are easily absorbed across the respiratory epithelium, so that inhalation is an exposure which may result in significant absorption and toxicity. Inhalation anesthesia is clinical application of this fact, while plumbism from inhalation of lead fumes is a clinical example.

CHAPTER 2 Laws describing the behavior of gases

An understanding of the physical laws describing the behavior of gases is basic to the study of respiratory physiology. Although this material is often relegated to an Appendix, we place it here in continuity because we consider it both essential and integral to the subject matter of this field. Respiration deals with gases, and gases obey physical laws. The student of respiration cannot escape from these laws but must develop a working knowledge of them if he is to understand respiratory physiology. The time and effort spent in mastering this chapter are a necessary investment that will yield rich rewards. The following presentation is an elementary review of the kinetic concept of gases.

KINETIC THEORY OF GASES

Four statements comprise the kinetic theory of gases.

1. A gas that fills a container or occupies a space is not continuous but, rather, consists of an enormous number of minute discrete particles, or molecules, that have mass.

2. Gas molecules are in a state of ceaseless, high-velocity, random motion. Because they move and have mass they have kinetic energy ($\frac{1}{2}$ mv^2). A gas, because of the incessant random motion of its individual molecules, completely fills all the available volume.

3. As a further result of this motion, gas molecules continually collide with each other and with the walls of a container. They rebound from these collisions without loss of energy (decreased velocity) and may thus be regarded as perfectly elastic. At relatively low pressure the distance between gas molecules is large compared with their own size, and their attraction for each other is negligibly small; they do not attract their own or other molecular species. Thus gas molecules exert force upon each other only when they collide.

4. The pressure (force per unit area) that a gas exerts is the summation of the impacts of its myriad, rapidly moving elastic molecules upon the confining walls of the container. The magnitude of the pressure is dependent upon the average kinetic energy and concentration of the gas molecules (molecules per unit volume). At a given temperature the product mv^2 is the same for all gases and, thus, at the same concentration, pressure is identical for all gases.

Although an oversimplification, the kinetic concept of an *ideal* gas, whose perfectly elastic, ceaselessly moving molecules neither occupy space nor attract each other, is useful in respiratory physiology. It predicts the behavior of *real* gases at low pressure, low concentration, or high temperature, and the set of physical laws that describe it. These laws apply to real gases very well at atmospheric pressure, but real gases deviate appreciably from ideal gas behavior as pressure and concentration increase. Under these conditions the volume occupied by the gas molecules themselves becomes significant and the molecules begin to attract each other. The following laws describe the behavior of gases under ordinary conditions of pressure, temperature, and concentration, in biologic as well as physical systems.

DIFFUSION AND GRAHAM'S LAW

Diffusion is the process by which matter moves from one part of a system to another as a result of random molecular motion. Fick derived equations that are mathematical statements of this process and that are termed his first and second laws. At relatively low pressure, gas molecules move independently of each other; however, they collide continually and rebound elastically with no preferred direction—sometimes toward a region of higher, sometimes lower, concentration. The motion of any single molecule can be described as a random walk. Although it is possible to calculate the mean square distance a gas molecule will travel in a given interval of time, it is impossible to predict in what direction it will move. Because there are more molecules in regions of higher concentration, random molecular motion results in a net transfer of molecules from regions of higher to regions of lower concentration. In the process pressure equalizes throughout the container. Diffusion in a mixture of gases is also a consequence of the continuous random movement of individual molecules and tends rapidly to equalize any local concentration differences that may exist. In certain ways diffusion is analogous to heat transfer by conduction—a process that also results from random molecular motion.

At any given temperature small molecules move faster, collide more frequently, and diffuse faster than large molecules. Since average kinetic energy, $\frac{1}{2}mv^2$, is the same for all gases at constant temperature, velocity increases as mass decreases. Graham's law states that the relative rates of diffusion of gases under constant conditions are inversely proportional to the square roots of the molecular weights of those gases.

Respiratory physiology involves both diffusion in gas mixtures and diffusion across membranes. Diffusion of gases across biologic membranes is affected by the solubility of the gas in the water of the membrane. This problem is discussed in the section on pulmonary diffusing capacity.

AVOGADRO'S LAW

Avogadro's law states that equal volumes of different gases at the same pressure and temperature contain the same number of molecules. This is consistent with the fact that the product mv^2 is the same for all gases at a given temperature. A molecule of hydrogen, a very light gas, takes up as much space as a molecule of krypton, a heavy gas. This is the theoretic basis for the volumetric determination of the composition of gas mixtures. Avogadro's number, 6.02×10^{23}, is the number of molecules in a mole, or in a mass in grams of substance equal numerically to its molecular weight. No matter how heavy the gas, a gram molecular weight occupies a gram molecular volume, or 22.4 L (STPD), and contains Avogadro's number of molecules. This volume applies strictly to an ideal gas. The gram molecular volume of CO_2, a real gas, is 22.26 L (STPD). Loschmidt's number, 2.687×10^{19}/cc, is the number of molecules of an ideal gas at 0° C and 760 mm Hg.

A further consequence of Avogadro's law is Gay-Lussac's law of combining volumes. If gases interact to form a gaseous product, the volumes of the reacting gases and the volumes of the gaseous products are to each other in simple proportions, which can be expressed by small whole numbers.

BOYLE'S LAW

Boyle's law states that, at constant temperature, the volume of a given quantity (number of moles) of any gas varies inversely as the pressure to which that gas is subjected. For an *ideal* gas changing from pressure P_1 and volume V_1 to pressure P_2 and volume V_2 at constant temperature, $P_1V_1 = P_2V_2$. Since gas molecules create pressure by colliding with the walls of a container, compressing the volume of a gas increases the number of molecules per unit volume, the number of impacts per unit area of container wall, and thus pressure. For a given gas, pressure is a function of the number of impacts and the velocity of the gas molecules; at constant velocity (constant temperature) the change in pressure is proportional to the change in volume.

Boyle's law is widely used in respiratory physiology. It is important for understanding the pressure changes in the lungs during the breathing cycle. It is also the basis of the plethysmographic method for measuring the volume of gas that remains in the chest at the end of expiration, as will be explained in a later section.

CHARLES' LAW

Gas expands as it warms and shrinks as its cools. Charles' law (also called Gay-Lussac's law) states that the volume of a given mass of any gas, the pressure remaining constant, is directly proportional to the absolute temperature. The change in volume is proportional to the change in absolute, or Kelvin, temperature. If V_1 and V_2 are volumes of the same mass of gas at corresponding absolute temperatures, T_1 and T_2, then:

$$\frac{V_1}{V_2} = \frac{T_1}{T_2}$$

On the absolute scale, mean respiratory tract temperature is 273 + 37° C = 310° K, whereas average body core temperature is 273 + 38° C = 311° K. If a person breathes into a 6° C (279° K) environment, his breath volume shrinks one tenth as a result of the temperature drop. Equations involving Charles' law are used to convert gas volumes measured at room temperature to the actual volume occupied by that gas saturated in the lungs at body temperature.

GENERAL GAS LAW

The general gas law is a composite statement of the laws of Charles, Boyle, and Avogadro for an ideal gas:

$$PV = nRT$$

where P is pressure, V is volume, n is the mass or number of molecules of gas, R is the gas constant (the numerical value of which depends upon the units in which the variables are expressed), and T is the absolute temperature. When pressure is expressed in atmospheres, volume in liters, and temperature in degrees absolute, the value of R is 0.082 liter · atmospheres · mole^{-1} · degree^{-1}.

Another statement of the general gas law for an ideal gas permits calculations for changing conditions:

$$\frac{P_1 V_1}{T_1} = \frac{P_2 V_2}{T_2}$$

where the subscript 1 indicates initial conditions of pressure, volume, and temperature, and the subscript 2 indicates the final conditions.

DALTON'S LAW OF PARTIAL PRESSURES

Barometric pressure is the pressure exerted by the weight of the gas in the atmosphere above the point of measurement. It varies with time as high or low pressure areas move through the atmosphere across the face of the earth; it decreases with altitude (see altitude-pressure table, p. 199, in the Appendix). The average barometric pressure (P_B) at sea level is 760 mm Hg. This is to say that the weight of the atmosphere above balances a column of mercury 760 mm high in a sealed evacuated tube.

The *partial pressure* or *tension* of a gas is the measurement or quantity upon which its chemical and physiologic actions depend. The pressure due to any particular gas, whether it is alone or in mixture with other gases, is termed its *partial pressure* or *tension*. Respiratory physiologists use the capital letter P followed by the subscript chemical symbol of any gas to denote its partial pressure; thus the partial pressure of nitrogen is written P_{N_2}.

The partial pressure of a gas depends upon the number of molecules in a given volume and upon the temperature. It is completely independent of the presence of other gases that may be simultaneously present in the same volume. Dalton's law of partial pressures states that the total pressure exerted by a mixture of gases is equal to the sum of the separate or partial pressure which each gas would exert if it alone occupied the entire volume. This fact is expressed in the following equation:

$$PV = V(P_1 + P_2 + P_3, \text{etc.})$$

For atmospheric air we can write:

$$P_B = P_{N_2} + P_{O_2} + P_{H_2O} + P_{CO_2}$$

where P_B is the barometric or ambient pressure and the terms on the right side of the equation represent the partial pressures of nitrogen,* oxygen, water vapor, and carbon dioxide, respectively.

*The term *nitrogen* in respiratory physiology is often used to mean nonabsorbable or "inert" gas. It usually includes small amounts of the rare gases such as argon, neon, and krypton (Table 2). The chemical and physiologic effects of "inert" gases cannot always be ignored. In gas chromatographic analysis, for example, argon is inseparable from oxygen—a fact that may cause appreciable error.

There is already considerable evidence that the "inert" gases are not inert in high concentration or chronic exposure. Nitrogen narcosis, xenon anesthesia, xenon combination with heme proteins, and the specific lethality of helium anoxia for various biologic systems are examples of the biologic effects of "inert" gases.

Similarly, for alveolar gas we can write:

$$P_B = P_{N_2} + P_{O_2} + P_{H_2O} + P_{CO_2}$$

It further follows that the fractional concentration of a gas in a mixture multiplied by the total gas pressure gives the partial pressure of the gas. Partial pressure = fractional concentration × total gas pressure. Thus we can obtain the partial pressure of O_2 in dry atmospheric air from its composition and the barometric pressure:

$$P_{O_2} = F_{O_2} \times P_B = 0.2095 \times 760 \text{ mm Hg} = 159 \text{ mm Hg}$$

where F_{O_2} is the fractional concentration of O_2 in dry atmospheric air and P_B is barometric pressure.

WATER VAPOR TENSION

The words *vapor* and *gas* are often used interchangeably. However, vapor is more frequently used for a substance which, although present in the gas phase, exists as a liquid or solid at room temperature. Gas, on the other hand, is more frequently used for a substance that exists in the gas phase at room temperature. Thus one speaks of water *vapor* but of nitrogen *gas*.

Vapor pressure is the pressure exerted when a solid or liquid is in equilibrium with its own vapor in the gas phase; for any given substance it is a function of temperature alone. The warmer a liquid the greater is its vapor tension.

When a gas comes into contact with water, a process of equilibration begins in which water (and all species of gas or vapor molecules) achieves a predictable, calculable distribution between the gas and liquid phases of the system. Water molecules evaporate into the gas until the rate at which they leave the liquid phase is equal to the rate at which they return from the gas phase. The rate at which the water molecules evaporate is a function of temperature, and the water vapor tension in the gas phase at equilibrium is also a function of temperature. *The par-*

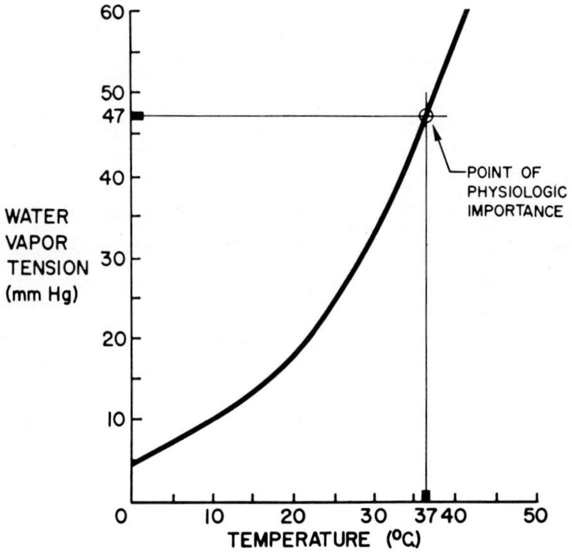

TEMP.	P_{H_2O}
20	17.54
21	18.65
22	19.83
23	21.07
24	22.38
25	23.76
26	25.21
27	26.74
28	28.35
29	30.04
30	31.82
31	33.70
32	35.66
33	37.73
34	39.90
35	42.18
36	44.56
37	47.07
38	49.69
39	52.44
40	55.32

Fig. 2-1
Exponential relationship between water vapor tension and temperature.

tial pressure of water vapor in a gas phase which is in contact and equilibrium with liquid water is a function of temperature alone, and does not depend upon the pressure as long as total pressure exceeds water vapor tension. Alveolar gas is saturated with water vapor at 37° C; its water vapor tension is therefore 47 mm Hg, regardless of the ambient pressure.

Fig. 2-1 shows the exponential relationship between temperature and water vapor tension and gives a table of values for the range of physiologic interest. This relationship is also termed the *absolute humidity curve.* Absolute humidity is the mass of water vapor present in a unit volume of the atmosphere; it is usually expressed in gm/M^3 or in terms of water vapor tension. The absolute humidity of alveolar gas at respiratory tract temperature is 47 mm Hg (P_{H_2O} = 47 mm Hg).

Relative humidity is the ratio of the quantity of water vapor actually present in the atmosphere to the quantity that would saturate at the existing temperature. It is also the ratio of the actual water vapor tension to the water vapor tension that would saturate at the existing temperature. If, at a certain temperature, the absolute humidity of a gas is 40 mm Hg and the relative humidity is 100%, then relative humidity would be 50% at an absolute humidity of 20 mm Hg and only 10% at 4 mm Hg. If the air cools, but the water vapor tension remains the same, relative humidity increases until it reaches the temperature at which it is 100%. This temperature, called the dew point, is the temperature at which condensation of water vapor in the air takes place.

Air is rarely completely dry, and gas within the body is always very damp. This dampness, or water vapor, occupies a portion of the gas phase and, therefore, is a portion of the total gas pressure. Water vapor obeys Dalton's law, exerting a pressure which is independent of that of the other gases present. For this reason the ambient pressure must be corrected for water vapor tension (P_{H_2O}) *before* dry gas pressures are calculated. At sea level on an average day the barometric pressure is 760 mm Hg. The total pressure of all gases in the lung expressed on a dry gas basis is, therefore, 760 mm Hg − 47 mm Hg = 713 mm Hg. If analysis of a sample of alveolar gas shows 5.60% CO_2 (dry gas basis) and if the corresponding barometric pressure is 760 mm Hg, then alveolar CO_2 tension is calculated as follows:

$$P_{A_{CO_2}} = F_{A_{CO_2}} \times (P_B - P_{A_{H_2O}})$$

$$P_{A_{CO_2}} = 0.056 \times (760 \text{ mm Hg} - 47 \text{ mm Hg}) = 40 \text{ mm Hg}$$

where $F_{A_{CO_2}}$ is the fractional concentration of carbon dioxide in the alveolar gas, P_B is the barometric pressure, and $P_{A_{H_2O}}$ is the alveolar water vapor tension. Note that fractional concentration of the gas on a *dry* basis is multiplied by total *dry* gas pressure. Note also that by use of the value 47 we are assuming normal respiratory tract temperature.

When water evaporates to form its vapor, heat energy is required to accomplish this change of state. This phenomenon, *evaporative cooling*, is of physiologic importance in temperature regulation by insensible water loss and panting. Latent heat of vaporization is the quantity of heat necessary to change a gram of liquid to its vapor without change of temperature and is expressed in cal/gm.

The Joule-Thomson effect is the cooling that occurs when a compressed gas is allowed to expand in such a way that no external work is done. This cooling is inversely proportional to the square of the absolute temperature.

DISSOLVED GAS AND HENRY'S LAW

Henry's law states that the quantity of a slightly soluble gas that dissolves in a liquid at a given temperature is very nearly directly proportional to the partial pressure of that gas in the gas phase. This statement holds only for gases that do not react chemically with the solvent. It therefore does not apply to such gases as CO_2 or NH_3. After chemical combination with a solvent or reaction with another solute, the chemically combined gas no longer contributes to partial pressure of the dissolved gas in physical solution.

At equilibrium the rate at which gas molecules leave the liquid is equal to the rate at which they enter the liquid. Gas in the liquid phase also has a partial pressure that is defined as equal to the partial pressure of the gas in the gas phase at equilibrium. Under equilibrium conditions the partial pressure of gas in the gas phase and that in the liquid phase are equal. Any change in the partial pressure of the gas, whether in liquid or gas phase, produces a corresponding change in the other phase until equilibrium is reestablished.

The solubility of a gas is the ratio of concentration of gas in the solution to its concentration in the gas phase above it. The concentration of dissolved gas must be carefully distinguished from its partial pressure, or tension.

The solubility of a gas depends also upon temperature. As temperature increases, solubility decreases. It is readily observed that bubbles of air come out of solution and form on the container wall before heated water is brought to a boil.

The total volume of a gas that dissolves in a given volume of liquid depends not only on the partial pressure of the gas but also on the solubility of the gas in the liquid. This relationship is expressed mathematically as follows:

$$\frac{\text{Volume of dissolved gas}}{\text{Volume of liquid}} = P \times C_s$$

where P is the partial pressure of the gas and C_s is the coefficient of solubility. The numerical value of the coefficient depends upon the units in which it is expressed. The Bunsen solubility coefficient, commonly used in the physical sciences, is expressed in liters (STPD) of dissolved gas per liter of liquid at 1 atm of gas pressure. In biologic sciences the solubility of a gas in body fluids is usually expressed in volumes percent*/millimeter of mercury gas pressure (vol %/mm Hg). The differing solubility of gases in a liquid is illustrated by comparing the solubility of O_2 dissolved in blood plasma (0.003 vol %/mm Hg) with that of CO_2 (0.063 vol %/mm Hg), a twenty-one–fold difference.

To determine the partial pressure of a gas in a liquid it is necessary to measure the concentration or pressure of the gas in an equilibrated gas phase. This is commonly done by allowing a small bubble of gas to remain in contact with a relatively large volume of the liquid (e.g., blood) at constant temperature until equilibrium with respect to gas tensions has been achieved. Partial pressure of the gas in the equilibrated gas bubble can then be determined.

The partial pressure of a gas is a measure of its tendency to escape from a system and is usually expressed in millimeters of mercury (mm Hg), or torr. Gas pressure is one of the factors that determines the availability, or effective "local concentration," of gas molecules for physicochemical reaction. The biomedical effects of any gas are thus a direct function of its *partial pressure,* or *tension,* not its *concentration.* Within a given system, pressure and concentration are related parameters and must *both* be considered in analyzing the dynamics of biomedical gas effects. Gas concentrations alone without simultaneous data for ambient pressure, or total gas pressure, are generally insufficient for biomedical purposes; a biomedically useful description of a gas must include either the partial pressure of that gas or the information necessary to calculate it. Henry's law is essential for understanding blood-gas transport, the movement of gases in body fluids, and the physiologic responses to varying inspired gas concentrations.

*It is conventional to express the amount of gas in blood in volumes percent. Volumes percent, symbolized *vol %,* is the volume in milliliters (STPD) of a gas dissolved in 100 ml of blood.

LAWS RELATING TO GAS FLOW

Viscosity, or internal friction, is the resistance within a fluid to change of shape, and is expressed in poises or dyne-sec/cm^2. Kinematic viscosity is the ratio of viscosity to density and is expressed in terms of a CGS unit, the stoke.

Viscosity may be pictured as the result of slippage between the adjacent concentric layers of a flowing gas. In molecular terms we may think of two adjacent moving layers of gas, slipping across each other. As gas molecules from the slower layer diffuse laterally into the faster moving layer, the latter will be slowed by the inertia of the slower molecules. This random lateral exchange of molecules accounts for the phenomenon of gas viscosity; it also explains why it takes a driving pressure to produce gas flow and why gas viscosity, contrary to that of liquids, increases with temperature.

During laminar flow, a fluid moves parallel to the walls of a conducting system at a rate that increases toward the center. Such flow is termed *laminar,* since the fluid may be thought of as moving in layers or lamina. Whether fluid flow is laminar or turbulent has important implications. In *laminar* flow the driving pressure varies *linearly* with flow rate; during *turbulent* flow the driving pressure varies as the *square* of the flow rate.

The driving pressure required to move gas through a tube is a function of gas viscosity, flow rate, and the length and radius of the tube. Poiseuille's law for laminar flow relates the various factors that determine the flow rate of fluids through a tube:

$$\text{Flow rate, or } \dot{V} = \frac{\pi \times \Delta P \times r^4}{8 \times L \times N}$$

where $\dot{V}$ is the rate of flow in cc/sec, ΔP is the pressure difference between the two ends of the tube, or driving pressure, in dynes/cm^2, r is the radius of the tube in cm, L is the length of the tube in cm, and N is the coefficient of viscosity in poises. The value of N for air is about 1.9×10^{-4} poises, or dyne-sec/cm^2. A pressure of 1 cm of H_2O is equivalent to 980 dynes/cm^2.

Reynolds found that the tendency to turbulent flow is dependent upon flow velocity, tube radius, fluid density, and fluid viscosity. He combined these variables to produce the following equation:

$$N_R = \frac{V \times 2r \times d}{N}$$

where N_R is Reynolds' number, V is average linear fluid velocity, r is internal tube or lumen radius, d is density of the flowing fluid, and N is absolute viscosity. If consistent units are used, the results are dimensionless. Note that Reynolds' number is directly proportional to the density of a flowing fluid. Reynolds' number is an expression of the tendency for a flowing fluid to degenerate from laminar into turbulent flow. When it is less than 2,000, flow tends to be laminar. Laminar equations apply only when Reynolds' number is less than 2,000.

The laws relating to gas flow find application in the study of air flow in the respiratory tract. In smooth, uniform, straight tubes, turbulent flow occurs only at high flow rates. However, the tracheobronchial tree is an irregularly branching system of tubes. Gas molecules must accelerate when moving through constricted segments of the airway, after being slowed by protrusions, when changing direction of flow, or after passing through eddy currents of turbulence. Such accelerations require pressure in proportion to the density of the gas and the square of the velocity of gas flow; they also favor turbulence.

During normal quiet respiration, gas flow in the airway is laminar in some regions, such as the bronchioles, and turbulent in others. The driving pressure is then the sum of two terms:

$$P = K_1\dot{V} + K_2\dot{V}^2$$

where P is the driving pressure, K_1 is a constant relating to gas viscosity, $\dot{V}$ is flow rate, K_2 is a constant relating to gas density, and $\dot{V}^2$ is the square of the flow rate. The laminar flow term, $K_1\dot{V}$, relates to dynamic viscosity and is independent of the density, whereas the turbulent flow term, $K_2\dot{V}^2$, relates to the density and kinematic viscosity.

The density of a gas changes in proportion to the absolute pressure. Increasing gas density favors turbulence, requiring increased driving pressure to maintain the same gas flow. The density of respired gas decreases with altitude and may also change greatly when artificial breathing mixtures are administered or in artificial chamber atmospheres.

With decreased gas density there is less turbulence associated with any given rate of gas flow, and in addition, less driving pressure is required for any turbulent flow that may be present. This effect of density is of considerable practical importance in the performance of tests of ventilatory capacity at altitude. For example, at the modest elevation of 1 mile (mean P_B = 628 mm Hg) the predicted values for tests of ventilatory capacity are estimated to be from 8% to 15% greater than at sea level.

Mixtures of 80% helium–20% oxygen have been used to reduce the work of breathing in patients with diffuse obstructive bronchopulmonary disease. It is interesting that this mixture decreases work by decreasing density, but increases work by reason of slightly increased viscosity. However, the *net* effect is decreased work during quiet breathing, but especially at higher ventilatory rates.

CALCULATIONS RELATING TO GAS VOLUME

From the general gas law it is readily seen that if we are to define a certain mass of gas or a certain number of gas molecules, then the volume of gas must be measured simultaneously with its corresponding pressure and temperature. This also permits volume measurements made in different environments to be compared.

In physiology it is customary to give the composition of a gas in terms of volumes percent (vol %). It is convenient to express the composition of respiratory gases as if they were dry because the basic chemical methods of gas analysis yield values on a dry basis and, further, because comparison of values for gas concentration is thus facilitated.

Physiologic measurements of gas volumes are customarily expressed in particular terms. For example, expiratory minute volume, $\dot{V}_E$, measured in a gasometer as expired vol/min at ambient temperature and pressure, saturated (ATPS)* is converted through multiplication by the appropriate factor to volume at standard temperature and pressure, dry (STPD) in calculation of O_2 uptake.* However, if it is the *anatomic space* from which a volume of gas came that is important, the gas volume is converted to volume at body temperature, ambient pressure, and saturated (BTPS).* Body temperature, ambient pressure, and dry (BTPD)* is used only occasionally as, for example, in calculation of FRC* in the open-circuit nitro-

*See Symbols and Abbreviations for Respiratory Physiology, p. 195.

Table 2
Normal composition of clean, dry atmospheric air near sea level*

Constituent gas and formula	Content (percent by volume)	Content variable relative to its normal	Molecular weight†
Nitrogen (N_2)	78.084	–	28.0134
Oxygen (O_2)	20.9476	–	31.9988
Argon (Ar)	0.934	–	39.948
Carbon dioxide (CO_2)	0.0314	‡	44.00995
Neon (Ne)	0.001818	–	20.183
Helium (He)	0.000524	–	4.0026
Krypton (Kr)	0.000114	–	83.80
Xenon (Xe)	0.0000087	–	131.30
Hydrogen (H_2)	0.00005	?	2.01594
Methane (CH_4)	0.0002	‡	16.04303
Nitrous oxide (N_2O)	0.00005	–	44.0128
Ozone (O_3)	Summer: 0 to 0.000007	‡	47.9982
	Winter: 0 to 0.000002	‡	47.9982
Sulfur dioxide (SO_2)	0 to 0.0001	‡	64.0628
Nitrogen dioxide (NO_2)	0 to 0.000002	‡	46.0055
Ammonia (NH_3)	0 to trace	‡	17.03061
Carbon monoxide (CO)	0 to trace	‡	28.01055
Iodine (I_2)	0 to 0.000001	‡	253.8088

*From U. S. standard atmosphere, Washington, D. C., 1962, Government Printing Office, p. 9.
†On basis of carbon-12 isotope scale for which $C^{12} = 12$.
‡The content of the gases marked with a double dagger may undergo significant variations from time to time or from place to place relative to the normal indicated for those gases.

gen wash-out method. The following volume conversions involving Charles' law, the temperature dependence of water vapor tension, and Dalton's law of partial pressures, are commonly used:

$$V_{STPD} = V_{ATPS} \times \frac{273}{(273 + T^{\circ}\ C)} \times \frac{(P_B - P_{H_2O}\ \text{at}\ T^{\circ}\ C)}{760}$$

$$V_{STPD} = V_{BTPS} \times \frac{273}{310} \times \frac{(P_B - 47)}{760}$$

$$V_{BTPS} = V_{ATPS} \times \frac{310}{(273 + T^{\circ}\ C)} \times \frac{(P_B - P_{H_2O}\ \text{at}\ T^{\circ}\ C)}{(P_B - 47)}$$

HOMOGENEITY AND COMPOSITION OF ATMOSPHERIC AIR

The composition of our atmosphere has changed greatly since the earth was formed 5 billion years ago. However, the rate of change has always been exceedingly slow until recently. Certain pollutants are now regularly present in detectable and increasing concentration. Local or regional abnormalities of atmospheric composition have developed around centers of pollution.

We pollute the air we breathe with impunity. We dump enormous quantities of wastes into it as if it were a gigantic sewer. We are truly the *effluent* society. Within the relatively short space of several generations we will convert the carbon in fossil fuels, which were half a billion years in the making, into CO_2.

For the present, Table 2 describes the generally homogeneous gaseous composition of our atmosphere up to an altitude of about 60,000 feet (18 km).

CHAPTER 3 Functional anatomy of the bronchopulmonary system

EMBRYOLOGIC DEVELOPMENT

The respiratory structures begin as an outgrowth from the primitive tube during the third week of gestation (3 mm embryo). The anterior wall of the foregut develops a longitudinal bulging ridge that pinches off from the main tube except at the cephalic end. It then separates from the foregut, resulting in the esophagus posteriorly and in the respiratory tube anteriorly. The lung bud continues to proliferate, branching, advancing, and producing the primary bronchial buds and the subdivisions of the bronchial tree. This outgrowth produces the epithelial lining and glands; the invaded mesenchyme produces the smooth muscle, connective tissue, and cartilage. During the fifth month of gestation the fetal lung looks like a gland, the bronchi resembling branching ducts connected to alveoli that resemble secretory units. After the expansion of the lungs and the establishment of air breathing, the epithelium stretches to form a thin layer that lines the alveoli.

There is evidence that ambient O_2 pressure affects lung development; low O_2 pressure increases, whereas high O_2 pressure decreases, the number of respiratory units in adolescent rat lungs.

STRUCTURE OF THE BRONCHOPULMONARY SYSTEM

The lungs are somewhat conical in shape and have an apex, a base, and three surfaces (Fig. 3-1). The cardiac fossa and the hilum are on the mediastinal surface. The hilum is a triangular depression containing lymph nodes where bronchi, blood vessels, and nerves enter to form the root of the lung. The diaphragmatic surface of the lung is concave.

The weight of the lungs depends upon the amount of blood and other fluids they contain but averages 1,100 gm for the adult male and 900 gm for the female. The right lung accounts for about 55% of total lung weight and function. The right lung has an upper, a middle, and a lower lobe, whereas the left lung has only an upper and a lower lobe. However, the left upper lobe has an upper division comparable to the right upper lobe and has a lower, lingular division comparable to the right middle lobe. The lobes are surrounded by the visceral pleura. The visceral and parietal pleurae on the right are entirely distinct from those on the left.

The tracheal cartilages form incomplete rings that are deficient posteriorly, where they are replaced by smooth muscle. The right main stem bronchus, wider and shorter than the left, is about 2.5 cm long; it follows the direction of the trachea more closely than does the left main stem bronchus. The left main stem bronchus is smaller in caliber but longer than the right, being nearly 5 cm long; it diverges from the direction of the trachea at a greater angle than does the right main

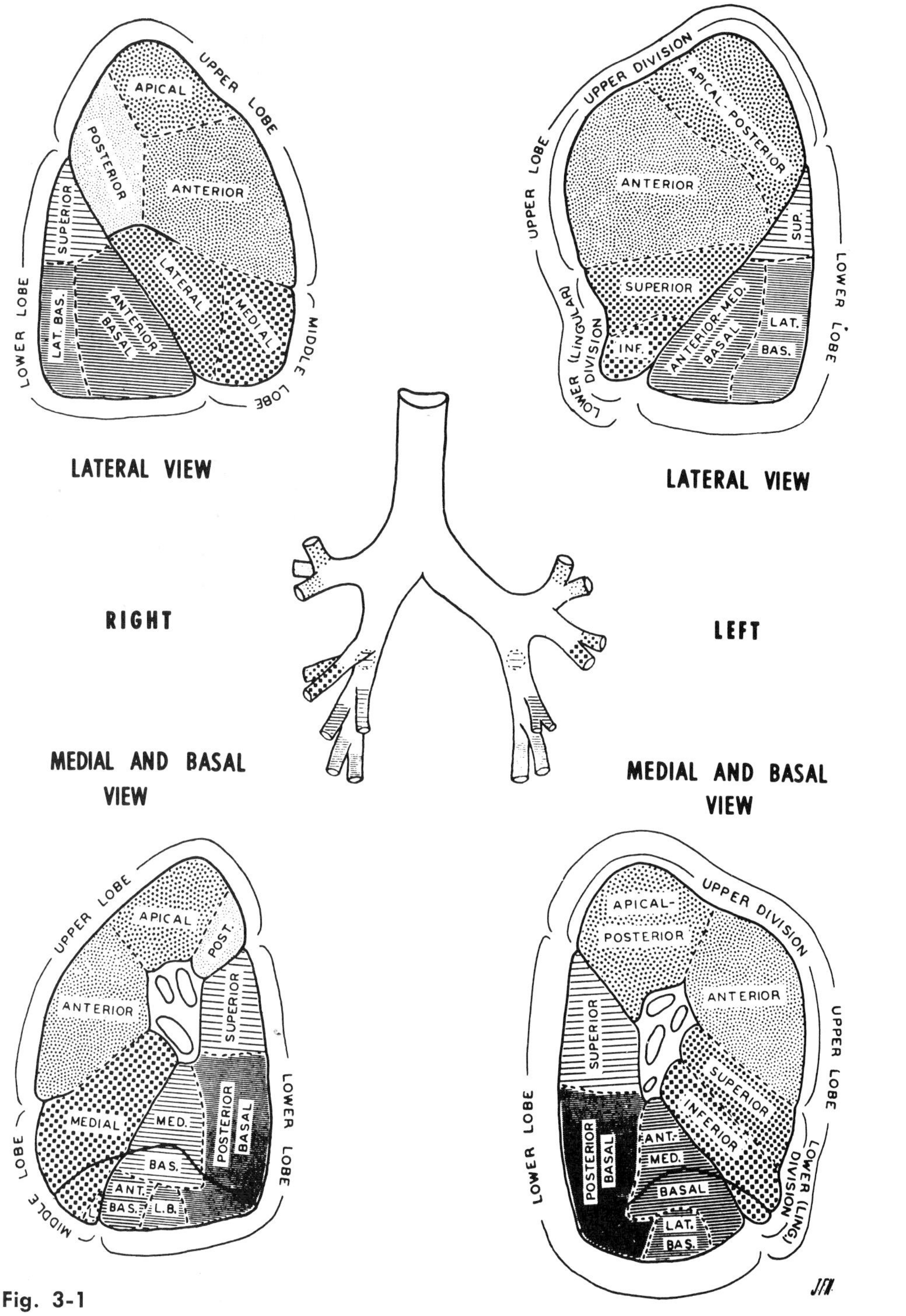

Fig. 3-1
Nomenclature of the bronchopulmonary segments according to Jackson and Huber. Bronchial branches are named by the pulmonary segments they supply. (From Huber, J. F.: J. Nat. Med. Ass. **41**:54, 1949.)

stem bronchus. Because of the verticality of the right main stem bronchus and its larger diameter, aspirated foreign bodies lodge more commonly in the right lung. The angle between the two major bronchi is somewhat larger in the female.

The right middle lobe bronchus is of relatively small caliber and length, and sometimes bends sharply near its bifurcation. It is surrounded by a collar of lymph nodes draining both middle and lower lobes and thus particularly subject to obstruction, recurrent infection, and atelectasis. Such partial or complete collapse of the right middle lobe is clinically termed *middle lobe syndrome* and, on occasion, requires surgical resection, or lobectomy.

The right and left main stem bronchi divide into lobar bronchi and these, in turn, subdivide by irregular dichotomy through twenty-three generations, finally arborizing into terminal bronchioles (0.6 mm in diameter), respiratory bronchioles (0.4 mm in diameter), alveolar ducts, atria, alveolar sacs, and alveoli. To describe this arborization, generations of airways are given a numerical order, beginning with the trachea as zero, and ending with the most peripheral airways. The first four orders of bronchi and their corresponding pulmonary segments are named according to position, providing a reference for radiographic, bronchoscopic, and physical findings. The smallest named units of lung structure are the bronchopulmonary segments, of which there are ten on the right and eight on the left. The Jackson and Huber terminology for the bronchopulmonary segments is widely used.

The first sixteen orders of bronchi merely conduct air and are supplied by the bronchial, rather than the pulmonary, arteries. As we move distally through the airway, there is a progressive loss of cartilage, mucus-secreting elements, and cilia. At order eleven, cartilage disappears and the airway is called a *bronchiole*. From this order on, radial traction of the lung (peribronchial radial traction) maintains airway patency. Scattered alveoli appear at the seventeenth through nineteenth generations, which are thus called transitional airways. The *terminal bronchioles* within the lung lobule, with a total cross-sectional area of 180 cm^2, are the last fully epithelialized and ciliated air passages. Alveoli increase and at order twenty their mouths form the entire wall of the airway, which is now called the *alveolar duct*. Although some alveoli arise from *respiratory bronchioles*, most arise from the alveolar ducts, which give rise either to single alveoli or to *alveolar sacs* containing two or more alveoli. Since the cross-sectional area of the trachea is 2.5 cm^2 and that of the alveolar sacs (not alveoli) is 11,800 cm^2, the cross-sectional area of the airway increases by a factor of 4,720 from trachea to alveolar sacs.

The *primary lobule* is the basic unit of bronchopulmonary structure; it consists of an alveolar duct and its dependent alveoli. The primary lobule or some multiple of it is a fundamental ventilation unit. The *secondary lobule* is that volume of lung bounded by connective tissue septa which arise from the pleura and extend into the lung; it is about 1 cm in diameter and includes ten to thirty ventilation-perfusion and diffusion units.

Nerves from the vagi and sympathetics form anterior and posterior plexuses at the lung hila and supply the bronchi and blood vessels.

The lung has two different circulations. The pulmonary circulation serves the respiratory function, and the bronchial circulation supplies the relatively high metabolic needs of the lung tissue itself. The pulmonary arteries accompany the bronchi in their arborization and finally terminate in a dense alveolar capillary network. The pulmonary veins arise mainly from alveolar capillaries and, to a lesser extent, from capillary networks of the alveolar ducts, bronchioles, and pleurae. Small veins coalesce into larger veins but generally follow an intersegmental course rather than that of the arteries and bronchi. Two large veins finally emerge from each lung to empty into the left atrium of the heart.

The bronchial circulation consists of relatively small systemic arteries that arise from the aorta, accompany the bronchi, and drain mainly into the pulmonary venous system. However, two bronchial veins form at the roots of the lungs, the right draining into the azygos vein and the left into the highest intercostal or accessory hemiazygos vein.

Small pulmonary arteries (not arterioles) divide into capillaries at the level of the respiratory bronchioles and alveoli. Pulmonary capillaries lie within the flat alveolar walls and do not bulge into the alveolar space; they have a total surface area of about 45 M^2. Pulmonary venules arise from the capillaries of the alveolar septa, the pleura, and the bronchial artery. In the healthy lung the bronchial and pulmonary systems anastomose only by way of the capillaries; capillaries of the bronchial circulation anastomose with those of the pulmonary circulation at the level of the respiratory bronchioles. However, the pulmonary artery alone supplies the respiratory bronchioles, the alveolar ducts, and the alveoli.

Microanatomy of the alveolocapillary region

The number of alveoli increases from 24 million at birth to 300 million by the age of 8 years, after which this number remains constant throughout life. In the human adult, alveoli measure about 0.2 mm in diameter and have a total surface area of 70 to 80 M^2. Adjacent alveoli are often interconnected by stomata called pores of Kohn, which are about 10 μ in diameter. As noted earlier, some alveoli arise directly from bronchioles.

Alveolar ductectasia is a change associated with aging that consists of enlargement of the lumina of alveolar ducts with broadening and decrease in depth of their subtending alveoli. The terminal alveoli also show broadening, decrease in depth, and enlargement of their mouths. These changes are greatest in the apices of the lung and are found in approximately 50% of individuals 60 to 80 years of age, more than 85% of those older than 80 years of age, but are not found in subjects less than 30 years of age.

Alveoli are lined by a thin, continuous epithelial layer. The existence of this *alveolocapillary membrane,* just below optical microscopic visibility, was first demonstrated by the electron microscope. These studies also revealed the intimate structure of the pulmonary alveolocapillary membrane. The alveolar surface is lined by a continuous, exceedingly thin (0.1 to 0.5 μ) squamous epithelium, the *pulmonary surface epithelium.* The normal alveolocapillary membrane consists of five layers (Figs. 3-2 to 3-5): (1) pulmonary surface epithelium, (2) superficial reticulin basement membrane (a framework with elastic fiber network and little collagen), (3) ground substance, (4) capillary reticulin basement membrane, and (5) capillary endothelial cell.

The pulmonary surface epithelium is a continuous membrane perforated only in places by cells desquamating into the alveolar spaces. The small (7 to 9 μ) discontinuities termed *alveolar pores of Kohn* may be formed by desquamating cells. The pulmonary surface epithelium is directly continuous with the epithelium of the terminal bronchioles. The superficial reticulin basement membrane of the alveolar wall is continuous with the basement membrane of the bronchiolar basement epithelium supporting the pulmonary epithelium. The capillary reticulin basement membrane supports the capillary endothelium and is continuous with the basement membrane beneath the endothelium of larger pulmonary blood vessels.

Text continued on p. 34.

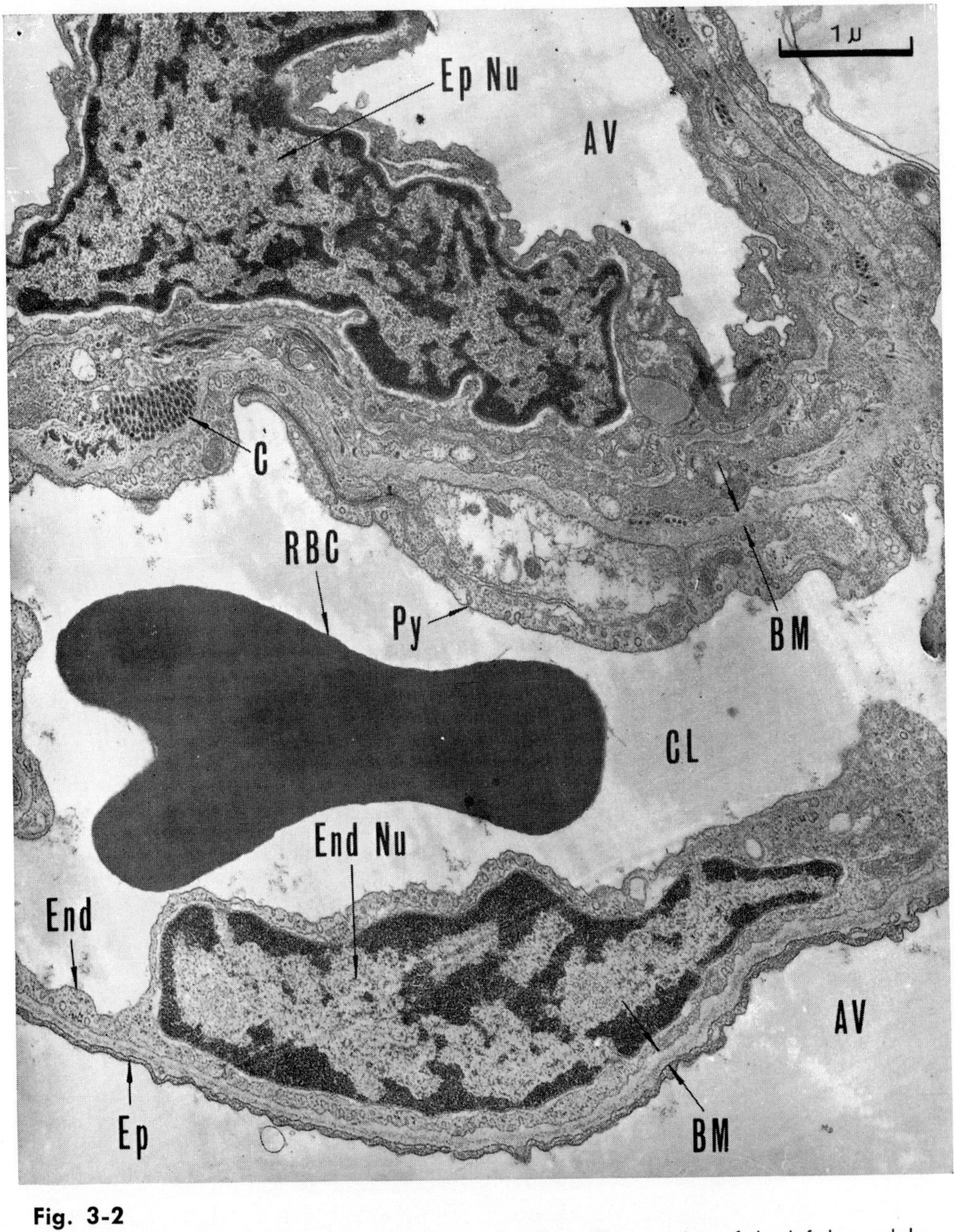

Fig. 3-2
Electron micrograph of the lung, showing the alveolocapillary region of the left lower lobe of a healthy 35-year-old man. **AV,** Alveolar space; **BM,** basement membrane; **CL,** capillary lumen; **C,** collagen (in cross section); **End,** endothelial cytoplasm; **End Nu,** endothelial nucleus; **Ep,** epithelial cytoplasm; **Ep Nu,** epithelial nucleus; **Py,** pinocytic vesicle; **RBC,** red blood cell. (Courtesy A. E. Vatter, Department of Pathology, Webb-Waring Institute, University of Colorado Medical Center, Denver, Colo.)

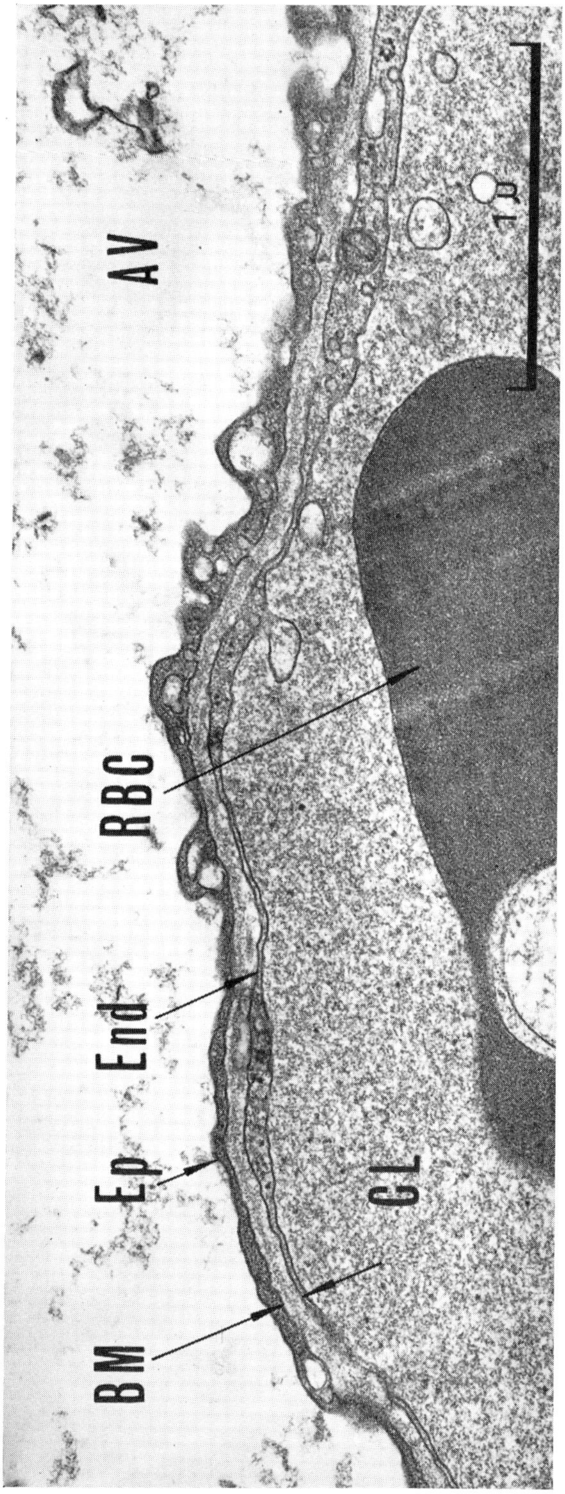

Fig. 3-3
Electron micrograph of the lung, showing the alveolocapillary region of the left lower lobe of a healthy 35-year-old man. **AV,** Alveolar space; **BM,** basement membrane; **CL,** capillary lumen; **End,** endothelial cytoplasm; **Ep,** epithelial cytoplasm; **RBC,** red blood cell. (Courtesy A. E. Vatter, Department of Pathology, Webb-Waring Institute, University of Colorado Medical Center, Denver, Colo.)

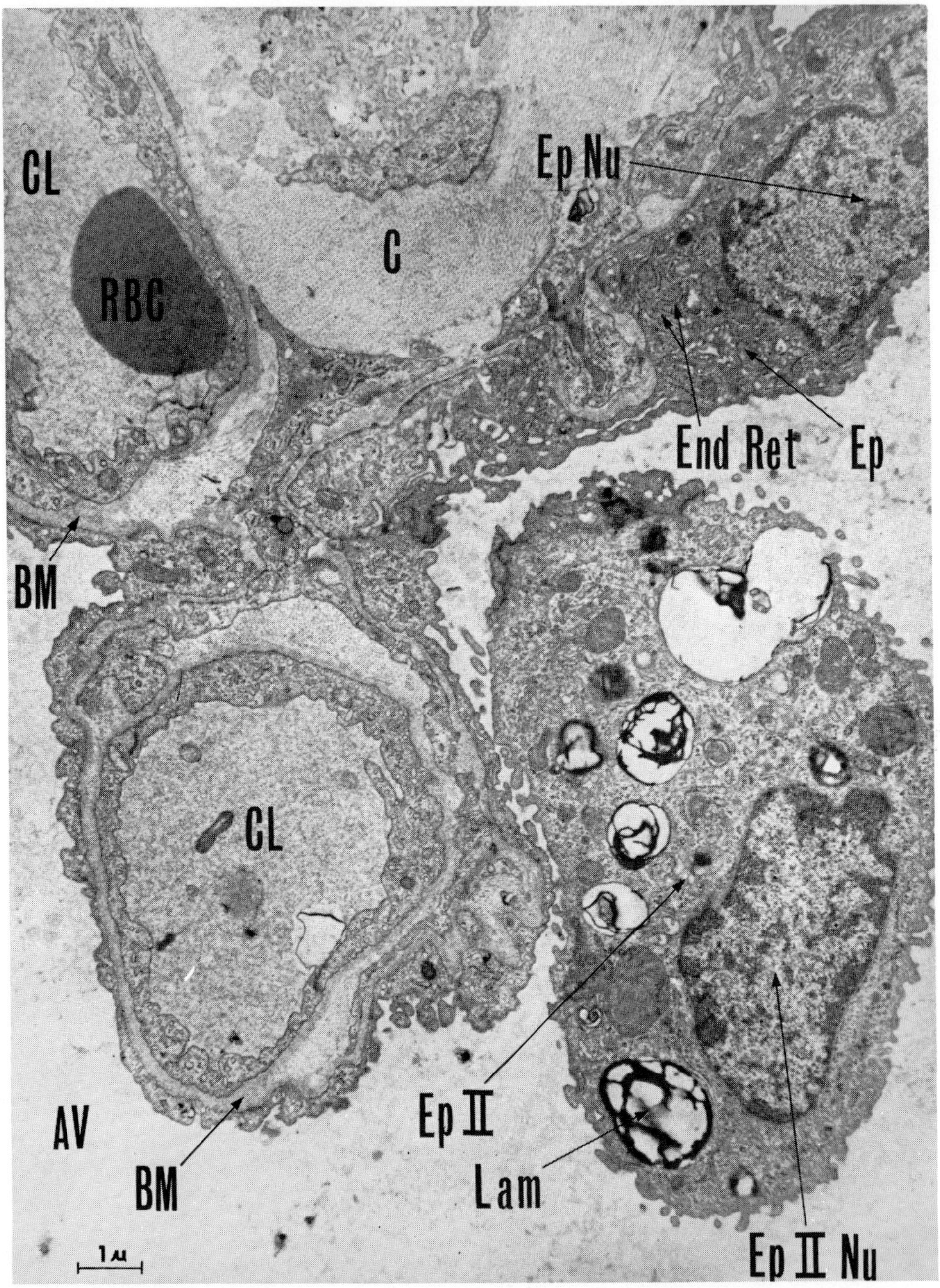

Fig. 3-4

Electron micrograph of the healthy human lung (specimen from the left lower lobe of a 74-year-old man), showing alveolocapillary structures with large epithelial (type B, type II) cell containing cytoplasmic laminar bodies. **AV,** Alveolar space; **BM,** basement membrane; **CL,** capillary lumen; **C,** collagen; **End Ret,** Endoplasmic reticulum; **Ep,** epithelial cytoplasm; **Ep Nu,** epithelial nucleus; **Ep II,** cytoplasm of alveolar epithelial cell, type II; **Ep II Nu,** nucleus of alveolar epithelial cell, type II; **Lam,** laminar body; **RBC,** red blood cell. (Courtesy Robert L. Hawley, Mercy Institute of Biomedical Research, Denver, Colo.)

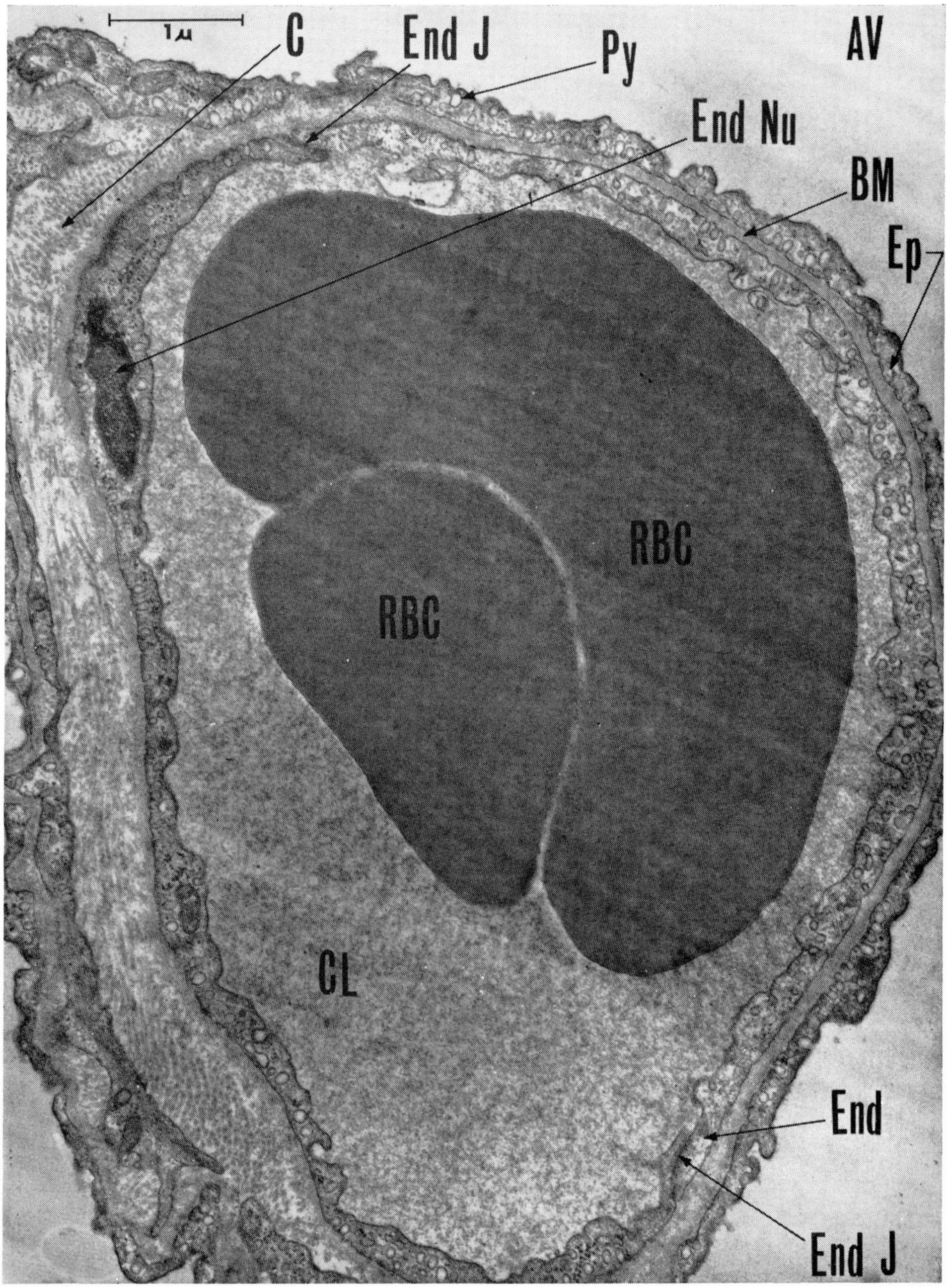

Fig. 3-5
Electron micrograph of the healthy human lung (specimen from the left lower lobe of a 74-year-old man), showing erythrocyte in a pulmonary capillary. **AV,** Alveolar space; **BM,** basement membrane; **CL,** capillary lumen; **C,** collagen; **End,** endothelial cytoplasm; **End J,** junction of two endothelial cells; **End Nu,** endothelial nucleus; **Ep,** epithelial cytoplasm; **Py,** pinocytic vesicle; **RBC,** red blood cell. (Courtesy Robert L. Hawley, Mercy Institute of Biomedical Research, Denver, Colo.)

The cells observed in normal pulmonary alveoli may be classified into seven distinct categories. The first category comprises alveolar epithelial cells, which form the pulmonary surface epithelium, also termed small, type A, or type I. The attenuated cytoplasm of this alveolar epithelial cell displays little or no affinity for histologic dyes. These squamous cells are incapable of phagocytosis.

The second category is a second type of alveolar epithelial cell of definite morphology, termed large, type B, or type II. These occur singly and contain interesting cytoplasmic laminar bodies. Klaus suggested that these structures may produce the alveolar surfactant that reduces surface tension at the alveolar interface. They may extend completely across an alveolar septum to border on two adjacent alveolar air spaces. Brooks has estimated that these cells occur in a ratio of 1/1 with the type I alveolar epithelial cell.

The third category of cells comprise alveolar macrophages, which occur in moderate numbers within the alveoli. In contrast to the alveolar epithelial cells, the cytoplasm of the alveolar macrophage shows definite affinity for a variety of histologic dyes. Alveolar macrophages, as the name implies, have pseudopods, exhibit ameboid motion, and are highly phagocytic scavengers. They are involved in pulmonary clearance of both viable and nonviable particles, ingesting exogenous, as well as endogenous, debris. Pulmonary cleansing mechanisms continually remove these cells, but some enter lymphatic channels, whence they proceed to regional lymph nodes. The total volume of the pulmonary alveolar macrophages is estimated to equal an organ the size of the thyroid gland. Heparin causes a migration of macrophages from pulmonary capillaries across the alveolocapillary membrane and into alveolar spaces. It has been found that BCG increases their metabolic activity even before phagocytosis occurs. In certain disease conditions, alveolar macrophages may form foam cells, dust cells, or heart failure cells. Alveolar macrophages can be obtained in nearly pure form by saline washing (pulmonary lavage) of rabbit lungs.

The four remaining categories include endothelial cells of the pulmonary blood capillaries, fibroblasts, histiocytes or septal macrophages, which are rare in normal lung, and migratory blood cells, which are normally present. Both granulocytic and lymphocytic cells leave the blood capillaries by diapedesis and enter the interstitial tissue of the alveolar septum. They are present in normal bronchial secretions. They penetrate the superficial reticulin membrane to pass between the pulmonary epithelial cells into the alveolar spaces, from which place they are continually removed by pulmonary cleansing mechanisms via the airway. The lung is thus a heterogeneous organ with respect to cell type; the study of individual cell types presents appreciable problems.

The alveolar walls contain a dense network of capillaries and reticular, collagenous, and elastic fibers. The alveolar septum consists of a connective tissue space supporting alveolar capillaries and containing collagen and elastic fibrils, fibroblasts, and occasional leukocytes and histiocytes.

AIRWAYS

Airway caliber changes

During spontaneous breathing there is a synchronous rhythmic fluctuation of bronchomotor tone, with airway constriction during expiration. In asthmatic patients this bronchial squeeze is accentuated and has been measured by intrabronchial balloons.

That part of the respiratory tract lying within the chest cavity is subject to intrathoracic pressure. When gas in the airway is only slightly below atmospheric pressure, but intrathoracic pressure is considerably lower (as during inspiration), the resultant transmural pressure dilates the airway. Since air flow is a function of the fourth or fifth power of the airway radius, flow is facilitated considerably by even small increases of airway caliber. During forced expiration the situation is reversed. High intrathoracic pressure increases transmural pressure, reducing airway caliber and increasing resistance to expiration.

Cough is an extreme example of high resistance to expiration. The cougher inspires, closes his glottis, performs a Valsalva maneuver, and then suddenly opens his glottis. The enormous transmural pressure collapses the lower trachea. The cartilaginous rings encircle two thirds to three fourths of the trachea; the balance is made up of soft tissue, or the pars membranacea. As air is expelled during cough, this soft tissue invaginates into the tracheal lumen, creating on cross section a crescent moon shape. This "barrel," the trachea, forms itself around the "bullet," the bolus, preventing air from escaping around it and thus conserving the full force of the explosive expiration for expulsion of the bolus.

Inspiration, in some circumstances, has another effect on airway caliber. During asphyxia, airway caliber decreases. Lung inflation dilates these airways, presumably through the agency of the slowly adapting pulmonary stretch receptors, the vagus, the brainstem, and the recurrent laryngeal nerve. A deep breath is perhaps the most potent bronchodilator known.

Warm and wet

Osmotically, the skin behaves as if it were a 9% or 10% salt solution. Fingertips wrinkle in sea water (about 3.5% salt) as the superficial cells swell with the water they absorb but do not pass on into the circulation. When relative humidity is below about 92%, water is lost insensibly from the skin to the air. However, when humidity is above this level, the skin is "drier" than the air and there is a water gain. Paradoxically, this insensible gain may occur at the same time that there is a sweat loss.

Unlike skin, the upper airways do not behave osmotically as a strong salt solution. Their water vapor tension is so slightly reduced that they could maintain about 99.5% relative humidity in adjacent quiet air. Contrary to views presented in older physiology texts, there is virtually no water loss from the lungs of normal mammals; the warm, wet upper airways lose water as they saturate the stream of inspired gas before it reaches the lungs.

The amount of water lost from the airways depends upon air temperature. On a cold winter day, a cold nose adds some water to the inspired air. A warm trachea adds still more water as the air column descends to warmer and warmer tracheal levels, and more air comes into contact with the wet airway walls. By the time the inspired air reaches the lower end of the trachea, it has come very close to respiratory tract temperature and is about 99.5% saturated with water vapor. Since the fluid lining the alveolar walls is not distilled water but contains dissolved materials, this fluid wets the inspired air no further.

During expiration, warm, wet alveolar gas flows past airway walls of progressively lower temperature. As this gas cools, it deposits moisture on these walls, including the cooler membranes of the nose, which may even drip as a result of this condensation. The wet stream of expired gas leaves the body at a temperature only slightly above that of the nose, but its water content is 100% of the maximum absolute humidity for that temperature. Much of this water appears as a small cloud as it condenses in the cold winter air.

As water evaporates during inspiration, it removes heat from the airway (evaporative cooling), but expiration with its attendant condensation returns a portion of this heat. The heat of vaporization varies with temperature but, in the example given, should be between 575 and 595 cal/gm of water evaporated or condensed.

PULMONARY CLEARANCE MECHANISMS

It is indeed remarkable that the normal lower respiratory tract is almost sterile since bacterial contamination by inspired air and aspiration of upper respiratory tract secretions are common occurrences. The ability of the lower respiratory tract to dispose of inhaled particulate matter involves the mechanisms of phagocytosis and ciliary activity. In peripheral lung, where the epithelium is devoid of cilia, alveolar macrophages and rich lymphatic networks trap and dispose of the small inhaled particles that impinge on the respiratory surfaces.

There is evidence that these mechanisms are impaired by cigarette smoke inhalation and by the use of alcohol (ethanol). Laurenzi found rapid clearance of *Staphylococcus aureus* from the lungs of mice after implantation by a precise aerosol system; the clearance curve was quantitative and exponential. He also showed that bacterial pathogens can be isolated from the bronchial secretions of patients with chronic bronchitis during periods of apparent well-being, suggesting that antibacterial factors which are effective in the normal bronchial tree are impaired in chronic bronchitis.

The mucus escalator

The total output of bronchial secretions in the healthy adult human being is estimated to be 100 ml daily. Normal bronchi contain two types of mucus-producing glands—the surface goblet cells, which react to irritation or chronic inflammation, and the submucosal glands, which are mixed serous and mucus in nature. The latter respond to vagal stimulation with increased mucus output. The submucosal bronchial glands atrophy after pulmonary denervation.

The composition of normal mucus is as follows: 95% water, 2% glycoprotein, 1% carbohydrate, less than 1% lipid, and 0.03% DNA. The glycoproteins, which average 1,000,000 molecular weight, are coiled polypeptide chains with saccharide side-chains, and determine sputum viscosity. Sputum viscosity can be decreased by hydration, increasing pH, increasing ionic strength, proteolytic enzymes (including papain, trypsin, and chymotrypsin), neuraminidase, and by rupture of S-S linkages, as with acetylcysteine, iodine, or iodinated tyrosine. Reid has distinguished the neutral and acid mucopolysaccharides and analyzed them to ascertain their neuraminic acid content. Sputum viscosity is a very important clinical consideration.

The protective function of the respiratory cilia is well established. Each ciliated epithelial cell bears approximately 275 cilia, and each cilium has nine peripheral and two central fibers anchored to basal corpuscles. Nerves do not supply the ciliated cells; their control mechanism remains unknown. The beat of the cilia, one after another, is rapid, coordinated, and unidirectional, continuously propelling a sheet of mucus (mucus blanket) from the lower respiratory tract upward toward the oropharynx at a rate of approximately 0.33 mm/sec or 2 cm/min. Here the mucus with its entrapped cells and inhaled particles, such as pollens and infectious particles, is eliminated by expectoration or by swallowing into the stomach, where normal gastric acidity and digestive processes render the material harmless.

The mucus produced by the goblet cells and mucus glands floats on a watery subphase layer of unknown origin. Cilia do not beat within the layer of viscous mucus but, rather, in the low viscosity watery medium, stroking the undersurface of the mucus. The physicochemical properties of this watery fluid affect the ciliary beat in a manner that remains unknown.

Mucociliary clearance, or transport, is effected by the mucus escalator. This function is optimal at normal P_{O_2}, whereas both hyperoxia and hypoxia impair it. Clearance is stimulated by cough and adrenergic bronchodilator drugs, such as epinephrine; it is impaired by drying (e.g., by heated but unhumidified indoor air during the winter) and by certain pollutants, such as cigarette smoke.

AIRWAY REACTIVITY

The airway reacts, actively or passively, to a variety of circumstances. The passive reactions are purely mechanical responses to changing transmural pressure. To understand the active responses of the airway one must know the physiology of its nerve and blood supply. Vagal and sympathetic efferent pathways innervate the conducting airways; sympathetic innervation is relatively less important than parasympathetic innervation. The pulmonary circulation perfuses the peripheral lung units, including terminal bronchioles and alveolar ducts, while the bronchial circulation perfuses conducting airways. Experimentally, bronchial artery injection allows better control of the distribution of a test material than aerosol inhalation.

The sympathetic neuron-effector junction is composed of the nonmyelinated termination of a postganglionic sympathetic neuron and the adjacent effector cell that it innervates. The adrenergic neuron synthesizes the catecholamine norepinephrine (the principal neurohumoral transmitter), stores it in small granules, and releases it in response to appropriate stimuli, such as nerve impulses or certain drugs. Epinephrine dilates the airway through an inhibitory action; this action is blocked by dichloroisoproterenol.

Laryngeal irritation reflexly constricts the airways. The afferent nerve fibers of this reflex are subepithelial in location and decrease in frequency from the larynx down to the respiratory bronchioles. Both afferent and efferent limbs are vagal. Stimulation of these subepithelial nerve fibers produces cough as well as bronchoconstriction. Laryngeal irritation increases total lung resistance, decreases anatomic dead space, but does not change lung compliance significantly; this suggests constriction of large conducting airways. Electric stimulation of cervical efferent vagus nerves causes similar changes.

Cough receptors are also termed *mechanoreceptors*. The receptors for this cholinergic reflex are located mainly in the upper airway. The rate of change of stimulus intensity is important for cough production; a transient stretch of the airways is a potent cough stimulus. The cough receptors are probably the slowly adapting receptors that are associated with the Hering-Breuer reflex.

Reflex cough and bronchoconstriction are produced by inhalation of sulfur dioxide (SO_2), inert dust of 1 to 6 μ particle size (e.g., charcoal), citric acid, histamine, and cold air. Atropine blocks the efferent limb of these cholinergic vagal reflexes, although a desire to cough persists because the afferents are unaffected.

Airway reactivity with respect to both cough and bronchoconstriction changes simultaneously. After acute tracheobronchitis reactivity to SO_2, citric acid, histamine, and cold is transiently increased; this increase is blocked by atropine. Age decreases the sensitivity of these receptors.

The initial condition of the airways is an important variable because a given change in caliber produces a larger effect when the airways are initially small. The synthetic isoproterenol, the prototype beta-adrenergic stimulator, is a widely used and potent bronchodilator; it is administered as both oral and sublingual tablets and by aerosol inhalation. Isoproterenol reverses vagal cholinergic reflexes. Rarely, the inhalation of pure isoproterenol precipitates severe bronchospasm; the mechanism of this paradoxical reaction remains unknown.

Histamine stimulates cough receptors by an autonomic reflex. Histamine inhalation produces a reaction resembling an asthmatic attack. As well as stimulating the reflex cholinergic bronchospasm, histamine acts locally to produce smooth muscle contraction. Injection of histamine into the pulmonary circulation decreases lung compliance, slightly increases total lung resistance, but does not decrease anatomic dead space, suggesting constriction of peripheral lung units. Anatomic studies, showing predominant constriction of the alveolar ducts, confirm this conclusion.

Serotonin (5-hydroxytryptamine) produces bronchoconstriction as well as increased pulmonary arterial pressure. Serotonin-secreting tumors (carcinoids) are sometimes misdiagnosed as asthma.

The inhalation of tobacco smoke causes both bronchoconstriction and bronchodilatation, as well as constriction of the bronchial arteries. These reactions are partly due to the ganglionic effects of nicotine but also involve local stimulation of vagal and sympathetic bronchopulmonary reflexes. Injection of nicotine into the bronchial artery produces acute bronchoconstriction, contralateral bronchoconstriction via vagal reflex, and vasoconstriction of the bronchial arteries, possibly via sympathetic nervous action. Heparin is reported to reverse cigarette smoke–induced airway constriction.

The airways of patients with chronic diffuse obstructive bronchopulmonary disease, especially asthmatics, are hyperreactive to a variety of stimuli. Asthmatic patients frequently suffer severe bronchoconstriction following inhalation of dusts, cold air, and performance of routine tests of ventilatory capacity, such as the maximal voluntary ventilation or forced expired vital capacity. The intensity of this reaction may equal that of their response to potent irritants. Airway resistance of asthmatics commonly decreases during mild to moderate physical exertion but increases in the immediate postexercise period. A careful medical history can often elicit such a sequence. Propranolol, a potent beta-adrenergic blocking agent, is contraindicated in asthma.

Airway reactivity to various stimuli is an insufficiently studied variable that probably plays a role in the pathogenesis of chronic diffuse obstructive bronchopulmonary disease.

CHAPTER 4 Lung volume and its subdivisions

The lung volume and its subdivisions are basically anatomic measurements; however, alterations in either absolute or relative size may reflect the effects of cardiopulmonary disease. The standard terminology for lung volume and its various subdivisions, or compartments, is given in Fig. 4-1. The term *volume* refers to one of the four primary (nonoverlapping) subdivisions of the total lung capacity; the term *capacity* refers to one of the four lung compartments that is measured by tests of pulmonary function. Each capacity consists of two or more primary volumes. Most of the lung subdivisions are measured from *resting midposition*—the respiratory level of a resting subject who is neither inspiring nor expiring; the thoracic forces tending to expand the chest balance the lung forces tending to contract it. Midposition defines a volume of gas in the lungs at the end of a spontaneous expiration.

Tidal volume (V_T) is the volume of gas added to, and then removed from, functional residual capacity with each breath; it is usually about 500 ml. Tidal volume comprises the volume entering the alveoli (300 to 400 ml) plus the volume remaining in the airway (150 to 200 ml) per breath. It increases with metabolic rate (O_2 consumption and CO_2 production) as, for example, in exercise. Tidal volume multiplied by respiratory frequency gives the rate of total pulmonary ventilation, a value that is usually expressed in L/min. During mild to moderate exercise, tidal volume increases largely by increase of the volume of gas in the lungs at the end of inspiration (at the expense of inspiratory reserve volume). During heavy exercise, tidal volume increases proportionately more by decrease of the volume of gas in the lungs at the end of expiration (at the expense of expiratory reserve volume).

Expiratory reserve volume (ERV) is the maximum volume of gas that can be expired at the end of a spontaneous expiration (from midposition); it measures reserve expiratory capability. Expiratory reserve volume reflects thoracic and abdominal muscle strength, thoracic mobility, and the balance of elastic forces that determine midposition at the end of spontaneous expiration.

Residual volume (RV) is the volume of gas that remains in the lungs at the end of a maximal expiration; it is the minimum volume of gas that the lungs can contain if both lungs and thorax are intact. It reflects the balance of elastic forces of lung and thorax, muscle strength affecting expiratory reserve volume, and the volume of extrapulmonary structures in the chest (heart, blood vessels, etc.).

Inspiratory reserve volume (IRV) is the maximum volume of gas that can be inhaled at the end of a spontaneous inspira-

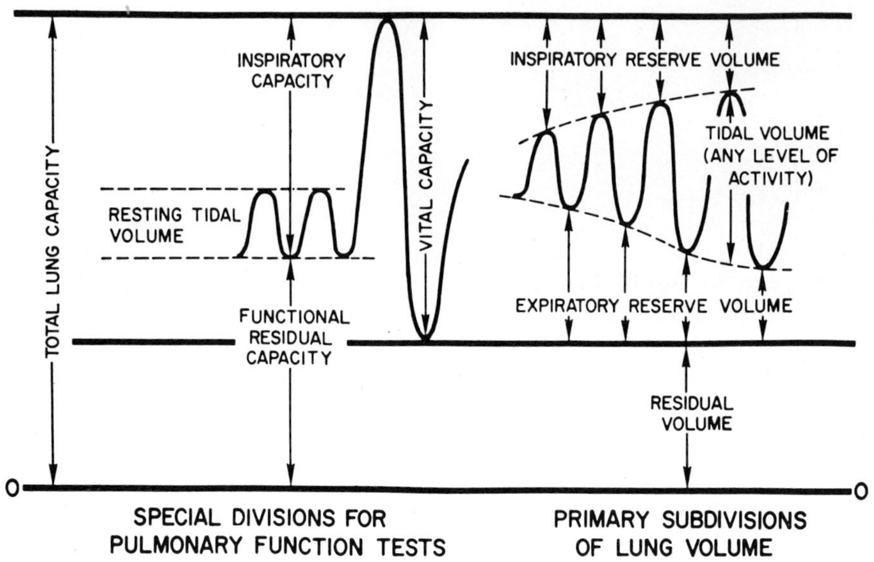

Fig. 4-1
Subdivisions of the lung volume. (Modified from Pappenheimer, J. R., et al.: Fed. Proc. **9:** 602, 1950.)

tion; it is the reserve available for increasing tidal volume. If midposition does not change, inspiratory reserve volume decreases as tidal volume increases. Inspiratory reserve volume reflects the balance between lung and chest elasticity, muscle strength, thoracic mobility, midposition, and tidal volume.

Beside division into the four primary lung compartments, the lung volume is also divided into four *capacities*. Although such a term seems logical, it is not customary to speak of an "expiratory capacity." Measured or calculated by standard technics, three of the capacities provide clinically useful information on the effects of various cardiopulmonary diseases.

Inspiratory capacity (IC) is the maximum volume of air that can be inhaled from midposition and comprises tidal volume plus inspiratory reserve volume. Midposition is a more reproducible level than is the peak of spontaneous inspiration; hence inspiratory capacity is used more commonly than inspiratory reserve volume.

Functional residual capacity (FRC) is the volume of gas remaining in the lungs at the end of a spontaneous expiration when lungs and chest are in midposition; it comprises expiratory reserve volume plus residual volume. Functional residual capacity is the lung volume in which gas exchange takes place. Its size is thus of considerable physiologic importance. During expiration and the ensuing respiratory pause, arterial blood O_2 content decreases as CO_2 content increases. Although detectable with a normal FRC, these fluctuations are small and often ignored. A small FRC results in larger respiratory fluctuations of arterial blood-gas composition as gas exchange proceeds during the period between successive inspirations. Conversely, a large FRC buffers the change of alveolar gas composition in response to changes of alveolar ventilation, inspired gas composition, or metabolic rate. For example, with increased FRC and initially high alveolar P_{CO_2} either increased alveolar ventilation rate or increased time is required to produce the same decrease of

P_{CO_2} as with a normal FRC. The rate at which lung gas composition stabilizes after an abrupt change in the composition of the breathing mixture depends upon FRC, respiratory frequency, tidal volume, and dead space.

Vital capacity (VC) is the maximum volume of gas that can be exhaled after the deepest possible inspiration. It consists of three subdivisions—inspiratory reserve volume, tidal volume, and expiratory reserve volume. Vital capacity limits the increase of tidal volume during maximal ventilatory effort. Although the term *vital capacity* is defined as just mentioned unless further qualified, there is frequent clinical use for *inspiratory vital capacity*. This is defined as the maximum volume of gas that can be inhaled after the fullest possible expiration. Although expiratory and inspiratory vital capacities are essentially equal in health, inspiratory vital capacity may be appreciably larger in patients who have diffuse obstructive bronchopulmonary disease.

In 1846 Hutchinson devised the first spirometer and described the compartments of the lung volume. He measured the vital capacity of 2,000 healthy males and of patients with various chest diseases, and he recognized that vital capacity increases with height and decreases with age. The average vital capacity of males is larger than that of females, a small difference due to sex remaining after correction for difference of body size. However, the two populations overlap. The vital capacity of young adults is roughly proportional to lean body mass.

Total lung capacity (TLC) is the maximum volume of gas that the lungs can contain; it is the sum of inspiratory capacity and functional residual capacity as well as the sum of vital capacity and residual volume. However, total lung capacity is not the volume of air available for gas exchange nor is it a measure of ventilatory capacity.

CHANGES IN LUNG VOLUME AND ITS SUBDIVISIONS

When a standing subject lies down in the supine position, the lung volume and its subdivisions change as blood shifts into the thorax and the weight of the abdominal viscera moves the hemidiaphragms toward the head. Vital capacity usually decreases slightly as a result of increased intrathoracic blood volume, although in some cases there is no measurable change. Application of tourniquets to the lower extremities prevents this decrease. Fig. 4-2 shows the expiratory shift of the respiratory level, or resting midposition. Functional residual capacity decreases with expiratory reserve volume as inspiratory reserve volume increases. Relative to total lung capacity the lungs are about one-half inflated during quiet breathing in the upright position but only about one-third inflated in the supine posture. Standing on one's head exaggerates these changes. Conversely, on standing erect the descent of the abdominal viscera allows the hemidiaphragms to assume a more inspiratory position, and FRC increases with ERV at the expense of IRV.

The pulmonary circulation contains 500 to 600 ml of blood, a volume that fluctuates slightly during the respiratory cycle. During inspiration there is a slight increase of thoracic blood volume and during expiration an equal decrease. A forced inspiratory effort (Müller maneuver) or forced expiratory effort (Valsalva maneuver) against a closed glottis produces much larger change. After deep inspiration a forced expiratory effort against the closed glottis squeezes out a volume of blood, leaving room for further inspiration. Such a Valsalva maneuver can increase vital capacity by 200 to 300 ml.

Age changes the lung volume and its subdivisions. As elastic lung recoil diminishes, the resting midposition shifts in the direction of inspiration, increasing residual volume and functional residual capacity

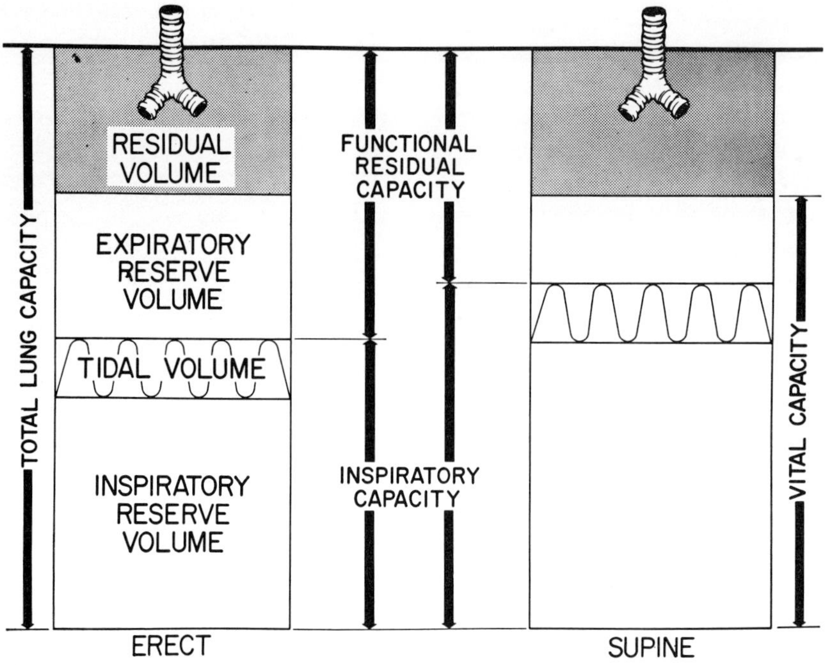

Fig. 4-2
Lung volume and its subdivisions. Diagram illustrates the importance of body position.

while decreasing vital capacity. The thoracic cage stiffens with age and chest mobility decreases. The greater FRC and decreased chest distensibility limit IC. Thus VC decreases slightly with age.

The ratio of residual volume to total lung capacity (RV/TLC) has considerable clinical significance; it is usually expressed as a percentage. Normal values range from 15% in young individuals to about 30% in the aged. Many writers give a value as high as 50% for older subjects; however, in our opinion this high value is the result of failure to distinguish between the effects of age and disease. Note that a change in this ratio may reflect a change of either RV or TLC, or both, and that proportionate change of both numerator and denominator in the same direction results in no change of the numeric value of the ratio.

The lung volume and its subdivisions may be very abnormal in patients with bronchitis-emphysema syndrome. Residual volume may increase by a factor of 2 or 3, and total lung capacity may be 150% or more of predicted. Since RV increases proportionately more than TLC, the ratio RV/TLC also increases; this ratio may reach 70% in severe cases.

Conditions producing pulmonary fibrosis and lung stiffness, such as tuberculosis, silicosis, and certain viral pneumonias, reduce TLC but somewhat increase RV. Thoracic deformity, whether congenital or acquired, reduces TLC and VC. A high proportion of patients who have severe thoracic deformity suffer from chronic alveolar hypoventilation, a condition that usually terminates in cardiopulmonary failure. Since no word existed meaning a condition of reduced thoracic volume, Slonim has proposed the neologism *stethomeiosis*.

MEASUREMENT OF LUNG VOLUME AND ITS SUBDIVISIONS

Since the lung volume and its subdivisions are essentially anatomic compart-

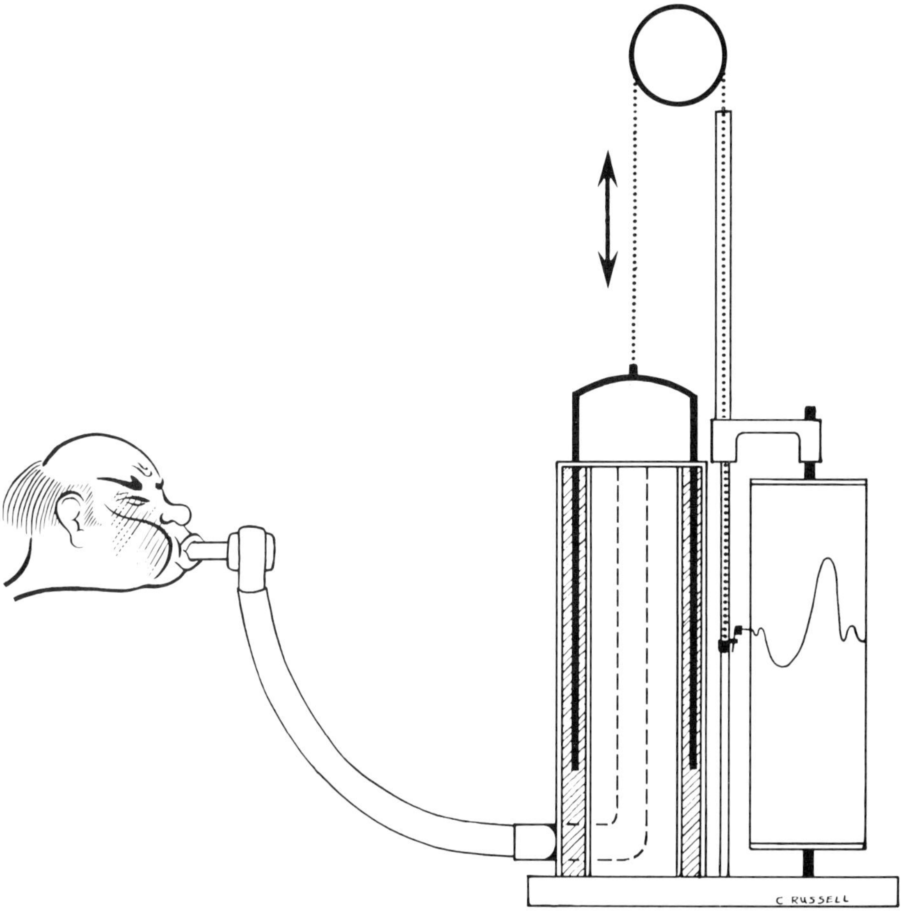

Fig. 4-3
A type of spirometer. Spirometers measure the volume of gas that the lungs inhale and exhale, usually as a function of time. They are used to measure the volume changes and flow rates of spontaneous breathing and various breathing maneuvers.

ments within the chest, their size is expressed in terms of gas volumes at body temperature, ambient pressure, and saturated with water vapor (BTPS). When they are measured or calculated by having a subject exhale into an external container or apparatus that is cooler than body temperature, the exhaled gas volume shrinks and loses water vapor. Such externally measured gas volumes are converted to volume at BTPS.

Some of the subdivisions, or compartments, of the lung volume are measured with a special gas volume recorder termed a *spirometer*. A commonly used type of spirometer is shown in Fig. 4-3. This instrument has a pen that writes on a rotating drum, inscribing a cartesian plot of spirometer gas volume versus time. When gas is blown into the spirometer, the bell rises, lowering the pen that is suspended over a pulley. As gas is inhaled from the spirometer the bell falls, raising the pen. As a result of the pulley, inspiration produces an upward, and expiration a downward, deflection on the spiro-

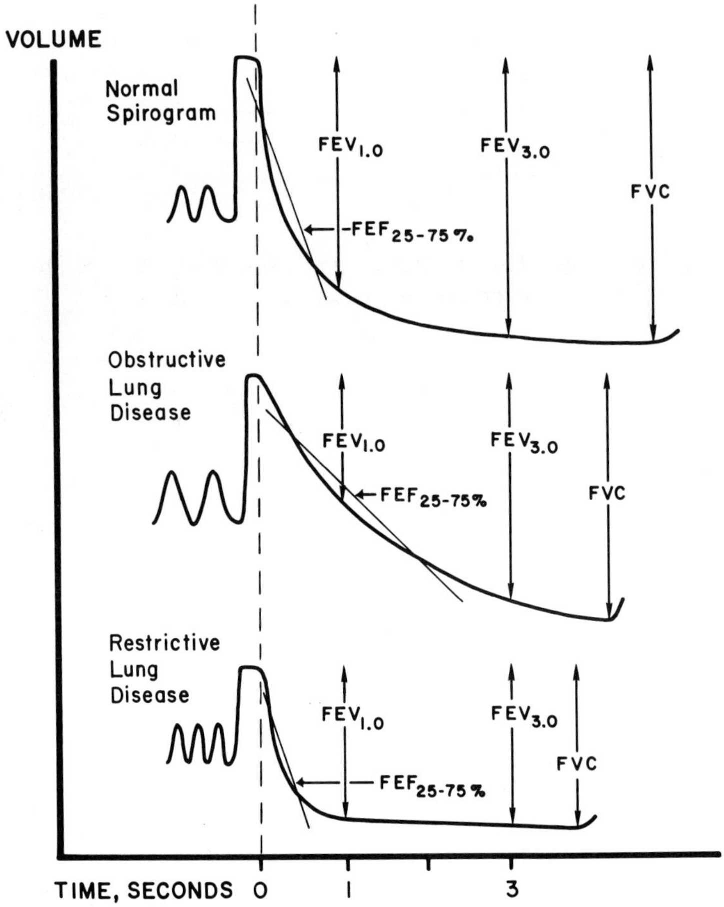

Fig. 4-4
Forced expiratory spirogram of a healthy subject (top), a patient with chronic diffuse obstructive bronchopulmonary disease (middle), and a patient with restrictive ventilatory impairment (bottom).

graphic record. Using the spirometer bell factor (the volume of gas per unit linear displacement, usually in ml/mm) we can calculate volume changes and thus tidal volume, inspiratory and expiratory reserve volumes, and vital capacity. A variety of spirometers are available for clinical use.

Spirometers also measure the capacity for dynamic changes of lung volume; that is, they measure the volumetric flow rate of gas into and out of the lung. The forced expiratory spirogram (Fig. 4-4) is a useful clinical tool for the evaluation of pulmonary function. Loss of ventilatory capacity is of two types: (1) reduced volume of gas that can be moved per breath (restrictive loss) and (2) reduced flow rate of gas during a breath (obstructive loss). Restrictive loss occurs in patients who have diminished lung or chest wall elasticity—the result, for example, of pulmonary fibrosis. Obstructive loss occurs in patients who have diffuse airways obstruction—the result, for example, of asthma or bronchitis-emphysema syndrome. Analysis and interpretation of the spirogram is discussed in Chapter 14.

Functional residual capacity, residual

volume, and total lung capacity cannot be measured with a spirometer because these compartments contain gas that cannot be expelled from the lungs. Any of three indirect methods are used to calculate them. The closed-circuit method involves the dilution of an inert, insoluble, foreign gas (usually helium) as it mixes with the gas in the lungs. The subject breathes into a sealed spirometer system of precisely known volume, containing a known initial concentration of helium. As the gas in the spirometer mixes with the gas in the lungs, helium concentration in the spirometer circuit gradually decreases to a new level. The following equation is then used to calculate the volume of gas in the lung at the beginning of the test:

$$V_L = (V_{Sp} \times \frac{He_{initial}}{He_{final}}) - V_{Sp} + C$$

where V_L is the initial lung volume; V_{Sp} is the spirometer volume; $He_{initial}$ is the initial concentration of helium in the spirometer; He_{final} is the final concentration of helium in both lung and spirometer; and C is a correction factor for change in volume due to N_2 "excretion," respiratory exchange ratio, and helium loss. The calculated gas volume must be converted from the basis of ATPS to BTPS. When this method is used, the initial lung volume is usually functional residual capacity, from which expiratory reserve volume is subtracted to obtain residual volume, or to which inspiratory capacity is added to obtain total lung capacity.

The open-circuit nitrogen wash-out method for determining functional residual capacity* involves measuring the N_2 concentration in alveolar gas. While the subject breathes pure O_2, the mixed expired gas is collected for a period of 7 minutes or more. From the volume of mixed expired gas and its N_2 concentration one can calculate the total volume of N_2 that was washed out of the lungs. Given this volume of N_2 and the initial and final alveolar N_2 concentrations, we can calculate the lung volume in which that volume of N_2 was contained. A correction is made for the volume of N_2 brought to the lungs by the blood from body stores.

A third method of measuring functional residual capacity uses a body plethysmograph, or "body box." The subject is placed within a gas-tight chamber of about 600 L, slightly smaller than a telephone booth. After temperature and humidity within the chamber have stabilized, the subject compresses the gas in his lungs by blowing against a pressure transducer. The volume changes within the sealed box produce corresponding pressure changes that are sensed by a second pressure transducer. The known initial ambient pressure, together with the measured pressure and volume changes, permit calculation of the total thoracic gas volume (V_{TG}). Both closed-circuit helium dilution and open-circuit nitrogen wash-out technics measure *communicating* gas volume. The body plethysmograph, on the other hand, measures *total* intrathoracic gas volume. Total thoracic gas volume is normally the same or slightly larger than FRC. In obstructive lung disease or pneumothorax there may be considerable difference.

In bronchospirometry a special endobronchial catheter separates the gas flows and volumes of the two lungs, permitting individual measurement of lung volumes, ventilation, and O_2 uptake. Normally, the right lung accounts for 55% and the left lung for 45% of volume, ventilation, and gas exchange.

*For further discussion of the open-circuit nitrogen wash-out method see Chapter 15.

CHAPTER 5 Mechanics of breathing

Breathing is the alternate inspiration and expiration of air into and out of the lungs. *Ventilation* is the volume of air moved into or out of the lungs per unit time, and is calculated as the product of breathing frequency (f) and tidal volume (V_T). Our definition of breathing does not include the process of gas exchange essential for effective breathing.

PATTERNS OF BREATHING

Several patterns of breathing are sufficiently significant and distinctive to be designated by special terms and discussed as entities. Certain abnormal patterns of breathing are described at the end of Chapter 12.

Eupnea is normal spontaneous breathing of which we are usually unaware. Ventilation satisfies metabolic demand. The frequency of breathing at rest is normally 13 to 17 breaths per minute with a tidal volume of about 500 ml (BTPS). Normal resting minute volume of breathing (ventilation) is thus about 7.5 L (BTPS)/min.

Hyperpnea is the increased pulmonary ventilation that matches an increased metabolic demand. For instance, muscular exercise increases pulmonary ventilation by increasing both breathing frequency and tidal volume. As a healthy trained subject exercises more and more intensely, pulmonary ventilation increases initially more by contributions from increased tidal volume than by contributions from breathing frequency; later, breathing frequency increases contribute proportionately more.

Hyperventilation also describes increased pulmonary ventilation but refers to ventilation that *exceeds* metabolic requirements. Hyperventilation is variously defined in terms of total pulmonary ventilation, alveolar ventilation, alveolar P_{CO_2}, or alveolar P_{O_2}. It may be produced by thoracic reflexes, conscious voluntary effort, or psychogenic factors (e.g., hysterical hyperventilation). In the healthy subject, alveolar hyperventilation decreases arterial blood P_{CO_2} and increases arterial blood P_{O_2}; hyperpnea does not.

Hypoventilation means underventilation in relation to the metabolic rate. For example, a total pulmonary ventilation rate of 8 L (BTPS)/min may be adequate at rest but constitutes hypoventilation during even mild exercise. As hyperventilation, hypoventilation is also defined in terms of total pulmonary ventilation, alveolar ventilation, alveolar P_{CO_2}, or alveolar P_{O_2}. Hypoventilation always increases alveolar P_{CO_2} and, when the inspired gas is air, is the *only* condition that does this. Hypoventilation is only one of several conditions that decrease arterial blood P_{O_2}. In bronchopulmonary diseases causing uneven distribution of inspired gas, some lung regions may be hyperventilated whereas others are hypoventilated.

Tachypnea is increased rate, or frequency, of breathing; it does not necessarily imply a change in total pulmonary ventilation. If total pulmonary ventilation does increase, tachypnea may occur with either hyperpnea or hyperventilation; if total pulmonary ventilation decreases due to concomitant decrease in tidal volume, tachypnea may actually occur with hypoventilation.

Dyspnea is difficult or labored breathing. It is defined as the uncomfortable subjective awareness of the desire for increased breathing. Dyspnea is thus a symptom, not a sign. Although usually associated with hypoventilation, it may be experienced during extreme hyperventilation (e.g., hysterical hyperventilation). The sensation of dyspnea is commonly related to abnormalities of pulmonary mechanics and seen in patients with reduced ventilatory capacity or cardiac insufficiency. Curiously, it is not directly related to chronic hypoxemia and hypercapnic acidosis. It is likely that a healthy trained subject does not experience true dyspnea even during the most extreme physical exertion.

Orthopnea refers to dyspnea that is experienced only in recumbency (usually supine) and is promptly relieved by assuming an upright position. It occurs in patients who have cardiac (left ventricular) insufficiency but is remarkably absent in patients with bronchopulmonary disease, even when associated with cor pulmonale.

Apnea is the absence or cessation of breathing, usually in the resting midposition. It connotes temporary cessation with the expectation that breathing will resume spontaneously. Apnea occurs during swallowing, after hyperventilation, as a result of trauma, and sometimes at birth. If breathing does not resume, the condition is termed *respiratory arrest.*

DEAD SPACE

The concepts of anatomic and physiologic *dead space* (V_D)* are essential to an understanding of alveolar ventilation. *Anatomic* dead space (inert-gas dead space) is the internal volume of all conducting (nongas-exchanging) airways, from the nose and mouth down to the respiratory bronchioles. *Physiologic* dead space is that portion of each tidal volume that does *not* exchange gas; it is a calculated quantity, not a topographic volume. In reality, inspired gas varies with respect to gas exchange from the extreme of full equilibrium with pulmonary end-capillary blood to the extreme of no gas exchange. We divide the volume of inspired gas between a theoretic dead space volume and a theoretic alveolar volume, both compartments having uniform composition, and express dead space volume as if only the two extreme conditions existed. It is an estimate of the volume of inspirate that would be returned to the atmosphere unchanged if all of the air undergoing gas exchange achieved complete equilibrium with pulmonary end-capillary blood. Physiologic dead space is thus a *theoretic* volume, comparable to the concept of *clearance* in renal physiology.

Anatomic dead space is calculated from measurements of expired volume per breath and the CO_2 concentrations of mixed expired gas and alveolar gas. Mixed expired gas, obtained by collecting the entire expired gas stream, is a mixture of alveolar gas with dead space gas. Since dead space gas has the composition of inspired air, it contains negligible CO_2. Using expired volume (V_E) and the fractional concentrations of CO_2 (F_{CO_2}) in the gas samples, the volume of gas coming from the alveoli per breath (V_{AT}) is calculated as follows:

$$(1)\ V_{A_T} = V_E \frac{F_{E_{CO_2}}}{F_{A_{CO_2}}}$$

Anatomic dead space is then calculated as follows:

$$(2)\ V_D = V_E - V_{A_T}$$

The anatomic dead space volume of an adult in milliliters is about equal to his

*See the Table of Symbols and Abbreviations for Respiratory Physiology in the Appendix.

ideal weight in pounds; it is closely related to body height. Although relatively constant, anatomic dead space is somewhat increased by lung inflation, during exercise, with age, and in pulmonary emphysema, a disease in which the lungs enlarge. It is decreased in the supine position and by pneumonectomy and tracheostomy because of the removal or bypass of some of the conducting airway. It may also decrease in asthma as a result of airway narrowing.

Physiologic dead space is calculated from measurements of mixed expired gas and arterial blood. Arterial blood P_{CO_2} is assumed to be in equilibrium with alveolar P_{CO_2} and to represent *mean* alveolar P_{CO_2}. This pressure is compared with the P_{CO_2} of mixed expired gas ($P_{E_{CO_2}}$). The P_{CO_2} of mixed expired gas that is saturated with water vapor is calculated as follows:

$$P_{E_{CO_2}} = F_{E_{CO_2}} (P_B - 47)$$

where P_B is barometric, or ambient, pressure and 47 is the water vapor pressure in mm Hg at 37° C. Substituting the pressure of CO_2 for fractional concentration of CO_2 and combining equations (1) and (2) earlier, we obtain:

$$(3)\ V_D = V_E - V_E \frac{P_{E_{CO_2}}}{P_{a_{CO_2}}}$$

When expressed for a particular gas, physiologic dead space may be defined as the number that must be used for V_D in the Bohr equation to relate tidal volume to arterial, inspired, and mixed expired gas tensions.

Physiologic dead space is more useful than anatomic dead space in assessing the effectiveness of pulmonary ventilation. When inspired gas and pulmonary capillary blood flow are both evenly distributed within the lung, gas exchange is optimal, alveolar gas is of uniform composition, and physiologic dead space is only *slightly* larger than anatomic dead space. However, in patients with diffuse bronchopulmonary disease these two may differ appreciably. The difference between anatomic and physiologic dead space has been termed *alveolar dead space* and is an index of uneven pulmonary blood flow; comparson with the anatomic dead space expresses the nonuniformity of $\dot{V}/\dot{Q}$ ratios in the lung. The concept of physiologic dead space is intimately related to the problem of ventilation-perfusion ratios.

Some prefer the term *total* dead space to *physiologic* dead space. The reasoning is as follows. In supine man* physiologic dead space is only slightly greater than anatomic dead space, a volume that, in health, may be thought of as the irreducible dead space. When physiologic dead space exceeds anatomic dead space appreciably in supine man, the difference is almost entirely *pathologic* and should not be included in the *physiologic* dead space. Under these conditions the conventional term *physiologic dead space* includes the pathologic alveolar dead space that results from disease, the physiologic alveolar dead space of upright man, and the anatomic dead space.

ALVEOLAR VENTILATION

Alveolar ventilation, also termed *effective ventilation,* is the volume of fresh air introduced into the gas-exchanging regions of the lung per minute. At the end of expiration the conducting airways (anatomic dead space) are filled with alveolar gas; this volume of gas returns to the alveoli at the beginning of the next inspiration but does not participate further in gas exchange. The effective volume of each inspiration is thus tidal volume minus dead space volume. Ventilation, or minute volume of breathing, is the product of volume per breath and breaths per minute. For total ventilation (volume expired per minute):

$$\dot{V}_E = V_E \times f$$

*Lung perfusion varies with body position.

and for dead space ventilation:

$$\dot{V}_D = V_D \times f$$

Alveolar ventilation is:

$$\dot{V}_A = \dot{V}_E - \dot{V}_D = (V_E - V_D)f$$

Dead space ventilation is the difference between total pulmonary ventilation and alveolar ventilation. Since the dead space of a given individual is relatively constant, changes in dead space ventilation are almost entirely due to changes in breathing frequency. Thus, if tidal volume remains unchanged, dead space ventilation increases as breathing frequency increases. Fig. 5-1 shows how breathing frequency and tidal volume affect total pulmonary ventilation, dead space volume and alveolar ventilation remaining constant. In chronic diffuse obstructive bronchopulmonary disease with increased dead space and airway resistance, it is even more economical to increase alveolar ventilation by increasing tidal volume than by increasing breathing frequency.

The ventilation equation

During a steady state of the circulation and respiration, the rate of metabolic CO_2 production equals the rate of CO_2 elimination:

$$\dot{V}_{CO_2} = F_{E_{CO_2}} \cdot \dot{V}_E$$

When air is breathed, respiratory dead space contains virtually no CO_2, so that all the expired CO_2 is a product of alveolar ventilation:

$$\dot{V}_{CO_2} = F_{A_{CO_2}} \cdot \dot{V}_A$$

Using the relationship

$$P_{A_{CO_2}} = F_{A_{CO_2}} (P_B - 47)$$

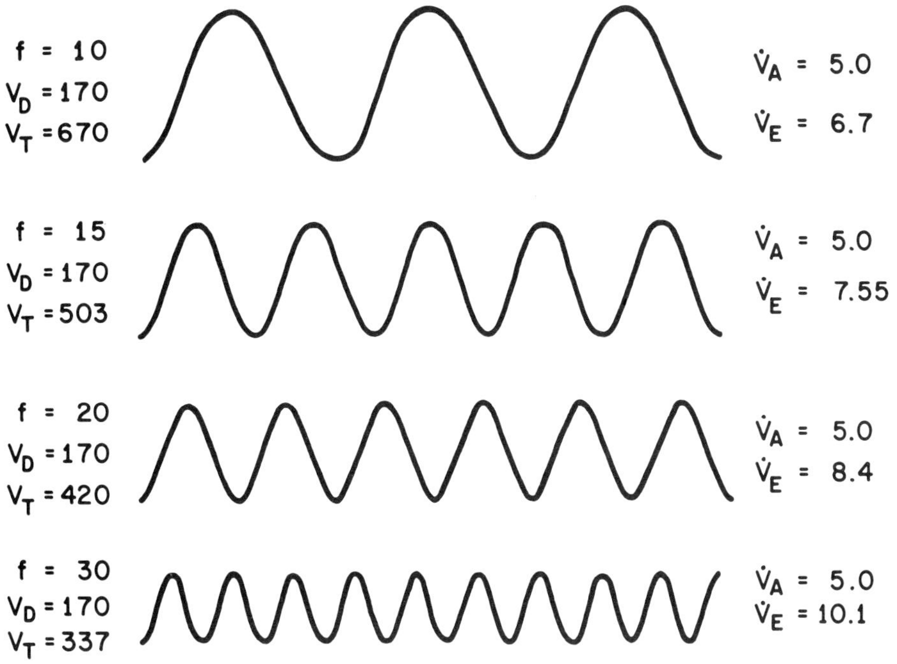

Fig. 5-1
Effect of changing breathing frequency and tidal volume on total pulmonary ventilation. Dead space volume and alveolar ventilation remain constant.

to substitute P_{ACO_2} for F_{ACO_2}, we obtain the following:

$$P_{ACO_2} \cdot \dot{V}_A = \dot{V}_{CO_2} (P_B - 47)$$

If activity level does not change, then $\dot{V}_{CO_2}$ remains relatively constant, and the graph of this equation is a rectangular hyperbola:

$$P_{ACO_2} \cdot \dot{V}_A = \text{Constant}$$

P_{ACO_2} and $\dot{V}_A$ are thus reciprocals. If a subject hyperventilates to such an extent that $\dot{V}_A$ is doubled, the P_{ACO_2} is halved. If he hypoventilates to such an extent that $\dot{V}_A$ is halved, P_{ACO_2} is doubled. This relationship is seen in Fig. 10-6 by comparing ventilation ratio with P_{CO_2}.

Since

$$R_S = \frac{\dot{V}_{CO_2}}{\dot{V}_{O_2}}, \text{ and } \dot{V}_{CO_2} = \dot{V}_{O_2} \cdot R_S$$

then $\dot{V}_{O_2} \cdot R_S$ can be substituted for $\dot{V}_{CO_2}$ in the ventilation equation, which then becomes:

$$\dot{V}_A \cdot P_{ACO_2} = \dot{V}_{O_2} \cdot R_S (P_B - 47)$$

INSPIRATION

Inspiration enlarges the chest cavity in all three dimensions. The external intercostal muscles are largely responsible for increases in two of these due to the shape of the thoracic cage and the oblique orientation of these muscles between the ribs. Descent of the two hemidiaphragms is responsible for expansion in the third dimension.

1. During inspiration the sternum and anterior portion of the thoracic cage are elevated, increasing the anteroposterior dimension of the chest. Due to the downward direction of the ribs from their origin and insertion this action has been called the "pump-handle" effect.

2. The ribs rotate outward. Due to their shape and angle of attachment this outward rotation increases the lateral dimension of the lower chest. This action has been called the "water-bucket-handle" effect.

3. Contraction flattens the normally convex muscular diaphragm. The hemidiaphragms descend into the abdomen, increasing the length of the thoracic cavity.

During hyperpnea or dyspnea the auxiliary muscles of inspiration come into play, assisting in the elevation of the anterior chest wall and increasing inspiratory volume by a small amount.

The visceral pleura on the surface of the lungs is in intimate contact with the parietal pleura that lines the inner wall of the chest cavity. As the chest wall moves out, this intimate pleural contact is maintained and the lungs move out with it. As the volume of the lung increases, gas pressure inside the lung decreases (Chapter 2, Boyle's law). If airways are patent, air moves from the outside where pressure is atmospheric, into the lungs where pressure is subatmospheric ("negative"). As inspiration continues, "negative" pressure is maintained within the lungs. At the end of inspiration the pressure equalizes between lung and atmosphere, and air inflow ceases.

Patients whose primary or ordinary accessory muscles of respiration are paralyzed, but whose head and neck muscles are not, can learn to "swallow" air rapidly into the lungs using the tongue and pharyngeal muscles. This method of breathing is sometimes called "frog-breathing" because the frog fills its cheeks with air, closes its orifices, and then contracts its buccal muscles, pushing air into its lungs. A better term is *glossopharyngeal breathing.*

EXPIRATION

The quiet expiration that follows a spontaneous normal inspiration is a passive process. The elastic recoil of the intrathoracic structures tends to decrease the volume of the thoracic cage; the ribs rotate downward and the hemidiaphragms relax. Decreasing lung volume compresses intrapulmonary gas, and if airways are patent, gas flows

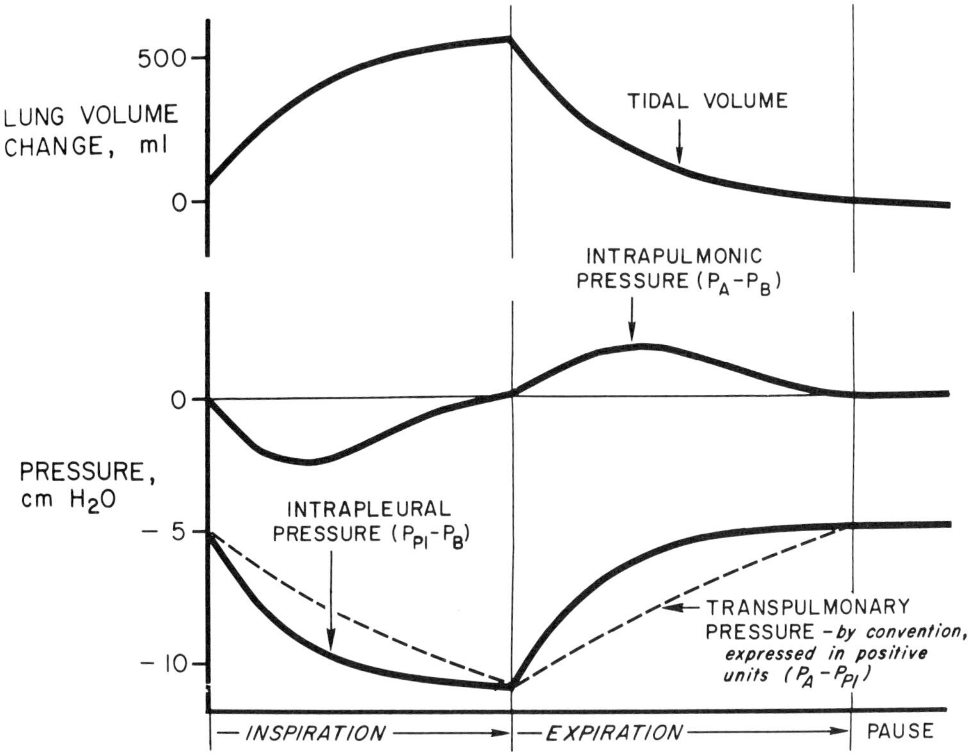

Fig. 5-2
Changes and interrelationships of lung volume, intrapulmonary pressure, intrapleural pressure, and transpulmonary pressure during a breathing cycle.

out of the lung toward the region of lower (atmospheric) pressure. At the end of expiration, relaxation forces have returned the lung-chest system to its resting level and the pressure within the lung is atmospheric. This completes the breathing cycle.

Although expiration is usually a passive process and relaxation forces are sufficient to restore the lung-chest system to resting midposition, a diminishing inspiratory muscle tone smooths expiration. Inspiratory muscles relax completely only near the end of quiet spontaneous expiration. The relationships among lung volume, intrapleural pressure, and intrapulmonary pressure for a normal spontaneous breath are shown in Fig. 5-2.

When expiration is active, internal intercostal muscles assist in returning the thoracic cage to end-expiratory level; the hemidiaphragms, forced by the abdominal muscles, move upward into the thorax faster and farther than they do during passive expiration.

RELAXATION FORCES

Both lungs and chest wall have elasticity and, in the intact thorax, each is deformed by the elastic pull of the other. If removed from the enclosing chest wall, the lungs contract to a much smaller size; freed from the opposing elastic force of the lungs, the chest expands to a larger volume. When lungs and chest wall are in normal relationship with their pleurae in contact and no external force applied, the resting lung volume reflects the balance between these two opposing elastic forces, functional residual capacity (Chapter 3).

Because the elastic forces of lungs and chest wall oppose each other, the interface between visceral and parietal pleurae (potential intrapleural space) is at subatmospheric ("negative") pressure. If this intrapleural interface develops a communication with the outside air or with intrapulmonary gas, gas moves into the "negative" intrapleural pressure region, creating an actual intrapleural space, or pneumothorax.

Breathing and body position both change intrapleural pressure. With trunk erect, gravity pulls the abdominal contents down, pushing out the abdominal wall. The hemidiaphragms descend and the volume of the chest cavity increases. During recumbency, gravity pulls the abdominal contents toward the head, decreasing the volume of the chest cavity and increasing intrapleural pressure.

RELAXATION PRESSURE CURVE

If a subject inhales moderately, closes the glottis, and relaxes the respiratory muscles, the pressure in the lungs exceeds

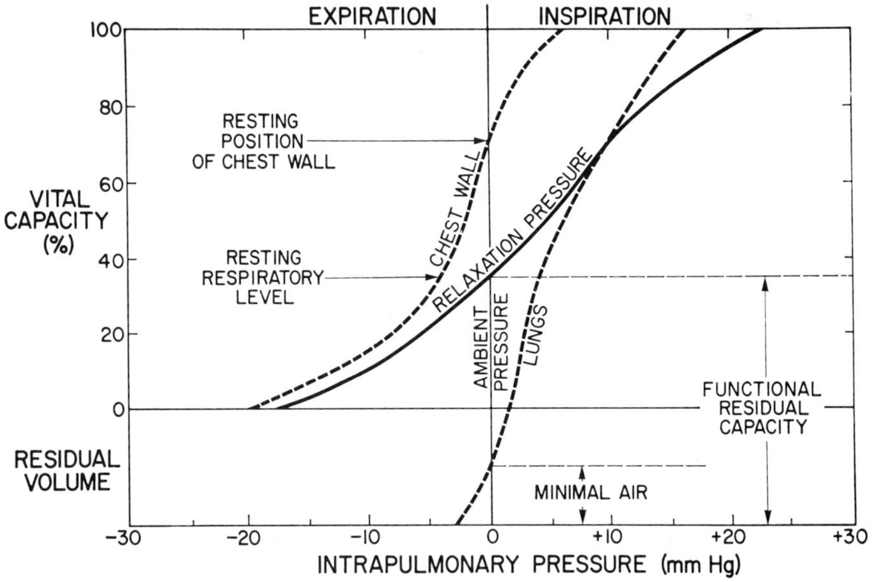

Fig. 5-3
The pressure-volume diagram of chest wall and lungs in healthy man: the relaxation pressure curve. The relaxation pressure curve (solid line) of the chest wall and lungs is the sum of its two components: the elasticity of the chest wall and diaphragm (dashed line on left), and the elasticity of the lungs (dashed line on right). The relaxation pressure curve crosses the ambient pressure or zero axis where lung elasticity exactly balances chest wall elasticity, thus indicating the resting respiratory level and defining the functional residual capacity. At about 70% of the vital capacity, relaxation pressure is due entirely to lung elasticity. At that level the lung curve intersects the relaxation pressure curve, and the chest wall curve crosses the ambient pressure on zero axis, thus indicating the resting position of the chest wall. Minimal air is defined by the level at which the lung curve intersects the ambient pressure or zero axis. (Redrawn from Rahn, H., Otis, A. B., Chadwick, L. E., and Fenn, W. O.: Amer. J. Physiol. **146:**161, 1946.)

atmospheric pressure; inflation increases the elastic recoil of the lung and decreases the opposing elastic force of the chest wall. If the subject inhales more deeply, closes the glottis, and relaxes, intrapulmonary pressure increases still further. However, if he exhales completely, closes the glottis, and relaxes, intrapulmonary pressure is subatmospheric; the deflationary elastic force of the lung is now less than the inflationary elastic force of the chest. A plot of an infinite number of such relaxation pressures against their corresponding lung volumes gives the *relaxation pressure curve* (Fig. 5-3).

The pressure at every point on this curve is the resultant of the elastic forces exerted by the lung and those exerted by the chest wall. At about 70% vital capacity the chest is the size it would assume if there were no lung elasticity pulling it in; at this volume* lung elasticity is solely responsible for the relaxation pressure. Above 70% vital capacity lung and chest

*The chests of patients who have lost lung elasticity approach this volume, accounting for the barrel-chest appearance of such individuals and their large functional residual capacity values. In extreme ectomorphs this effect is more difficult to observe because the barrel chest resembles the normal-sized chest of average individuals.

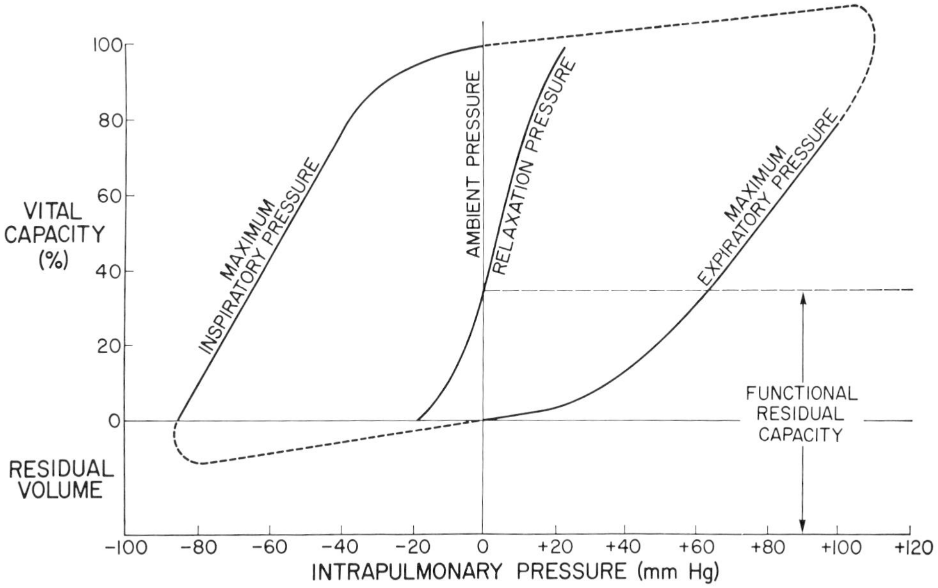

Fig. 5-4

The pressure-volume diagram of chest wall and lungs in healthy man. On the vertical axis 100% vital capacity represents maximum inspiration, and 0% vital capacity represents maximum expiration at ambient or zero intrapulmonary pressure. The diagram shows the pressures that are developed passively (relaxation pressures) and those that can be developed actively (maximum pressures) at various lung volumes. Where the lung is maximally expanded with high intrapulmonary pressure (dashed line in right upper corner), there is danger of lung rupture. Where intrapulmonary pressure is lowest (dashed line in left lower corner), there is extreme dilatation of blood vessels and danger of hemorrhage. (Redrawn from Rahn, H., Otis, A. B., Chadwick, L. E., and Fenn, W. O.: Amer. J. Physiol. **146:**161, 1946.)

forces are no longer antagonistic but operate additively to give the relaxation pressure curve.

MAXIMUM PRESSURE CURVES

The relaxation pressure curve results from passive elastic forces of the lung and chest. However, it is only part of a larger picture that includes maximum inspiratory and expiratory pressure curves (Fig. 5-4). These maximum curves indicate the limits within which ventilation must occur. We commonly exert maximum or submaximum expiratory pressure against a closed glottis (Valsalva maneuver) while straining at stool, during childbirth, or lifting. The maximum expiratory pressure attainable varies with the lung volume at which the pressure is exerted. The larger the initial lung volume the greater is the pressure that can be exerted; the smaller the initial lung volume the more subatmospheric ("negative") is the maximum inspiratory pressure (Müller maneuver). Obviously, further inspiratory efforts are without effect at full inspiration, just as further expiratory efforts are without effect at full expiration.

The maximum pressure curves are the resultant of active muscle forces (intercostal and diaphragmatic during a Müller maneuver and abdominal during a Valsalva maneuver) and the passive elastic forces of the lung and chest; that is, the maximum Valsalva maneuver at full inspiration is due partly to passive elastic forces (relaxation pressure) and partly to active forces (mostly abdominal muscle). By subtracting the relaxation pressure curve from the maximum expiratory pressure curve, we obtain a muscle length-tension diagram.

The great pressure, usually exceeding 100 mm Hg, of a maximum Valsalva maneuver impedes systemic venous return to the right heart. If continued longer than 10 or 15 seconds, cardiac output and, consequently, cerebral blood flow diminish greatly and unconsciousness may occur.

COMPLIANCE

Compliance is a measure of the distensibility of the chest and/or lungs—the ease with which lung volume is changed. It is expressed in units of liters (BTPS) of lung volume change per cm H_2O pressure change. Greater compliance means a larger volume change per unit pressure change. For calculating the compliance of the total lung-chest system we use the pressure difference (ΔP) between airway pressure and atmospheric pressure.

For calculating *lung* compliance (C_L) we use *transpulmonary* pressure—the pressure difference (ΔP) between alveolar pressure and intrapleural pressure. During normal quiet breathing, lung compliance is about 0.2 L (BTPS)/cm H_2O. With lungs and chest wall intact the total lung-chest compliance is about 0.1 L (BTPS)/cm H_2O, half that of lungs or chest alone. Fig. 5-3, with intrapulmonary pressure on the horizontal axis and lung volume (percent vital capacity) on the vertical axis, shows that a larger pressure change is required to produce a given volume change in the combined system than in either lungs or chest wall alone.

Compliance of the bronchopulmonary system is a measure of its elasticity, the resistance to deformation (strain) produced by an applied force (stress). Truly elastic bodies have a linear relationship between applied force and resulting deformation, or length (Hooke's law). If we substitute change in pressure for change in force, and change in volume for change in length, a pressure-volume curve for the bronchopulmonary system can be plotted. This elasticity curve is the relaxation pressure curve (Fig. 5-3), a measure of the *static* compliance of the system. Bronchopulmonary diseases affect lung compliance primarily, whereas chest wall compliance (C_W) is affected by obesity and by diseases of thoracic nerves, muscles, bones, and joints. However, lung compliance appears to have more medical relevance than chest wall compliance.

Determinants of lung compliance

Surface tension. Surface tension is a phenomenon at a liquid-gas interface. The property is due to the attractive forces, or cohesion, between molecules at the boundary of the liquid and to their specific orientation. The attractive forces between liquid molecules at the surface are greater than those between liquid and gas. The result is a net force exerted in the plane of the boundary that acts to preserve the integrity of the surface of separation and to resist rupture of the surface film of the liquid. This net force of attraction, or surface tension, tends to contract an exposed liquid surface such as a drop (one surface) or bubble (two surfaces) to the smallest possible area, minimizing the surface area to volume ratio. Surface tension is expressed in dynes/cm or ergs/cm^2.

Laplace's law. The surface tension of a soap bubble on the end of a tube tends to collapse the bubble, compressing the gas inside with a certain pressure if collapse is resisted. Laplace's law states that the pressure within a spherical liquid drop or bubble is directly proportional to the surface tension and inversely proportional to the radius; the equation that describes this relationship for a drop (one surface) is as follows:

$$P = \frac{2T}{r}$$

where P is pressure in dynes/cm^2, T is surface tension in dynes/cm, and r is radius in cm. For a bubble (two surfaces) the relationship is as follows:

$$P = \frac{4T}{r}$$

As surface tension increases or as radius decreases, the pressure required to maintain the volume of a bubble increases. If we interconnect two bubbles with the same surface tension but different radii, that with the smaller radius (r_1) will empty into that with the larger radius (r_2) because P_1 is greater than P_2 (Fig. 5-5). The

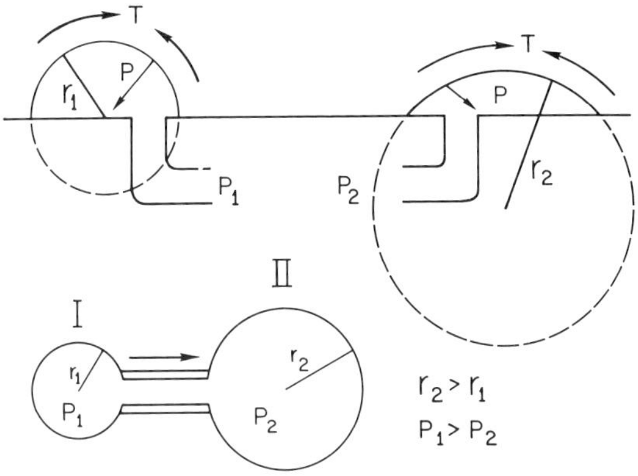

Fig. 5-5
Pressure-radius relationship for two bubbles of different size but having equal surface tension. Bubble I, with smaller radius **(r)**, has a higher pressure **(P_1)** and will empty into bubble II when they are interconnected.

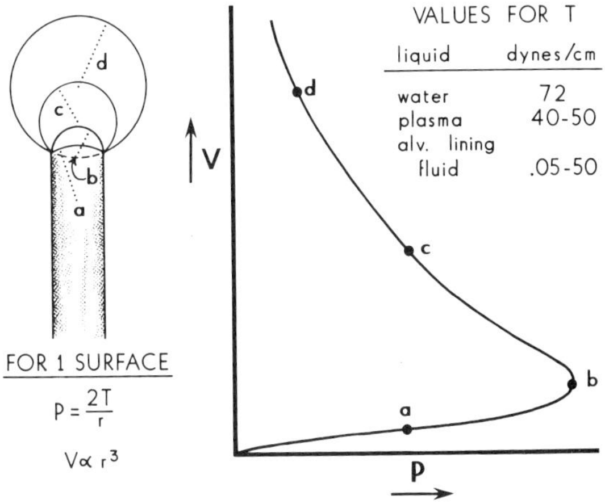

Fig. 5-6
Pressure-volume relationship of a bubble of radius **b** on the end of a tube. Surface tension is constant.

minimum radius and, therefore, maximum pressure is reached when the diameter of the bubble equals the diameter of the supporting tube. Since the volume of a spherical bubble is proportional to the cube of its radius, volume is a nonlinear function of the internal pressure. Fig. 5-6 shows this relationship for a bubble at the end of a tube. The Laplace relationship for a drop (one surface) is relevant for respiratory physiology because the liquid lining the pulmonary alveoli has one gas-liquid boundary.

Compliance, an important biophysical characteristic of the lungs and chest, is due to the elasticity of the connective tissue of airways, lungs, and blood vessels and to the surface tension of the alveolar gas-liquid interface. We can isolate the effect of elasticity by removing the gas-liquid interface and, thus, the surface tension component. An excised de-aerated lung, suspended in saline to cancel the weight of the filling liquid, inflates with saline much more easily than the same lung suspended in air can be inflated with air. Fig. 5-7 compares the pressure-volume relationship for an excised lung during inflation with air to that during saline inflation. Since saline inflation abolishes the gas-liquid interface without changing elastic recoil, the curve on the left is compliance due to elasticity alone and that on the right is compliance due to both elasticity and surface tension.

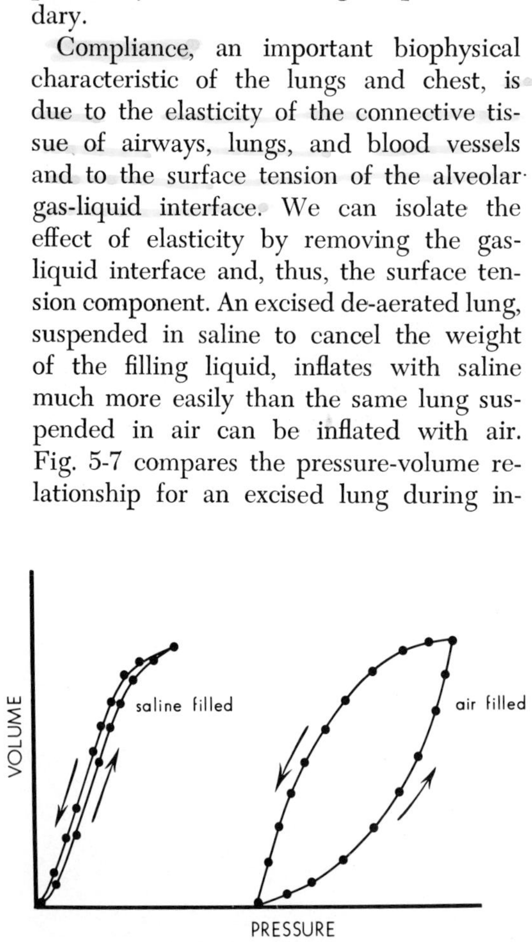

Fig. 5-7
Static pressure-volume curves of saline-filled and air-filled excised lungs, demonstrating the effects of elastic forces (left) and elastic plus surface tension forces (right) on static compliance of the lung.

Measuring lung compliance

Transpulmonary pressure, the difference between intrapleural pressure and alveolar pressure, is used to calculate lung compliance. To obtain intrapleural pressure the subject swallows a balloon on the end of a small catheter. The slightly inflated balloon is positioned in the lower third of the esophagus to measure intraesophageal pressure; this pressure is assumed to be equal to intrapleural pressure. Alveolar pressure is momentarily equal to ambient pressure at the end of inspiration and expiration. Thus, at these two points, intrapleural pressure is equal to transpulmonary pressure (Fig. 5-8), and we can use these two intrapleural pressures to calculate compliance.

Dynamic lung compliance is calculated by dividing the lung volume change during a tidal breath by the simultaneous intrapleural pressure change. A normal compliance curve is shown in Fig. 5-8. A 1 L lung volume change associated with a 5 cm H_2O transpulmonary pressure change gives a lung compliance (C_L) of 1.0 ÷ 5, or 0.2 L (BTPS)/cm H_2O. The loop generated by a continuous plot of pressure versus volume during a single breath is due to the changing pressure-volume relationship during inspiration and expiration.

Elastance

Elastance is the transpulmonary pressure change (ΔP) required to produce a unit change of lung volume (ΔV); it is thus the reciprocal of compliance. Since a transpulmonary pressure change of 5 cm H_2O normally produces a 1 L volume change, lung elastance is 5.0 ÷ 1.0, or 5 cm H_2O/L (BTPS). In one sense elastance is anal-

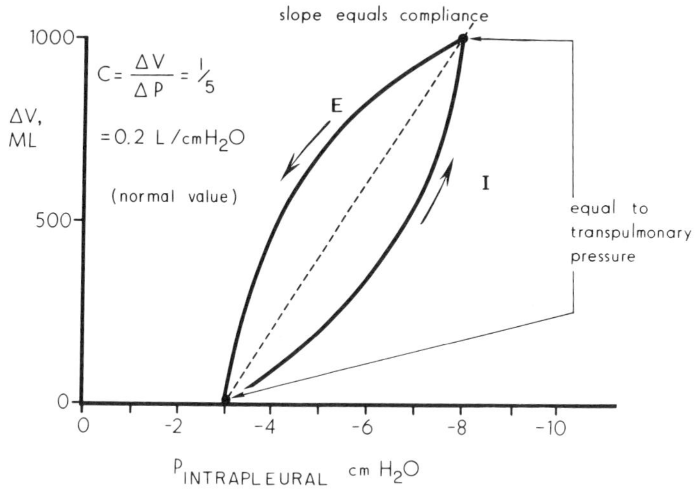

Fig. 5-8
Pressure-volume curve. Dynamic compliance of the lung is calculated from such a curve.

ogous to the resistance of an electric circuit; total resistance of a series of electric resistances is the algebraic sum of the individual resistances. Similarly, the total elastance of the lung-chest system is the sum of the individual elastances:

$$El_T = El_L + El_W$$

Lung elastance and chest wall elastance are normally about equal; the total elastance of the lung-chest system is about twice that of the lung alone:

$$El_T = 5.0 + 5.0 = 10 \text{ cm } H_2O/L \text{ (BTPS)}$$

ALVEOLAR PRESSURE–VOLUME RELATIONSHIP

Fluid lines the alveoli, and the surface tension at the gas-liquid interface affects alveolar filling. Thus the alveolar pressure–volume relationship involves both alveolar surface tension and alveolar elasticity. This complex relationship is shown in Fig. 5-9. Surface tension effect predominates when alveoli are small, and elastic forces predominate when alveoli are inflated. In the process of opening a collapsed alveolus, pressure increases steadily, overcoming alveolar surface tension until

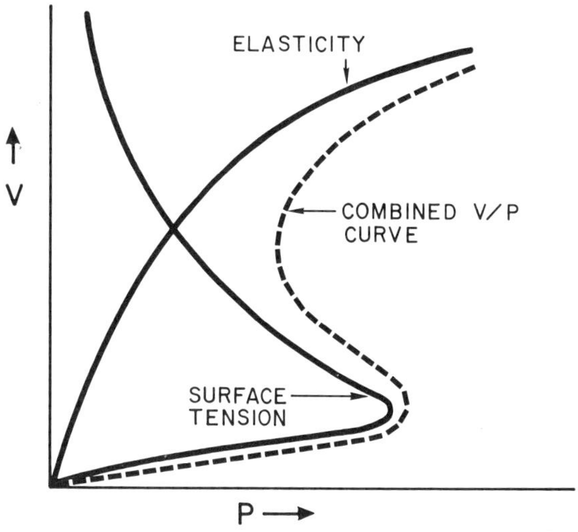

Fig. 5-9
Theoretic pressure-volume curve for an alveolus that has unchanging surface tension. The combined curve is the sum of the elasticity curve and the surface tension curve.

alveolar radius equals that of the alveolar duct; any further pressure increase will snap the alveolus open. The pressure necessary to reach this point, termed *critical opening pressure*, is determined primarily by alveolar surface tension and by the

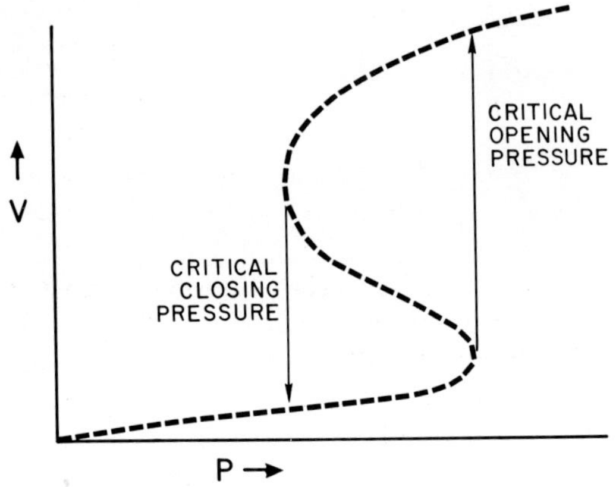

Fig. 5-10
Pressure-volume curve for an alveolus that has unchanging surface tension, showing the "critical opening pressure" and the "critical closing pressure."

diameter of the alveolar duct. Beyond this pressure, elasticity is the chief determinant of the pressure–volume curve. In the process of closing an open alveolus, the pressure-volume relationship initially reflects alveolar elasticity, but as volume continues to decrease, surface tension becomes the more important factor. The point at which further pressure decrease allows the alveolus to collapse is called *critical closing pressure.* Fig. 5-10 shows these two critical points.

The pressure-volume relationship during alveolar inflation differs from that during deflation. Thus, at a given pressure, inspiratory alveolar volume differs from expiratory alveolar volume, the lung reflecting its recent history with respect to volume change; this characteristic is termed *hysteresis.*

PULMONARY SURFACTANT

All open alveoli are exposed to the same airway pressure on the inside and to the opposing intrapleural pressure on the outside. The difference, or transpulmonary pressure, is thus essentially the same for all open alveoli regardless of their size. Laplace's law, as well as other pressure-volume considerations, suggests that as transpulmonary pressure increases, large alveoli should get larger, small alveoli should get smaller, and collapsed alveoli should never open; indeed, small alveoli should empty into larger alveoli and tend to collapse. How does the lung inflate evenly if the only factors involved are alveolar elasticity and a fixed surface tension? The relatively even distribution of ventilation within the lung implies that some other factor is operating. The identification and solution of this problem is one of the most fascinating chapters in the history of respiratory physiology.

A chemical substance in the alveolar lining fluid varies surface tension as alveolar volume changes—*pulmonary surfactant.** Strictly speaking, the plural, pulmonary *surfactants* is preferable because there is a family of phospholipid surfactants; for simplicity we will call them *pulmonary surfactant.* The lung synthesizes fatty acids and incorporates them into phospholipids such as dipalmitoyl lecithin. Lecithin, which is present in the highest concentration and is thus the most important surfactant, must contain two saturated fatty acid residues to exhibit surfactant properties. Pulmonary phospholipids are probably synthesized within the type II epithelial cells and secreted into the alveoli, where they become a part of the lining layer. The surface-active lecithin has a relatively short half-life of 14 hours. The fate of the phospholipids is unknown, although there is evidence that macrophages play a role in their removal from the lining. It is likely that the entire metabolic cycle, from synthesis to removal, occurs within the lung.

The surfactant molecule has a *hydrophobic end* (water insoluble) and a *hydrophilic end* (water soluble). It thus remains

*Detergents also decrease surface tension; however, they differ from surfactants in that they are entirely soluble in the liquid phase and thus do not change the surface tension as surface area changes.

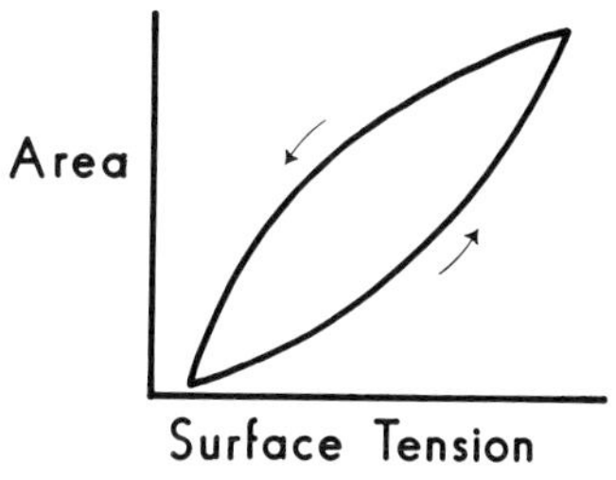

Fig. 5-11
Idealized curve for the area versus surface tension relationship of normal lung extract with surfactant.

at the gas-liquid interface oriented so that the polar (hydrophilic) portion of the molecule is in the liquid phase and the nonpolar (hydrophobic) portion is in the gas phase. The interruption of the surface by surfactant molecules decreases surface tension. The surface tension of the alveolar lining fluid, which might otherwise be about 72 dynes/cm (the surface tension of water), is reduced to a *mean* tension of 20 to 25 dynes/cm. As the boundary area containing pulmonary surfactant contracts, surface tension falls; as it expands, surface tension increases. Decreased surface area increases the number of surfactant molecules per unit area, decreasing surface tension; increased surface area decreases surfactant concentration, increasing surface tension. This effect promotes alveolar stability. The resistance of the boundary to compression is related to the surface density (number of molecules per unit area) of surfactant; as the boundary contracts, it offers progressively greater resistance to further compression. This effect also promotes alveolar stability.

The surfactant effect of lung washings or lung extracts can be demonstrated with a Wilhelmi balance. In this apparatus surface tension is continuously measured as a slowly moving barrier changes the area containing surfactant. Fig. 5-11 shows an idealized curve for the area-surface tension relationship of an alveolar extract. As area is first decreased and then increased a hysteresis loop is recorded, presumably due to a change in the orientation of surfactant molecules as their concentration changes. However, the significance of this hysteresis is not fully understood.

Since alveolar surface tension decreases more rapidly than alveolar radius, small alveoli enlarge with even less pressure than large alveoli; since transpulmonary pressure is essentially equal for all lung units, pulmonary surfactant increases lung compliance and favors even distribution of inspired gas. Surfactant has significance for alveolar liquid balance. If alveolar surface tension were as high as that of serum, approximately 55 dynes/cm, the alveoli would be edematous. A high surface tension favors movement of liquid from pulmonary capillaries and interstices into alveolar spaces and may cause alveolar collapse. The low surface tension of healthy lungs, an essential element in the balance of forces, including colloid osmotic pressure and capillary hydrostatic pressure, favors alveolar dryness. The movement and spread of surfactant molecules and the concomitant movement of the hypophase may also have significance for alveolar clearance and alveolar configuration.

Surfactant deficiency

Deficiency of pulmonary surfactant impairs lung function, decreasing compliance and causing uneven distribution of inspired gas. Various conditions interfere with the normal production of surfactant or favor its inactivation:

1. Hypoxia.
2. Acidosis.
3. Abnormalities of pulmonary circulation, such as embolism and vascular congestion.
4. Atelectasis.
5. Pulmonary edema (the accumulation of fluid in interstitial and alveolar spaces).

6. Extracorporeal circulation (cardiopulmonary bypass).
7. Hyperoxia. In the usual clinical setting O_2 is administered in relatively low concentration with frequent interruption necessitated by patient activity and nursing care. However, long-term administration of O_2 in excessive concentration can aggravate the distribution and diffusion problems of patients with bronchopulmonary disease. Surfactant deficiency may be involved in these adverse effects.
8. Pulmonary lavage.
9. Aspiration of various foreign materials, including hydrocarbons.
10. Drowning.
11. Respiratory distress syndrome of the newborn infant.

RESISTANCE TO BREATHING

Biophysical components of resistance to breathing

Resistance means opposition to motion. Because motion involves friction, resistance occurs in any moving part of the respiratory system. Resistance to breathing involves the dynamic forces required to initiate and maintain gas flow through the airways during the breathing cycle. Total respiratory resistance consists of airway resistance plus pulmonary-tissue resistance plus chest-wall resistance. Gas flow during breathing is opposed by the following: inertial forces, viscous resistance, and airway resistance.

Inertial forces. A force must be applied to a gas to start it in motion or, once in motion, to change its velocity or direction. The force required to overcome this inertia is related to the mass of the gas and to the acceleration imparted. Physiologically, inertia is a negligible fraction of the resistance to breathing.

Viscous resistance. The viscous component of resistance to breathing is due to tissue friction during inspiration and expiration. The pleurae are moistened with a serous secretion that facilitates the movements of the lungs in the chest. Despite this fact, viscous resistance is primarily due to movement of parietal and visceral pleura and friction between pulmonary lobes as the shape of the thorax changes. In healthy persons viscous resistance is approximately 20% of the total resistance to breathing.

Airway resistance. The airway component includes friction between gas molecules and the walls of the airways plus the internal friction between gas molecules themselves (viscosity); at rest it constitutes the remaining 80% of total respiratory resistance. At a given flow rate the magnitude of the airway resistance component depends on the flow regime (whether gas flow is laminar or turbulent) and on the anatomy of the airways (length, radius, and bifurcation geometry).

Viscosity (internal friction) is the resistance within a fluid to flow (change of shape), and is expressed in *poises*, or dyne $\times$ second $\times$ cm^{-2}. Kinematic viscosity is the ratio of viscosity to density and is given in *stokes*. When flow is laminar, we may visualize viscosity as the friction between adjacent concentric layers of flowing gas. As gas molecules from the slower moving outer layers diffuse laterally into the faster moving inner layers, the inertia of the slower molecules retards the latter. This random lateral exchange of molecules accounts for the phenomenon of gas viscosity and also explains why gas viscosity, contrary to that of liquids, increases with temperature.

Laminar gas flow

As gas flows slowly and steadily through a straight, smooth, rigid, large-caliber, cylindric tube, a laminar (streamlined) flow pattern develops. Friction between the gas molecules and the wall of the tube retards the outer layer of gas, while this layer, in turn, retards the gas layer next inside. Thus we may think of concentric layers of gas flowing parallel to the wall of the tube at linear flow rates that increase toward the center. Such a laminar flow pattern has a parabolic velocity profile. Poiseuille's law relates the factors that determine laminar gas flow through a smooth unbranched tube of fixed dimensions:

$$\dot{V} = \frac{\pi r^4 \Delta P}{8L\eta}$$

where $\dot{V}$ is volumetric flow rate, r is tube radius, ΔP is driving pressure (pressure difference between two arbitrary points in the tube), L is tube length, and η is gas viscosity.

All these factors are variables except for $\pi/8$, which is constant. $\dot{V}$ is a function of r^4; tube radius profoundly affects flow rate. If all other factors remain constant, doubling tube radius increases gas flow by a factor of 16. A slight decrease of airway caliber caused by secretions, edema, or bronchoconstriction increases airway resistance greatly; to maintain the same flow rate requires a correspondingly great increase in driving pressure. Poiseuille's equation also shows that flow rate is inversely related both to tube length (L) and to the viscosity (η) of the gas. Other factors remaining constant, volumetric flow rate is a linear function of, and proportional to, driving pressure; Poiseuille's law for a laminar flow regime (character) may then be simplified:

$$\Delta P = K_1 \times \dot{V}$$

The constant K_1 incorporates dynamic gas viscosity as well as tube length and radius.

Turbulent gas flow

When the molecules of gas flowing through a tube reach a critical *linear* velocity, the character of flow changes. Concentric layers no longer slide smoothly over adjacent layers, and the orderly laminar flow pattern degenerates into eddy currents and turbulence. Gas now tends to advance along the tube at the same velocity at the center as it does at the periphery. This transition from a laminar flow pattern to chaotic turbulent flow is a function of density, linear flow velocity, viscosity, and tube radius. A Reynolds' number (N_R) (Chapter 2 and Appendix, Respiratory Calculations) greater than 2,000 generally indicates turbulent flow.

Density times velocity expresses momentum, whereas diameter divided by viscosity relates to viscous forces. The flow regime of a flowing fluid thus depends essentially on Reynolds' number, a ratio of inertial effects to viscous forces. When inertial effects increase to a critical level, instability results and the flow pattern degenerates into chaotic turbulence. The equation that relates driving pressure to volumetric flow rate during turbulence is as follows:

$$\Delta P = \frac{fL}{4\pi^2 r^5} \times \dot{V}^2$$

where f is a friction factor that incorporates the roughness of the tube surface as well as Reynolds' number. As N_R increases (1) f becomes less dependent on it and (2) density becomes increasingly important whereas viscosity becomes less so. Reynolds' numbers of 10,000 occur in the trachea during exercise. The other symbols in this equation have the same meaning as those in Poiseuille's equation. If all other conditions remain constant, the relationship between driving pressure and the resultant volumetric flow rate for a turbulent flow regime is as follows:

$$\Delta P = K_2 \times \dot{V}^2$$

The constant K_2 incorporates *f* (a function of density relative to viscosity—the reciprocal of kinematic viscosity) as well as tube length and radius.

During expiration, increased linear flow velocity changes the flow regime from a laminar pattern in the bronchioles to turbulent flow in the large airways. A mixed flow regime obtains during quite spontaneous breathing. The following equation, combining the separate equations for laminar and turbulent flow, relates driving pressure to resultant volumetric flow rate:

$$\Delta P = K_1 \times \dot{V} + K_2 \times \dot{V}^2$$

The first term of the right-hand member of the equation is for laminar flow and the second term is for turbulent flow. Note that laminar flow relates to dynamic viscosity, whereas turbulent flow relates to kinematic viscosity.

Airway resistance

Airway resistance is the ratio of driving pressure to the resultant volumetric flow rate; its units are cm $H_2O \times L^{-1} \times sec^{-1}$. For a healthy adult, airway resistance values range from 2 to 3 cm $H_2O \times L^{-1} \times sec^{-1}$ measured at an arbitrary flow rate of 0.5 L/sec; this is a flow rate usually achieved in quiet breathing during both inspiration and expiration. If airway resistance were measured at a higher arbitrary flow rate of, for example, 1.0 L/sec, normal values would be higher.

Airway resistance is always less during inspiration than during expiration. Airway resistance decreases with increasing lung volume. The expanding lung exerts radial traction on the airways within, increasing airway caliber. Further, the more "negative" intrapleural pressure increases transpulmonary pressure, dilating airways; during expiration intrapleural pressure rises toward intrapulmonary pressure, decreasing airway-distending pressure. Airways lengthen during inspiration and shorten during expiration; however, inspiratory airway lengthening cancels only a small fraction of the resistance decrease associated with increasing airway caliber. Similarly, during expiration airway shortening affects resistance only slightly.

Linear airflow velocity depends on volumetric flow rate as well as airway caliber. At increased linear velocity, turbulence increases and a greater driving pressure is then required to maintain the same volumetric flow rate; resistance also increases. Where turbulence exists, airway resistance is a nonlinear function of volumetric flow rate as well as driving pressure.

Factors that decrease airway caliber increase airway resistance, sometimes greatly. These factors include bronchial secretion, edema, vascular congestion of the mucosa, and constriction of bronchial smooth muscle (bronchoconstriction) from chemical (e.g., histamine) or parasympathetic (vagal) stimulation.

A less obvious cause of increased airway resistance is loss of lung elasticity. Increased lung compliance decreases transpulmonary (distending) pressure; intrapleural pressure more closely approximates intrapulmonary (alveolar) pressure. The diameter of small airways decreases, increasing airway resistance.

Factors that limit expiratory flow rate

Expiratory flow rate is limited by airway resistance, transpulmonary pressure, and intrapulmonary pressure (Fig. 5-12). As gas flows through an airway, the pressure diminishes steadily along the stream. During *forced* expiration, the expiratory flow rate at which intrapleural pressure becomes "positive" depends on transpulmonary pressure (a function of lung compliance) and the airway resistance. Compliance and airway resistance thus interact to determine the point of reversal of transmural pressure. If this pressure reversal occurs in peripheral airways, these airways, unsupported by cartilage, tend to collapse. If the resistance of small, peripheral airways increases, the pressure drop is greater along these less well-supported airways and they tend to collapse at a modest expiratory flow rate. This flow-limiting ("check-valve") mechanism produces the characteristic plateaus in the isovolume pressure-flow curves of healthy subjects. In pulmonary emphysema this effect is exaggerated

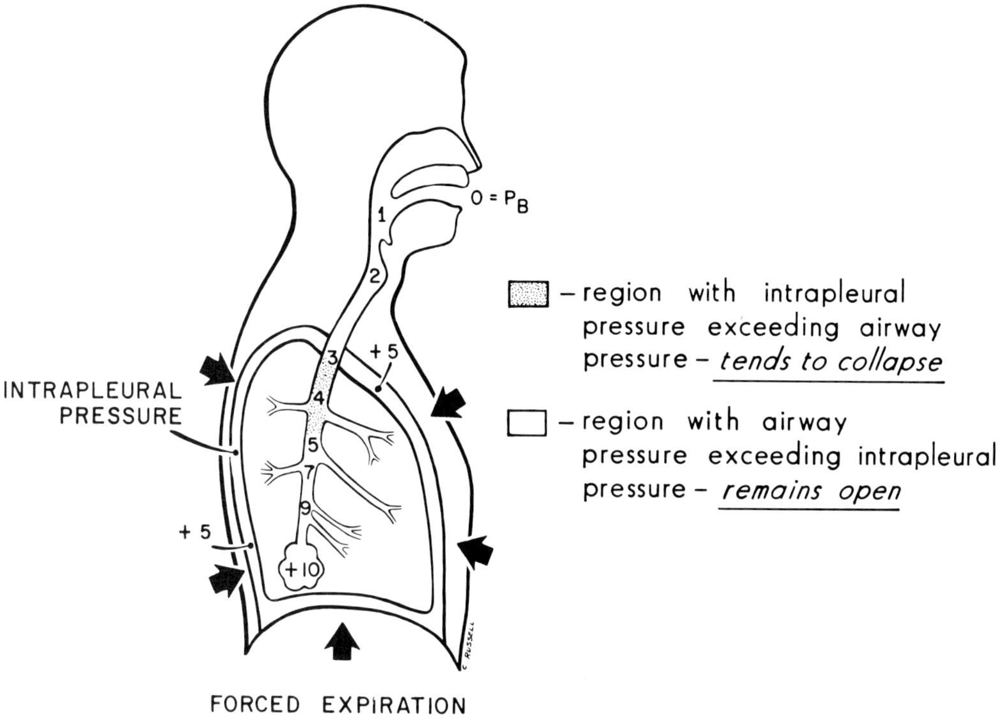

Fig. 5-12
Mechanism that limits maximal expiratory flow rate. Forced expiration increases intrapleural pressure, reversing transpulmonary pressure relationship. This reversal collapses nonrigid airways to produce an expiratory "check-valve."

by loss of lung elasticity and by airway collapsibility, so that air enters the lung with relative ease but is trapped during expiration behind a segment of bronchial collapse.

WORK OF BREATHING

Breathing involves muscular work. During inspiration, as muscles increase the volume of the thorax, elastic tissue is stretched and deformed and surface tension is overcome, creating a subatmospheric intrapulmonary pressure so that air flows into the lungs. Work is necessary to overcome the factors that resist lung inflation. This work of breathing is generally expressed in two ways—mechanical work and metabolic work.

Mechanical work of breathing

Physical work is defined as force times distance. The work of inspiration is expressed in terms of pressure change (ΔP) times volume change (ΔV) in units of cm H_2O-liters rather than kilogram-meters. In Fig. 5-13 the total work of quiet inspiration (sum of all shaded areas) is divided into the work required to overcome elasticity (approximately 65%) and the nonelastic work required to overcome friction (about 35%). About 80% of the nonelastic work is used to overcome airway resistance, whereas 20% is used to overcome the viscous resistance of the lung. Quiet spontaneous expiration is passive and the work required is recovered from energy stored in the lung-chest system during the preceding inspiration. The rest of the stored energy is transformed into heat and thus wasted. When expiration is active, more work is done per breath.

As compliance decreases or as resistance increases, the work of breathing increases. Fig. 5-14 illustrates the work of breathing in health, in restrictive lung disease (with decreased compliance), and in obstructive lung disease (with increased resistance).

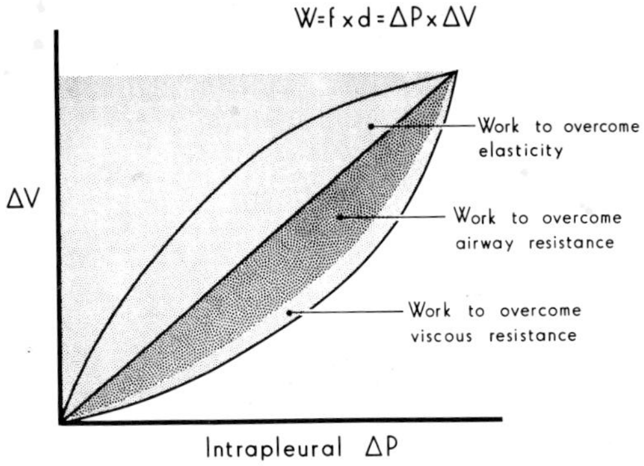

Fig. 5-13
Work of inspiration (total shaded area) consists of the work to overcome elasticity plus airway resistance plus viscous resistance. As work is done to overcome elasticity during inspiration, energy for the succeeding passive expiration is stored in the system.

Metabolic work of breathing

The work of breathing appears more meaningful to a physiologist when expressed in metabolic terms. It is calculated as the *additional* O_2 consumption required for breathing multiplied by the mechanical equivalent for O_2 consumption, expressed in units of ml (STPD) of O_2/L of ventilation. The metabolic cost is low during quiet breathing but increases steadily as ventilation increases. Fig. 5-15 shows this relationship.

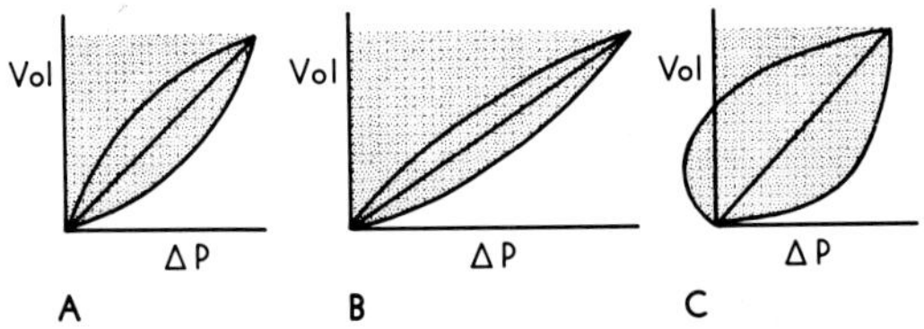

Fig. 5-14
Analysis of the work of breathing (shaded areas) for a healthy subject **(A)**, a patient with restrictive ventilatory impairment **(B)**, and a patient with chronic diffuse obstructive bronchopulmonary disease **(C)**.

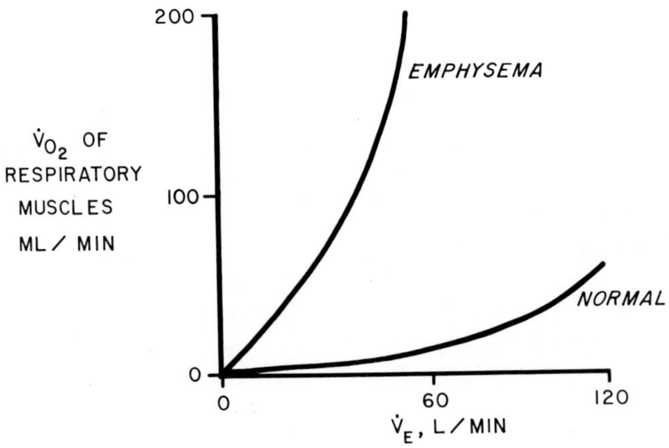

Fig. 5-15
Relationship of oxygen cost of breathing to expiratory minute volume for a healthy subject and for a patient with bronchitis-emphysema syndrome. (After Campbell, E. J. M., Westlake, E. K., and Cherniack, R. M.: J. Appl. Physiol. **11**:303, 1957.)

Energy cost of breathing

Obstructive lung disease increases the cost of breathing. In severe cases the O_2 cost of increased ventilation exceeds the additional O_2 provided by the increased effort. Thus a patient with advanced emphysema may actually supply less O_2 to his metabolizing tissues as a result of increasing pulmonary ventilation, aggravating hypoxemia. Furthermore, such increased work of breathing may produce extra CO_2 at a rate in excess of the patient's ability to eliminate it, aggravating hypercapnic acidosis.

We cannot measure the O_2 consumption of the respiratory muscles directly. We estimate the O_2 cost of breathing by measuring total O_2 consumption at several different levels of pulmonary ventilation. Assuming that the O_2 consumption increments represent the metabolic cost of additional ventilation at each level, the O_2 cost of breathing at rest is estimated by extrapolation of the curve to the O_2 consumption axis (control ventilation). By this method the O_2 cost of resting breathing is usually found to be 0.5 to 1.0 ml (STPD) of O_2/L of ventilation. The efficiency of breathing is calculated in percent as 100 times the work output per metabolic cost or as 100 times the mechanical work per metabolic work. The mechanical efficiency of breathing is approximately 10% and is thus similar to that of other mechanical work done by the body.

CHAPTER 6 Pulmonary circulation

The cardiovascular system consists of the heart, which functions as a variable output pump, and the blood vessels, which also react adaptively to changing physiologic conditions. The primary function of the cardiovascular system is to circulate the blood—transporting O_2 and nutrients to the metabolizing body tissues and removing CO_2 and the end products of metabolism. In addition, blood plays an important role in immune processes and in the transport of various chemical mediators, or hormones. For all of this the continuous, efficient, and adaptive performance of the heart is essential.

The total blood volume constitutes slightly less than one tenth of the body weight. The cardiac output, or volume of blood that passes through the heart in 1 minute during rest, is nearly equal to the total blood volume. In response to physical activity, fever, or certain emotions, cardiac output increases. This is accomplished by some combination of increased cardiac rate and increased stroke output, the product of which is cardiac output.

The circulatory system consists of two rather different segments—the *pulmonary* circulation and the *systemic* circulation—which are connected in series. The systemic circuit is a high-resistance circuit with a large pressure difference between its arteries and veins, whereas the pulmonary circuit, which accommodates the same blood flow, normally offers only slight resistance. The pulmonary blood flow is distributed to a *single* organ, whereas the systemic circuit supplies *numerous* organs that have various functions; pulmonary blood volume is considerably less than systemic blood volume. The capacity of the pulmonary vascular bed is estimated to be about 500 ml, but it varies appreciably in response to changing physiologic conditions; the capacity of the pulmonary capillary bed is estimated to be about 100 ml. Because the pulmonary circulation is a low-pressure, low-resistance vascular system in series with the systemic circulation, the flow through one system is identical with the flow through the other over any appreciable period of time, unless there are abnormal vascular communications (shunts) in the heart or lungs.

During diastole the venous blood flows from the right atrium through the tricuspid valve to fill the right ventricle, a process that is facilitated by atrial contraction. During systole, pressure increases within the right ventricular cavity, the tricuspid valve closes, and blood is ejected through the pulmonic valve into the main pulmonary artery. The variable volume of blood that remains in the ventricle after systole is termed its *residual volume.*

The main pulmonary artery divides into right and left branches, and each of these divides further, closely paralleling the arborization of the airway. Anatomically, the pulmonary vasculature does not normally contain the muscular type of arteriole that is the stopcock of the systemic circulation. The terminal branches of the pulmonary artery enter directly into dense alveolocapillary networks. In the alveoli, pulmonary capillary blood is separated from alveolar gas by a remarkably thin, continuous, submicroscopic layer of tissue, termed the *alveolocapillary membrane.* This membrane was first demonstrated by electron microscopy.

Mixed venous blood enters the pulmonary capillaries and, prior to exit, is fully arterialized by diffusion of CO_2 and O_2 across the alveolocapillary membrane. Oxygenated arterial blood then flows into the pulmonary venous system, which, in turn, empties into the left atrium via the four pulmonary veins. Paradoxically, the pulmonary artery contains mixed venous blood, whereas the pulmonary veins contain arterial blood.

It is estimated that a red blood cell (subject at rest) is exposed to alveolar gas during its passage through a pulmonary capillary for less than 1 second. The process of alveolocapillary diffusion by which mixed venous blood P_{O_2} achieves near equilibrium with alveolar gas P_{O_2} was studied by Bohr. If we make several simplifying assumptions, the process of alveolocapillary equilibration (diffusion) as blood flows through the pulmonary capillary is described by the *Bohr integration.*

Technics for study of the human pulmonary circulation have developed rapidly since 1929 when Forssmann performed the first right heart catheterization (on himself). This technic was subsequently developed and applied by Cournand for the study of pulmonary hemodynamics of human subjects in health and disease. Much basic physiologic information has been gained in this way, and excellent technics for diagnosis of cardiopulmonary diseases are now available.

When a subject is asked to inhale deeply during right heart catheterization, and the cardiovascular catheter is advanced in the pulmonary artery until it wedges in a small branch, the forward flow of blood in that particular ramification is obstructed and an end pressure is recorded, termed the *pulmonary artery wedge pressure.* This pressure reflects the pulmonary venous or left atrial pressure. The vertical level of the particular pulmonary artery branch in which the catheter tip is wedged has obvious hydrostatic importance. In making pressure measurements the level of the catheter tip with respect to the left atrium must be noted. In practice it is sometimes difficult to achieve an *unobstructed* wedge position of the cardiovascular catheter. Freedom from obstruction is usually judged from the facts that (1) a blood sample can be withdrawn (usually highly saturated), (2) the intravenous fluid can flow through the wedged catheter, and (3) the typical pulmonary arterial pressure-pulse contour is absent.

Total pulmonary blood volume can be estimated from analysis of dye dilution curves after injections into the pulmonary artery and left atrium. Pulmonary capillary blood volume can be calculated from measurements of the diffusing capacity of the lung for carbon monoxide at different alveolar P_{O_2}'s. Pulmonary arterial circulation time can be measured by an ether plethysmographic technic, and the pulmonary arterial blood volume can be calculated as the product of mean transit time and pulmonary blood flow. The validity of this measurement depends upon the fact that the exchange of gaseous ether takes place almost wholly at the alveolocapillary level and not to any significant extent at a precapillary level. Pulmonary venous volume can be calculated by subtracting the sum of the pulmonary arterial blood volume and pulmonary capillary blood volume from the total pulmonary blood volume.

PULMONARY BLOOD FLOW

In the absence of circulatory shunts, right ventricular output is exactly equal to pulmonary blood flow. The direct Fick method for determination of pulmonary blood flow is the reference standard for other methods. The Fick principle can be applied to any flowing stream of fluid that an indicator either enters or leaves, provided the *rate of entry or exit* of the indicator together with its *concentrations* on both sides of the site of entry or exit can all be measured. The fluid flow rate during any given period of time equals the quantity of indicator entering or leaving the stream during that same period of time, divided by the difference between the indicator concentration before and after the site of entry or exit. A basic requirement of the Fick principle is that the indicator must be thoroughly mixed with the flowing stream at each of the two sampling sites.* Therefore, in measuring pulmonary blood flow, blood samples for analysis must be obtained beyond the two ventricles, which in the absence of circulatory shunts serve as mixing chambers for the entire bloodstream. This requires a right heart catheterization.

After right heart catheterization is accomplished the catheter tip is placed in the pulmonary artery for withdrawal of the mixed venous blood sample. An indwelling arterial needle is inserted into a systemic artery such as the brachial, radial, or femoral artery. A steady state of rest of the circulation and respiration is approached as closely as possible. Mixed expired gas is collected over a precisely timed interval. Samples of systemic arterial and mixed venous blood are slowly and simultaneously drawn at a constant rate from the two sources, midway during the expired gas collection. Because blood O_2 content fluctuates constantly and during exercise or hyperventilation may do so greatly, blood samples must be withdrawn slowly and at a constant rate over a period of 10 seconds, or preferably longer, so that a *time* average sample is obtained. Cardiac output is calculated as follows:

$$\text{Cardiac output (L/min)} = \frac{O_2 \text{ uptake (ml/min, STPD)} \times 1/10}{\begin{matrix}\text{Arterial blood} \\ O_2 \text{ content} \\ \text{(vol \%)}\end{matrix} - \begin{matrix}\text{Mixed venous} \\ \text{blood } O_2 \text{ content} \\ \text{(vol \%)}\end{matrix}}$$

The distribution and regulation of pulmonary blood flow is a subject of great importance about which much remains to be learned. With trunk erect the apices of the lungs of resting healthy persons are not perfused because pulmonary arterial pressure is too low. Perfusion improves during mild exercise and is ample during recumbency. The remarkable homeostatic coordination of ventilation with perfusion may involve the direct effects of the respiratory gases, O_2 and CO_2, on the pulmonary vasculature.

To study this problem, Krahl injected India ink into the right heart of the rabbit. The surface of the lungs showed well-delineated areas of perfusion or no perfusion. Fear or adrenaline injection increased the areas of perfusion, whereas vagal stimulation or acetylcholine injection restricted the areas of perfusion. Krahl accounted for these observations by showing that pulmonary blood vessels of 30 to 50 μ diameter contain muscle bundles that act as sphincters. These beautiful experiments have important implications for the distribution and regulation of pulmonary blood flow.

Lung inflation and pulmonary perfusion

As already noted, pulmonary arterial pressure is not sufficient in the normal

*Oxygen is a suitable indicator for the direct Fick method because the pulmonary rate of O_2 uptake and blood O_2 concentrations are readily measurable. Furthermore O_2 uptake is a relatively stable on-going process that is not unduly sensitive to various slight, moment-to-moment cardiopulmonary fluctuations as, for example, is the process of CO_2 output.

resting, erect, sea level dweller to perfuse the upper portions of the lungs. However, it appears that perfusion of these areas is assisted by lung inflation. Riley has devised an analogy to explain this assistance. Groups of alveoli, or lobules, are clustered together to form a small globular mass. Each such mass touches other similar masses; however, there are spaces between these masses just as there are spaces between pingpong balls stored in a basket. These spaces are occupied, in part, by pulmonary blood vessels of various intermediate sizes. Each globe increases in size during inspiration but retains its globular shape. When this occurs, the spaces between the masses increase in volume, increasing the space between adjacent globes. The pressure in the blood vessels within these spaces decreases, sucking up pulmonary artery blood from more dependent areas. Quiet breathing is generally not of sufficient volume to promote perfusion of the lung apices in the erect person; however, deep breathing, such as the hyperpnea of exercise, is.

According to Permutt, the small blood vessels that cause resistance to flow are closely surrounded by alveolar pressure. There are two implications of this close association between the small pulmonary vessels, including arterioles, and alveolar pressure: first, it allows the direct exchange of respiratory gases between alveoli and small blood vessels; second, the transmission of alveolar pressure to the small blood vessels influences the pressure-flow patterns throughout the lungs. Experimental evidence suggests that both factors are of significance in regulating pulmonary blood flow.

The lung scan is a clinical technic for study of the distribution of the pulmonary circulation. This procedure can reveal abnormalities of the pulmonary arterial distribution pattern, or obstructive lesions that may not be seen in the usual roentgenogram, such as pulmonary emboli. Radioiodinated (I^{131}), macroaggregated human serum albumin is injected intravenously to be arrested in the pulmonary capillaries. Scanning technics are then used to give a picture of the distribution of the pulmonary blood flow. Although the procedure obstructs the pulmonary capillaries, it is quite safe and the macroaggregated albumin is quickly removed. Serial injections may be safely done at intervals of several days to follow the course of a changing pulmonary lesion. Microscopic study of the distribution of these aggregates gives further support to the concept that pulmonary capillaries alternately open and close.

Angiocardiography is another technic for clinical study of the pulmonary circulation. A radiopaque contrast medium is injected immediately upstream from the cardiovascular region to be studied, and high-speed serial roentgenograms are made in rapid succession from one or more directions. This technic yields information about the pulmonary artery and its larger branches, including location, size, shape, and patency.

PULMONARY ARTERIAL PRESSURE

Confusion often arises because of failure to distinguish clearly among the different pressure measurements that can be made in a stream of fluid flowing through a tube. It is necessary to distinguish *driving* pressure, *lateral* pressure, *end* pressures (coming and going), and *transmural* pressure.

Hemodynamic analysis of the pulmonary circulation is complicated by the same factors that complicate study of the systemic circulation:

1. Blood vessels are not rigid tubes.
2. Blood vessels are not of uniform caliber.
3. Blood vessels are not perfectly straight.
4. Blood vessels branch irregularly.

Table 3
Typical hemodynamic values for the pulmonary as opposed to systemic circulation

		Pulmonary circulation	Systemic circulation
Arterial pressure (mm Hg)	Systolic	25	125
	Diastolic	8	80
	Mean	12	95
Capillary pressure (mm Hg)		6-9	25
Blood flow (L $\times$ min^{-1} $\times$ M^{-2})		3.1	3.1
Calculated total vascular resistance index (dynes $\times$ sec $\times$ cm^{-5} $\times$ M^{-2})		100-200	1,800
Blood volume (ml)		500	5,000

5. Blood flow is pulsatile, not steady.
6. Blood is a nonhomogenous, non-newtonian liquid.

The pulmonary circulation lies within the thoracic cavity, where it is subject to the intrathoracic pressure which it reflects immediately and with great fidelity. The intrathoracic pressure changes that occur during respiration, cough, and Valsalva and Müller maneuvers are readily detected by pressure-sensing devices placed within the pulmonary artery or veins. Such pressure increases are uniformly applied and thus tend to support the pulmonary vessels, rather than causing disruptive stress. Vagal receptors in the pulmonary conus sense increased transmural pressure and reflexly decrease blood pressure and heart rate.

The mean pulmonary arterial pressure at rest is about one eighth of the systemic arterial pressure. The pulmonary vascular bed is relatively distensible and readily accommodates increased blood flow and volume. Exercise increases pulmonary arterial pressure slightly because flow increases relatively more than resistance decreases. Following unilateral pulmonary artery ligation, pulmonary arterial pressure increases transiently but returns to a normal level after a short time. A comparison of typical hemodynamic values for the pulmonary as opposed to systemic circulation is given in Table 3.

Pulmonary arterial hypertension can result from four different pathophysiologic conditions: (1) increased pulmonary arterial blood flow and volume, as in left-to-right circulatory shunts; (2) increased resistance of the pulmonary vasculature or of the venous side of the pulmonary circulation, as in rheumatic mitral valvular disease; (3) hypoxia, with or without acidosis, as at altitude; and (4) massive loss or obstruction of the pulmonary vascular bed, as in thromboembolic disease.

PULMONARY VASCULAR RESISTANCE

Resistance is a *calculated* quantity that actually consists of several separate components. The concept includes all factors that cause a pressure loss along the intravascular course of the flowing bloodstream. The chief components of total calculated resistance are viscosity and density of the blood, and length and cross-sectional area of the vascular segment under study.

Resistance may also be defined as the impedance to blood flow through a given segment of the circulation; this may be a total circuit, such as the systemic or pulmonary circuit, a region, such as the hand, or an organ, such as the brain. Resistance is generally expressed in terms of pressure loss per unit of blood flow.

Although there is no general agreement on the exact anatomic location or physiologic basis of vascular resistance, the concept has practical value. The resistance of multiple pipe systems in hydraulics can be calculated by analogy to Ohm's law. The simplest formula for calculating resistance is as follows:

$$\text{Resistance} = \frac{\text{Arterial mean pressure gradient (mm Hg)}}{\text{Blood flow (ml/sec)}}$$

Aperia's formula treats the hemodynamic data so as to give the result in CGS values:

$$\text{Resistance (dynes} \times \text{sec} \times \text{cm}^{-5}) = \frac{(P_1 - P_2) \times 1{,}330}{\text{Blood flow}}$$

where R = resistance, $(P_1 - P_2)$ = pressure loss across the resistance bed in mm Hg, and Blood flow = blood flow through the resistance bed in ml/sec. The pressure drop across the resistance to be calculated must be determined. Usually, both entrance and exit pressures are measured. The exit pressure for the systemic circuit is so unrelated to the entering pressure that in practice it is often disregarded. However, in the pulmonary vascular bed this is certainly not the case, and the actual pressure gradient must therefore be measured.

Resistance is calculated from measurements of arterial blood flow and blood pressure; since these are subject to considerable error, the calculated resistance will be correspondingly in error. Small changes in resistance may therefore be of no significance. Changes in calculated resistance cannot be interpreted without consideration of arterial pressure changes and, in the pulmonary circuit, alterations of pulmonary venous pressure, as well. Changes in resistance may result from the distending effect of the inflow or exit pressure, or, conversely, a change in the

Table 4

Calculation of typical normal values* for pulmonary vascular resistance

	High	Low
Cardiac index ($cc \times min^{-1} \times M^{-2}$)	3,100	3,100
Pulmonary arterial mean pressure (mm Hg)	15†	12†
Pulmonary artery mean wedge pressure (mm Hg)	9	6
TPVRI Range: 309-386 Mean: 348	$\frac{15 \times 1{,}330 \times 60}{3{,}100} =$ 386 dynes × sec × cm^{-5} × M^{-2}	$\frac{12 \times 1{,}330 \times 60}{3{,}100} =$ 309 dynes × sec × cm^{-5} × M^{-2}
PARI Range: 77-232 Mean: 154	$\frac{(15\text{-}6) \times 1{,}330 \times 60}{3{,}100} =$ 232 dynes × sec × cm^{-5} × M^{-2}	$\frac{(12\text{-}9) \times 1{,}330 \times 60}{3{,}100} =$ 77 dynes × sec × cm^{-5} × M^{-2}

*Assume typical normal values for healthy man at supine rest.

†Pulmonary arterial mean pressure increases with altitude.

state of the vascular bed may be masked by alteration in the distending pressure. Other hemodynamic factors remaining equal and unchanged in a given subject, changes in calculated resistance are presumed to reflect changes in vascular cross-sectional area. However, a decrease in calculated resistance may be due either to increased vascular distention by higher entering pressure or to actual vasodilatation. Another problem that arises in interpreting resistance values is the variable effect of body size. As in the case of cardiac output, the validity of using body surface area to "take out" body size as a variable is subject to discussion.

Total pulmonary vascular resistance index (TPVRI) is a calculation of the vascular resistance from the pulmonary artery to the left ventricle, whereas pulmonary arteriolar resistance index (PARI) is a calculation of the vascular resistance from the pulmonary artery to a pulmonary vein. The word *arteriolar* is used here loosely because, first, vessels comparable to the thick-walled, heavily muscled systemic arterioles are not found in healthy lung* and, second, the vascular segment involved comprises precapillary, capillary, and postcapillary blood vessels. Table 4 shows calculation of typical normal values for pulmonary vascular resistance.

To make meaningful calculations it is necessary to measure the blood flows correctly and, when shunts are present, to use the *appropriate* flows in the resistance formula.

*However, such vessels often develop after prolonged, severe pulmonary arterial hypertension.

Total pulmonary vascular resistance, TPVR (dynes × sec × cm^{-5}) =

$$\frac{\left[\begin{array}{c}\text{Pulmonary arterial}\\ \text{mean pressure}\\ \text{(mm Hg)}\end{array}\right] \times 60 \times 1{,}330^{*}}{\begin{array}{c}\text{Cardiac output}\\ \text{(cc/min)}\end{array}}$$

Total pulmonary vascular resistance index, TPVRI (dynes × sec × cm^{-5} × M^{-2}) = TPVR/BSA (M^2)

Pulmonary arteriolar resistance, PAR (dynes × sec × cm^{-5}) =

$$\frac{\left[\begin{array}{c}\text{Pulmonary arterial}\\ \text{mean pressure}\\ \text{(mm Hg)}\end{array} - \begin{array}{c}\text{Pulmonary artery}\\ \text{mean wedge}\\ \text{pressure}\\ \text{(mm Hg)}\end{array}\right] \times 60 \times 1{,}330^{*}}{\begin{array}{c}\text{Cardiac output}\\ \text{(cc/min)}\end{array}}$$

Pulmonary arteriolar resistance index, PARI (dynes × sec × cm^{-5} × M^{-2}) = PAR/BSA (M^2)

*1,330 (mercury density × acceleration due to gravity) is used in this formula to convert pressure from units of mm Hg to CGS units of dynes/cm^2. This value varies slightly with temperature (mercury density varies with temperature), altitude, and latitude (acceleration due to gravity, g, varies both with altitude and latitude).

The important comparison of TPVRI with PARI is facilitated by calculation of percent of predicted for each as follows:

$$\text{Percent of predicted} = \frac{\text{Value obtained from cardiac catheterization data (found)}}{\text{Typical normal mean value (predicted)}} \times 100$$

Clinically, the comparison of PARI with TPVRI provides important information as to *where* the circulatory resistance is located. Calculations of PARI both *before* and *after* exercise, O_2 breathing, and injection of certain drugs provide important information as to whether pulmonary vascular resistance is fixed or reversible.

In clinical practice, chronic obstruction of the pulmonary circulation results from either diffuse constriction or obliteration of small pulmonary blood vessels or, in the left atrium, from thrombus, tumor, or mitral valvular disease. A third situation is the intense pulmonary vascular constriction that intervenes secondarily when pulmonary capillary pressure rises to edema-threatening levels. This occurs in mitral stenosis or high-flow, left-to-right shunts, in which latter case it is termed an *Eisenmenger reaction.*

Also of clinical interest is the fact that development of increased peripheral vascular resistance and consequent arterial hypertension can mask a pressure gradient across a pulmonic or aortic cardiac valve, so that both diagnostic pressure gradient and cardiac murmur disappear. The value of this hemodynamic fact is apparent.

A serious pulmonary condition of newborn infants has been variously called respiratory distress syndrome, hyaline membrane disease, and as more understanding of the mechanism has accumulated, *pulmonary hypoperfusion syndrome.* The basic functional abnormality, as implied by the name, is pulmonary hypoperfusion. A reflex pulmonary vasoconstriction, which tends to preserve blood flow to the brain, heart, and placenta at the expense of flow to other organs, develops in response to hypoxemia, acidosis, hypothermia, or hypovolemia. This type of response to stress has survival value. However, in the fetus and newborn infant the ductus arteriosus is patent, so that flow to alveolar capillaries is seriously diminished by the pulmonary vasoconstriction, and ischemic damage may occur in the lungs. Rational therapy is aimed at relieving the constriction of the pulmonary vascular bed. Acetylcholine infusion has been used to decrease pulmonary vascular resistance, thereby increasing pulmonary blood flow and decreasing dead space:tidal volume ratio and arterial P_{CO_2}.

Alveolar pressure and pulmonary vascular resistance

The fluid analogy of Ohm's law is

$$\text{Pressure drop} = \text{Flow} \times \text{Resistance}$$

widely applied in physiology. When applied to the pulmonary circulation, it reads as follows:

$$\text{Pulmonary vascular resistance} = \frac{\text{Pulmonary arterial mean pressure} - \text{Pulmonary venous mean pressure}}{\text{Cardiac output}}$$

However, the transmural pressure across the alveolar wall (alveolar intrapulmonary pressure minus intrathoracic pressure) can become great enough under certain conditions to interfere significantly with pulmonary capillary flow. When this happens, should the preceding equation be calculated as shown, or should the pressure drop be taken as pulmonary arterial pressure minus alveolar transmural pressure? Permutt concluded that in calculating the resistance to flow of a river containing a waterfall, it is meaningless to calculate it from the river source to the bottom of the waterfall. When high alveolar transmural pressure is the cause of increased resistance to flow in the pulmonary capillaries, the flow downstream from the alveoli to the pulmonary vein is a waterfall. In this situation the equation should read as follows:

$$\text{Pulmonary vascular resistance} = \frac{\text{Pulmonary arterial mean pressure} - \text{Alveolar transmural pressure}}{\text{Cardiac output}}$$

PULMONARY VASCULAR REACTIVITY

Although the autonomic nerve supply of the bronchopulmonary system is an obvious anatomic feature, pulmonary blood vessels are relatively unresponsive to it. The pulmonary vasculature is also relatively unresponsive to various drugs that exert powerful effects on systemic blood vessels. The effects of changes in O_2 and CO_2 tensions on the pulmonary vasculature are *opposite* to the effects of these gases on the systemic circulation. Hypoxia is a potent constrictor of the pulmonary vascular bed, whereas increased P_{O_2} tends to dilate these vessels. This reactivity of the pulmonary vasculature to changing respiratory gas tensions may be an important homeostatic factor in maintaining optimal ventilation-perfusion relationships in the lung.

Clinically, the effect of hypoxia on the pulmonary vasculature may result in serious elevation of pulmonary arterial pressure with consequent increase of right ventricular work. The mechanism is of importance in chronic mountain sickness, as well as in patients with pulmonary insufficiency and cor pulmonale. High altitude disease of cattle ("brisket disease") involves the same mechanism. Harvey demonstrated that hypoxia and acidosis exert a synergistic vasoconstrictor effect on the pulmonary vasculature. Gomez has proposed an equation to describe this combined action:

$$P = K + aH + bS + \omega HS$$

where P is pulmonary arterial mean pressure in mm Hg, K, a, b, and ω are coefficients, S is arterial oxyhemoglobin unsaturation in percent, and H is H^+ concentration in mμEq/L. In view of this synergism it is difficult to evaluate the degree to which increased calculated pulmonary vascular resistance depends upon structural changes and the degree to which it depends upon potentially reversible factors. Acute O_2 administration, although relieving hypoxia, simultaneously decreases alveolar ventilation, thereby increasing acidosis and maintaining pulmonary vasoconstriction.

A great deal of research has yielded a relatively few drugs that have potent effects on the pulmonary circulation. Silove, holding blood flow rate constant in the isolated lobe of newborn calf lung, found that isoproterenol consistently produces pulmonary vasodilatation, whereas norepinephrine has a variable vasoconstrictor effect that depends upon the initial conditions of P_{O_2} and pH. Serotonin (5-hydroxytryptamine) constricts both bronchi and the pulmonary vasculature, increasing pulmonary arterial pressure. Intravenous nicotine administered to anesthetized, intact dogs causes a significant rise in pulmonary arterial pressure. Experimental evidence suggests pulmonary vasoconstriction as the mechanism. Nicotine stimulation of the aortic body also produces pulmonary vasoconstriction. Fritts showed that the pressor response to hypoxia of normal subjects is abolished by an infusion of acetylcholine. Tolazoline (Priscoline), like acetylcholine, decreases pulmonary arterial pressure in many patients in whom it is initially elevated.

Intravascular injection of small volumes of autologous hemolyzed blood produces a prompt, marked increase of pulmonary arterial pressure in experimental animals. Injection of small doses of ADP causes a similar reaction, together with decreased platelet count and formation of platelet and fibrin thrombi.

DETECTION OF VENOUS-TO-ARTERIAL CIRCULATORY SHUNTS

Central shunts can be defined as abnormal communications between the two sides of the circulation. Advances in thoracic surgery have made the accurate preoperative diagnosis of circulatory shunts a matter of practical concern. Shunt detection and estimation are important aspects of the diagnosis of cardiopulmonary diseases. Shunts are of three types with respect to direction of shunt flow: (1) right-to-left, or venous-to-arterial, (2) left-to-right, and (3) bidirectional. Shunt detection is basically detection of flow, and all methods of detection or semiquantitation involve either simultaneous withdrawal and analysis of blood samples for O_2 content from various parts of the circulation, or the injection or inhalation of various indicator substances.

Venous-to-arterial shunts produce arterial hypoxemia because a certain fraction of the mixed venous blood bypasses the alveolar gas. Pulmonary arteriovenous fistula is an example of such a vascular abnormality. In bronchiectasis, large abnormal shunts between the bronchial and pulmonary arteries have been described by Lindskog and Liebow. The O_2 method for detection of venous-to-arterial circulatory shunts is described on p. 191.

If Kr^{85}, an inert radioactive gas,* is dissolved in saline or blood and injected intravenously, the proportion of the injected dose that appears in the systemic arterial blood is a measure of pulmonary venous-to-arterial shunting. This relatively insoluble, foreign, radioactive gas is almost completely cleared from the blood during a single passage through the pulmonary capillaries of *ventilated* alveoli, so that radioactivity appearing in the systemic circulation must have come from shunted blood. Kr^{85} injection has been combined with a conventional indicator-dilution curve by dissolving the gas in solutions of indocyanine green dye. After making certain assumptions, the proportion of the cardiac output shunted from right to left can be calculated. This calculation gives values for venous-to-arterial *pulmonary* shunt and does not include shunts of other types. It is the most specific method available.

Hydrogen is also used to detect right-to-left shunts. Hydrogen-saturated saline or blood is injected through a cardiac catheter placed in the right heart. The hydrogen is detected by a platinum electrode placed in a systemic artery. Another method involves the injection of indocyanine green dye into the right side of the circulation and sampling from the left side via a systemic artery. A densitometer system, such as is commonly used for cardiac output, records the concentration of indicator in the arterial blood and also measures the appearance time of injections made at various locations within the right heart. Angiocardiography can also be used to detect and localize shunts. Radiopaque contrast medium is injected in the right heart and observed as it appears in the left heart.

*Kr^{85} is a radioactive isotope of krypton which has a 10.3-year half-life, has a 20:1 air-to-water partition coefficient, and emits 672 KEV beta with only 0.65% gamma.

CHAPTER 7 Blood-gas transport

HEMOGLOBIN

The transport of molecular O_2 within the circulatory systems of vertebrates is greatly facilitated by the hemoglobins—pigments that are remarkably adapted to their function. Hemoglobin increases blood O_2 content and capacity for any given loading pressure (P_{O_2}), whereas its intraerythrocytic location prevents the drastic colloid osmotic effect that would otherwise result if 15 gm % of protein were free in the plasma.

Ferrohemoglobin and ferrihemoglobin

Human erythrocytes are normally in the shape of biconcave discs; they consist of about one-third hemoglobin. Each of the four heme groups in the normal adult hemoglobin molecule (Hb A) has a polypeptide chain. These chains are of two types—alpha, which has 141 amino acid residues, and beta, which has 146 residues; each half-molecule of hemoglobin thus contains almost 300 amino acid residues.

Hemoglobin consists of a protein globin, and a ferrous-protoporphyrin complex, ferroheme. Its iron content is 0.335% to 0.340%, and its molecular weight of about 67,000 corresponds to the presence of four hemes per molecule. Oxygen and carbon monoxide combine with ferrohemoglobin in the ratio of one gas molecule per ferroheme. The oxidation of ferroheme to ferriheme by the loss of one electron produces ferrihemoglobin, a derivative that combines with a number of anions but not with O_2 or CO. These reactions are reversible, the globin being unaffected in each case, and each of the compounds has a characteristic absorption spectrum. Ferrohemoglobin and ferrihemoglobin are also called hemoglobin and methemoglobin, respectively. The stable complex of the cyanide ion with methemoglobin, cyanmethemoglobin, finds use both as a standard in hemoglobinometry and in the treatment of cyanide poisoning. Since the various compounds of hemoglobin differ with respect to chemical and physical properties, erroneous results may be obtained from analysis of blood samples containing hemoglobin that is partially oxidized to ferrihemoglobin, denatured, or converted to another hemoglobin compound. Such changes may occur during the course of an analysis.

Methemoglobin is produced in nitrite poisoning and in toxic reactions to oxidant drugs.* Congenital methemoglobinemia is the result of a deficiency of diphosphopyridine nucleotide diaphorase; hereditary methemoglobinemia with and

*The aniline breakdown products of certain local anesthetics, such as the toluidine derivative prilocaine (Citanest), produce methemoglobin and, when given in large doses, may even cause visible discoloration of the skin and mucous membranes. However, such methemoglobinemia is not clinically serious unless hypoxia or methemoglobinemia already exists and is readily corrected by intravenous administration of methylene blue.

without mental retardation has been described. Hereditary methemoglobinemia is due to an inherited defect in the enzyme-controlled reducing mechanism of the red blood cell, permitting accumulation of methemoglobin and resulting in heterogeneity with respect to the oxidation state of the heme iron after the hemoglobin molecule has been completely synthesized. A form of inherited methemoglobinemia has been described in which the globin moiety is apparently affected.

Carbon monoxide combines avidly with both hemoglobin and myoglobin, the respiratory pigment in "red" muscle cells. Its affinity for hemoglobin is about 210 times (Haldane number) as great as that for O_2. Carboxyhemoglobin, also called carbon monoxyhemoglobin, occurs in the blood of smokers and of individuals exposed to the exhaust fumes of internal combustion engines. The blood of firemen who have just attended a blaze may contain large amounts of carboxyhemoglobin. Carbon monoxide is very slowly oxidized in the body to CO_2. A small amount of CO is formed as a product of hemoglobin catabolism. Certain plants, for example, ocean kelp *(Nereocystis luetkeana)*, produce CO in abundance.

Xe^{133} is a radioactive isotope with a half-life of 5.27 days and gamma emission of 81 kev that is used as an indicator for study of inspired gas and pulmonary blood flow distribution, as well as for determination of cardiac output. The gamma emission of Xe^{133} is readily detectable, yet sufficiently soft that relatively large doses produce little tissue damage. It is therefore of interest that xenon combines chemically with both hemoglobin and myoglobin, occupying a specific site in each molecule.

The biochemical structure and physiologic function of hemoglobin are intimately related. The enzymatic removal of a single histidine residue from the terminal end of the beta chain of globin (remote from heme) results in a pigment having a hyperbolic oxyhemoglobin dissociation curve, whereas removal from the alpha and beta chains of only five amino acid residues increases its affinity for O_2 fifty times and eliminates the Bohr effect.

Fetal hemoglobin

Körber, in 1866, discovered that the hemoglobin from human placental blood is more resistant to denaturation by alkali and by acid than the hemoglobin of adult blood. It is now known that this pigment is fetal hemoglobin, or Hb F. Other species also have a fetal and an adult form of hemoglobin. The hemoglobin of a newborn infant is a mixture of fetal and adult forms. Fetal hemoglobin is present in the blood of normal infants for some months beyond the expected lifespan of the red cells in the peripheral circulation at birth. Replacement of fetal by adult hemoglobin may be complete by the end of the first year of postnatal life; however, fetal hemoglobin persists beyond infancy in some types of severe, chronic anemia. The structure of fetal hemoglobin is an inherited characteristic, and its properties are characteristic for a given species. The control of its synthesis appears to differ from that of the normal and abnormal adult hemoglobins since a patient may have fetal hemoglobin in addition to two of the inherited adult forms. A small amount of fetal hemoglobin may be present in all nonanemic adults, and elevated amounts are produced under the stress of acquired as well as congenital anemia; thus the production of this form is not restricted to the fetal period of life.

Abnormal hemoglobins

Considerable progress has been made in studying the genetics and biochemistry of normal hemoglobin (Hb A) synthesis. The discovery by Linus Pauling of the genetically determined biochemical abnormality of sickle cell hemoglobin (Hb S) opened up a new field in molecular biology. Hereditary variations of hemoglobin polypeptides are prototypes of abnormal protein synthesis. Within a relatively brief time, more than thirty abnormal hemoglobins have been described that differ from normal hemoglobin by a single amino acid residue in the alpha or beta chain. All but one can be explained on the basis of a single base change in the corresponding structural gene. One abnormal hemoglobin, termed *Lepore*, is the result of unequal crossing-over between beta and delta loci. Hemoglobins H and Barts are multimers of normal polypeptide chains, not hemoglobin variants. Unlike fetal hemoglobin, the abnormal hemoglobins are very similar structurally and chemically to hemoglobin A. An individual with two abnormal hemoglobin alleles, like or unlike, has no hemoglobin A in his red blood cells. Like hemoglobin A the abnormal hemoglobins are present in very low concentration at birth.

Before a hemoglobin is accepted as a new form and given a letter designation, characterization by electrophoresis with both the moving boundary and zone technics at different pH's, chromatography, solubility, spectrophotometry with visible and ultraviolet light, and denaturation by alkali and cold are usually necessary.

Pauling demonstrated that the hemoglobin in sickle cell anemia is electrophoretically abnormal and that the hemoglobin in individuals with sickle cell trait, an asymptomatic condition, is a mixture of the abnormal form with normal adult hemoglobin. A single abnormal gene induces the synthesis of this abnormal hemoglobin. He originally suggested that sickling is due to the chemically abnormal hemoglobin molecule, which, upon deoxygenation, aggregates into rods and twists the erythrocyte out of shape. Deoxygenated sickle cell hemoglobin is less soluble than deoxygenated normal hemoglobin or either type of oxyhemoglobin. The abnormality of Hb S is genetically determined—glutamic acid is replaced by valine at the sixth position in each of the two beta polypeptide chains. It has been suggested that this substitution creates a hydrophobic intramolecular bond that changes the configuration in such a way that molecular stacking occurs.

Reduced ferrohemoglobin is paramagnetic, whereas oxyhemoglobin and carboxyhemoglobin are diamagnetic. Normal human erythrocytes do not orient themselves in a magnetic field. However, deoxygenated sickled erythrocytes in a magnetic field of 3.5 kilogauss orient themselves with their long axes perpendicular to the magnetic lines of force, suggesting that Hb S molecules are linearly arranged.

OXYGEN TRANSPORT

Blood carries O_2 in two ways: (1) in physical solution as O_2 dissolved in the aqueous phase and (2) in a loose reversible chemical combination with hemoglobin, as oxyhemoglobin. In both cases the amount of O_2 held depends upon the O_2 tension, or loading pressure, to which the blood is exposed.

Dissolved oxygen

Dissolved O_2, also termed O_2 in physical solution, comprises little more than 1% of the total blood O_2 content under ordinary physiologic conditions. The amount of O_2 dissolved in blood is directly proportional to the P_{O_2} to which it is exposed (Fig. 7-1). Henry's law implies that, at constant temperature, the amount of dissolved O_2 depends on the solubility coefficient (C_S) of O_2 in blood and is a linear function of P_{O_2}. Since the solubility coefficient for O_2 at 38° C is 0.003 vol %/mm Hg, arterial blood that has a P_{O_2} of 95 mm Hg contains about 0.29 vol % dissolved O_2. When a healthy subject breathes pure O_2 at sea

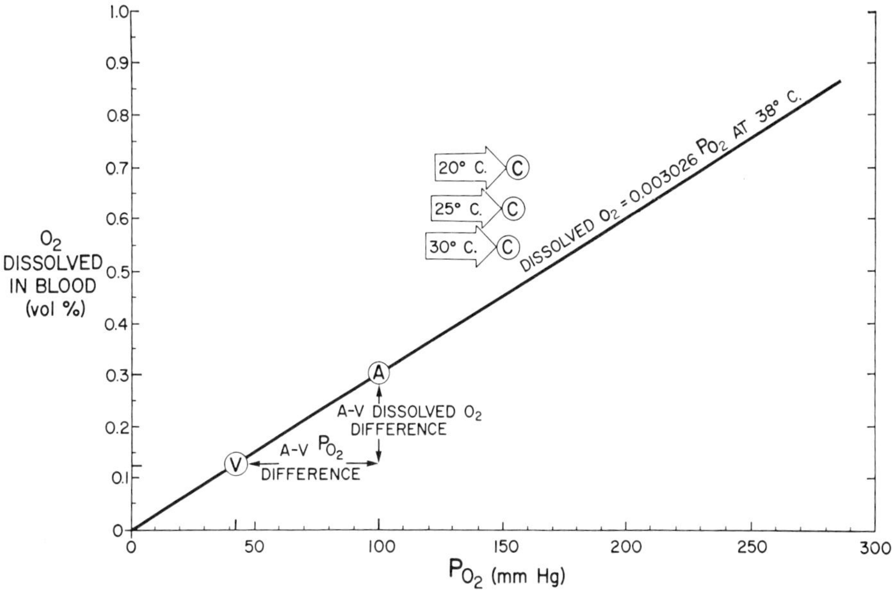

Fig. 7-1
Oxygen dissolved in blood at 38° C as a function of P_{O_2}. For use in "correction" of various blood samples for dissolved O_2 content in calculation of oxyhemoglobin saturation. Typical normal points are given for arterial, Ⓐ, mixed venous, Ⓥ, and air-equilibrated capacity, Ⓒ, blood samples at sea level.

level, alveolar P_{O_2} rises toward a theoretic maximum of 673 mm Hg, arterial P_{O_2} exceeds 600 mm Hg, and dissolved O_2 approaches 2 vol %. It is possible, but usually not of practical importance, to distinguish the fraction of dissolved O_2 that is in the blood plasma from the remainder that is dissolved in the aqueous phase within the blood cells.

Hyperbaric chambers increase total pressure to several times atmospheric pressure. During hyperbaric oxygenation, the concentration of dissolved O_2 increases proportionately in accordance with Henry's law and may then comprise a significant fraction of the total blood O_2 content. A subject breathing pure O_2 at 3 atm pressure has an alveolar P_{O_2} of approximately 2,000 mm Hg, and his arterial blood contains about 6 vol % of dissolved O_2. This amount of dissolved O_2 would theoretically satisfy the O_2 requirements of a subject at rest. However, the toxicity of O_2 at high pressure limits the medical use of hyperbaric oxygenation to treatment of certain conditions by experts.

In homothermic animals, temperature is not ordinarily a physiologically important variable affecting gases dissolved in blood, except during febrile or hypometabolic states such as hypothermia or hibernation. However, in certain poikilothermic species, temperature is indeed an important variable, and for aquatic forms it may be a variable affecting the dissolved O_2 content of the aquatic environment as well as blood O_2 content. The effect of temperature on the dissolved O_2 content of whole blood is illustrated by the following data from Table 5. At a P_{O_2} of 760 mm Hg, whole blood contains 2.32 vol % of dissolved O_2 at 38° C, whereas it contains 3.29 vol % at 22° C.

In this regard the ice fish *(Chaenocephalus aceratus)* is an interesting example of vertebrate adaptation involving

Table 5
Dissolved oxygen in whole blood at various temperatures*

Temperature (° C)	Dissolved O_2 ml/100 ml blood P_{O_2} = 760 mm Hg (vol %/atm)	Dissolved O_2 ml/100 ml blood/mm Hg P_{O_2} (vol %/mm Hg)
20	3.44	0.00453
22	3.29	0.00433
24	3.12	0.00411
26	3.00	0.00395
28	2.85	0.00375
30	2.73	0.00359
32	2.61	0.00343
34	2.52	0.00332
36	2.41	0.00317
38	2.32	0.00305
40	2.23	0.00293

*From Dittmer, D. S., and Grebe, R. M., editors: Handbook of respiration, Philadelphia, 1958, W. B. Saunders Co., p. 7.

the relationship of dissolved O_2 to temperature. These fish attain a length of about 2 feet and are almost completely devoid of scales. They are truly anemic in that they virtually lack both red blood cells and hemoglobin. The Antarctic Ocean water in which they live remains near 0° C throughout the year. The body temperature of this poikilothermic animal is approximately that of the surrounding frigid water, so that tissue metabolic demand for O_2 is low, whereas the low water temperature permits a good concentration of dissolved O_2.

It is interesting to compare the concentrations or pressures of various substances taken up and then released by the blood in arterial blood samples with their concentrations or pressures in mixed venous blood samples. Such differences are termed *arteriovenous differences.* Given normal values for a healthy subject at rest: cardiac output equals 5.63 L/min, O_2 uptake equals 240 ml (STPD)/min, and arterial blood total O_2 content equals 18.97 vol %. The Fick equation relates these factors as follows:

$$\dot{Q} = \frac{\dot{V}_{O_2} \times 1/10}{C_{a_{O_2}} - C_{\bar{v}_{O_2}}}$$

$$5.63 = \frac{240 \times 1/10}{18.97 - 14.71} = \frac{24}{4.26}$$

Thus, in healthy man at rest the amount of O_2 extracted from the blood by the tissues (arteriovenous blood O_2 difference) is about 4 vol %; in contrast the arteriovenous difference for dissolved O_2 is about 0.18 vol %, or 4.5% of the total O_2 extracted.

Oxygen combined with hemoglobin

From the foregoing it is apparent that the amount of O_2 dissolved in blood or plasma is insufficient for tissue needs even at rest, and certainly does not constitute the kind of reservoir required for intermittent physical activity, during which tissue O_2 demand may suddenly increase fifteen to twenty times. In the resting subject more than 95% of the O_2 delivered to the tissues is transported in combination with hemoglobin, and during exercise this value may exceed 99%. The

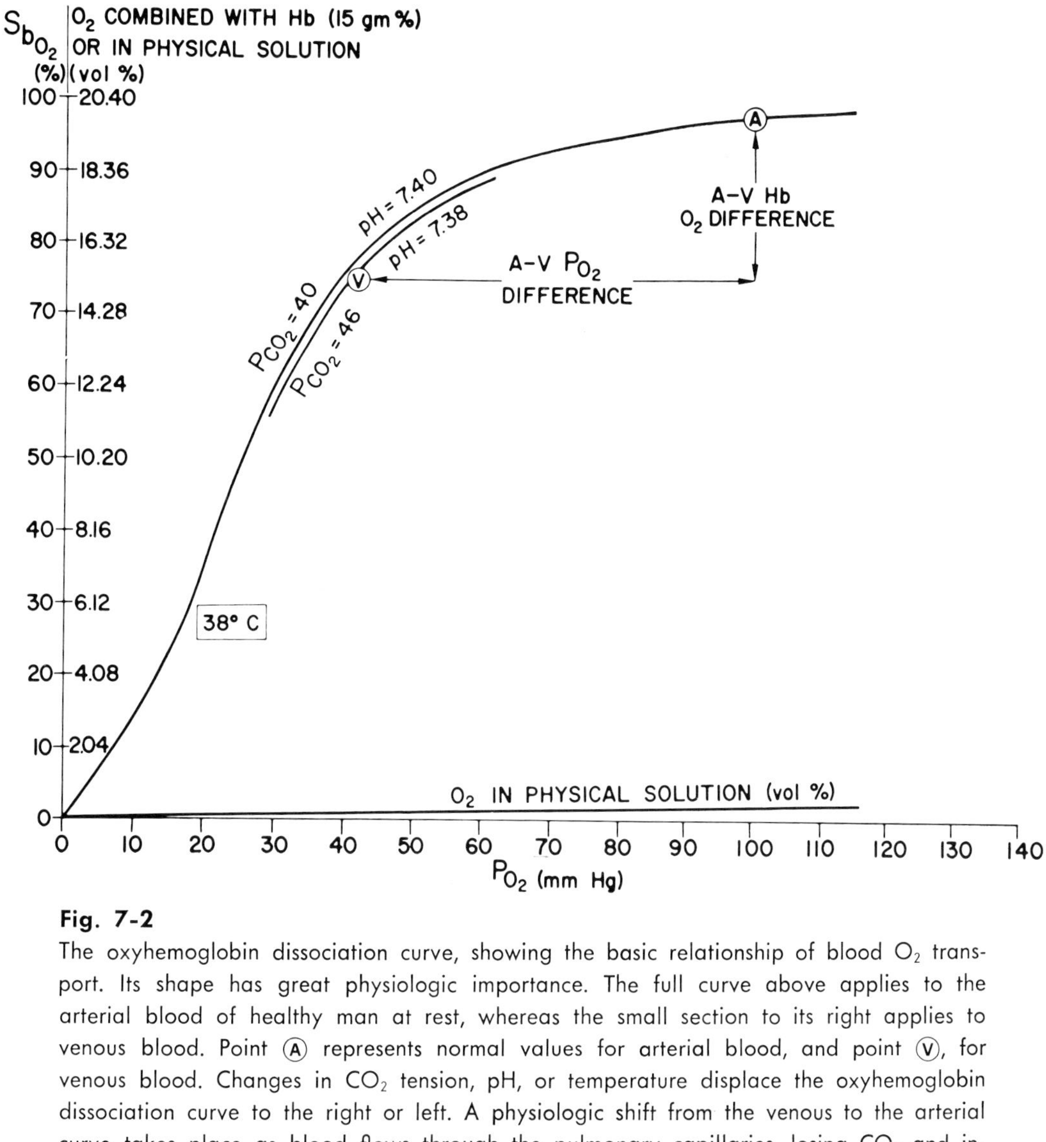

Fig. 7-2
The oxyhemoglobin dissociation curve, showing the basic relationship of blood O_2 transport. Its shape has great physiologic importance. The full curve above applies to the arterial blood of healthy man at rest, whereas the small section to its right applies to venous blood. Point Ⓐ represents normal values for arterial blood, and point Ⓥ, for venous blood. Changes in CO_2 tension, pH, or temperature displace the oxyhemoglobin dissociation curve to the right or left. A physiologic shift from the venous to the arterial curve takes place as blood flows through the pulmonary capillaries, losing CO_2 and increasing in pH. The reverse shift occurs as blood flows through the systemic capillaries. Note that this effect, termed the Bohr shift, facilitates O_2 uptake in the lungs and O_2 dumping in the tissues. Note also the relatively small amount of O_2 carried by the blood in physical solution in the physiologic range of O_2 tension.

loading, transport, and unloading of O_2 are some of the physiologically significant functions of the remarkable pigment of vertebrate blood—hemoglobin.

Each molecule of hemoglobin contains four sites for combination with molecular O_2. Avogadro's law, defining the number of molecules per unit volume of gas, together with the molecular weight of hemoglobin, implies that 1 gm of hemoglobin can combine chemically with a maximum of 1.36 ml (STPD) of O_2. One hundred milliliters of blood containing 15 gm of hemoglobin can combine with 15 × 1.36 = 20.4 ml (STPD) of O_2. The amount of O_2 actually combined with hemoglobin depends upon blood P_{O_2}, since oxygenation is a reversible process that depends upon the P_{O_2} to which the hemoglobin is exposed. Unlike dissolved O_2, the amount of O_2 combined with hemoglobin is *not* linearly related to P_{O_2} but is described by an S-shaped curve that slopes steeply between 10 and 50 mm Hg P_{O_2} and a nearly flat portion between 70 and 100 mm Hg P_{O_2} (Fig. 7-2).

The unique shape of this oxyhemoglobin dissociation curve is an important example of physiologic adaptation. The relatively flat portion above 70 mm Hg ensures the oxygenation of most hemoglobin despite wide variations in alveolar (and therefore arterial) P_{O_2}. On the other hand, the steep portion of the curve between 10 and 50 mm Hg P_{O_2} assures unloading of large amounts of O_2 in the systemic capillaries in response to small tissue P_{O_2} decrements. The dissociation curves of various hemoglobins, including fetal hemoglobins and myoglobins, are beautiful examples of adaptation to environment.* As a result of the shape of the oxyhemoglobin dissociation curve, patients with initial hypoxemia from pulmonary insufficiency respond to altitude with relatively large decreases of arterial blood O_2 content and saturation.

Oxygen pressure versus oxygen content

The question is often asked concerning whether arterial blood O_2 *pressure* or *content* is more important for normal body function. The answer must be that they are *both* important. These two factors are inseparable aspects of the same thing, and each is related to a different aspect of O_2 supply. Oxygen pressure difference promotes diffusion of O_2 across membranes and into cells. Further, tissue P_{O_2} provides an input to the homeostatic mechanism regulating O_2 delivery.

Gas pressure is one of the factors that determines the availability, or effective "local concentration," of gas molecules for physicochemical reaction. The effects of any gas are thus a *direct* function of its *partial pressure,* not its concentration. The significance of P_{O_2}, as contrasted with O_2 content, depends further on the fact that this intensive factor can be detected by physiologic sensors anywhere within the system and that the information thus obtained can be used in a feedback control system.

Oxygen content, or concentration, determines *how much* O_2 can be transferred to the cells without producing a physiologically significant P_{O_2} decrease. At rest with a normal arteriovenous blood O_2 difference, mixed venous P_{O_2} remains above 30 to 40 mm Hg. If arterial O_2 content is low, as in anemia or carbon monoxide poisoning, tissue P_{O_2} decreases to hypoxic levels when arteriovenous blood O_2 difference is only 4 vol % even though arterial blood P_{O_2} is normal.

Blood O_2 *pressure,* or P_{O_2}, is measured directly by means of an O_2 electrode. Blood O_2 *content* is measured in several ways. The manometric method of Van Slyke and Neil measures total whole blood O_2 content (O_2 combined with Hb plus dissolved O_2). Blood O_2 *capacity* is the O_2 content of a blood sample that has been exposed to a sufficiently high P_{O_2} so that all the hemoglobin is combined with O_2. Total O_2 content of the saturated capacity blood sample is then determined in the Van Slyke manometric apparatus. The dissolved O_2 content is subtracted from the total O_2 content of both content and capacity blood samples, giving the

*The hemoglobin of the llama, an animal that is adapted to high altitude, has a dissociation curve considerably to the left of human adult hemoglobin; llama hemoglobin is 50% saturated at 19 mm Hg P_{O_2}.

O_2 combined with Hb for each. If the O_2 *actually* combined with hemoglobin is divided by the O_2 *capable* of combining with hemoglobin (content minus its dissolved O_2 divided by capacity minus its dissolved O_2), multiplication of this fraction by 100 gives oxyhemoglobin saturation in percent. Blood O_2 saturation (oxyhemoglobin saturation) is best calculated from analyses of O_2 content and capacity; however, it can be measured with oximeters of both spectrophotometric and reflectance type. These instruments are useful where rapid analysis of many blood samples is necessary, as during cardiac catheterization, but are less accurate than the chemical methods that are required to calibrate them. Reflectance oximeters, in particular, tend to give falsely high values for oxyhemoglobin saturation, the magnitude of the error depending upon the O_2 pressure difference between blood sample and room air as well as the duration of blood sample exposure. Excessive familiarity with these instruments without concomitant thorough indoctrination in the proper anaerobic technic for handling blood samples can ruin laboratory personnel for careful work.

Factors affecting oxygen transport by hemoglobin

Since a gram of hemoglobin can combine with 1.36 ml (STPD) of O_2, blood O_2 content depends not only on P_{O_2} but also on hemoglobin concentration. Increased hemoglobin concentration increases blood O_2 content at any given P_{O_2} (Fig. 7-3). To eliminate hemoglobin concentration as a variable we plot P_{O_2} against oxyhemoglobin saturation in percent rather than against blood O_2 content. A curve

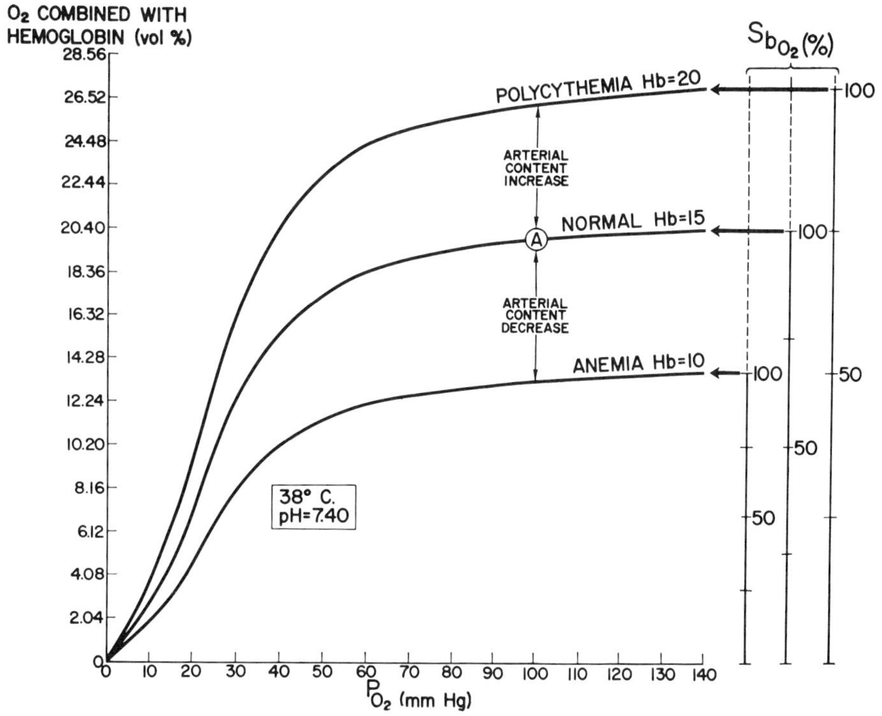

Fig. 7-3
Oxyhemoglobin dissociation curve in anemia and polycythemia.

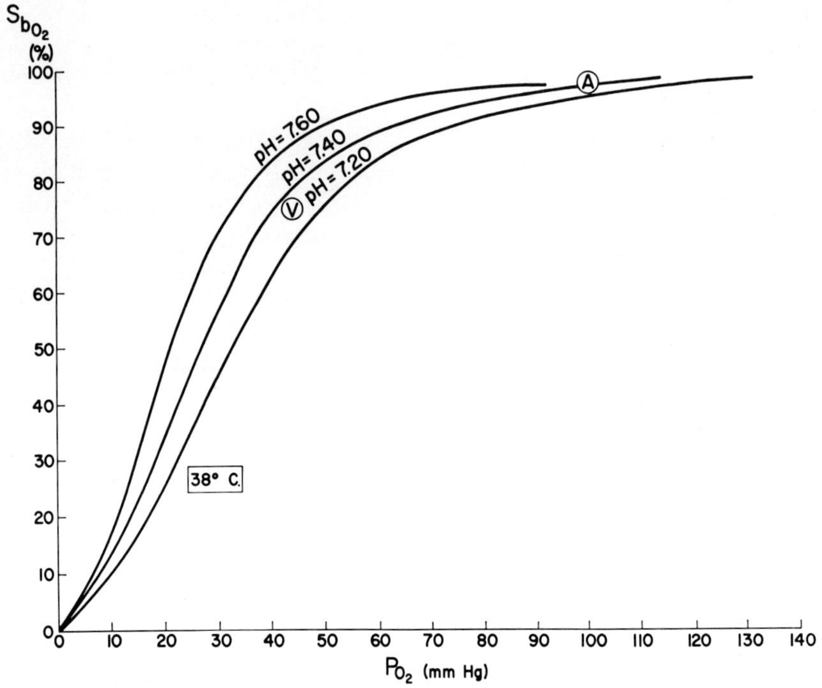

Fig. 7-4
Effect of pH on the oxyhemoglobin dissociation curve.

presented in terms of oxyhemoglobin saturation reveals the effects of factors such as pH or temperature on the affinity of hemoglobin for O_2. Temperature increase, as well as pH decrease, decreases hemoglobin affinity for O_2 (Figs. 7-4 and 7-5); thus, at a given P_{O_2}, hemoglobin is less saturated with O_2. These shifts in the oxyhemoglobin dissociation curve release O_2 in regions of high metabolism, high O_2 consumption, high CO_2 production, and increased local temperature.

Oxygen delivery rate

Oxygen delivery involves the processes of uptake and release of O_2 by hemoglobin in the erythrocyte and is influenced by many factors such as P_{O_2} gradient, P_{CO_2}, pH, temperature, and concentrations of various electrolyte and nonelectrolyte substances. Oxygen delivery is studied by means of the polarographic method, which measures O_2 concentration in solution. When erythrocytes are near the dropping mercury electrode in the polarographic circuit, the electrode is a cathode on which all O_2 diffusing to its surface is instantly reduced and thus removed from solution. The dropping mercury electrode is thus comparable to an O_2-consuming living cell. The resulting polarographic diffusion current is directly proportional to the P_{O_2} of the solution. With blood, however, an *excess current* is observed, which is taken as a measure of the process

$$\text{Oxyhemoglobin} \longrightarrow \text{Hemoglobin} + O_2$$

and considered to reflect the *oxygen delivery rate.* The diffusion current of blood divided by the diffusion current of a solution at the same P_{O_2} gives a ratio called *relative oxygen delivery rate.* Dissociation constants for oxyhemoglobin have been calculated using such measure-

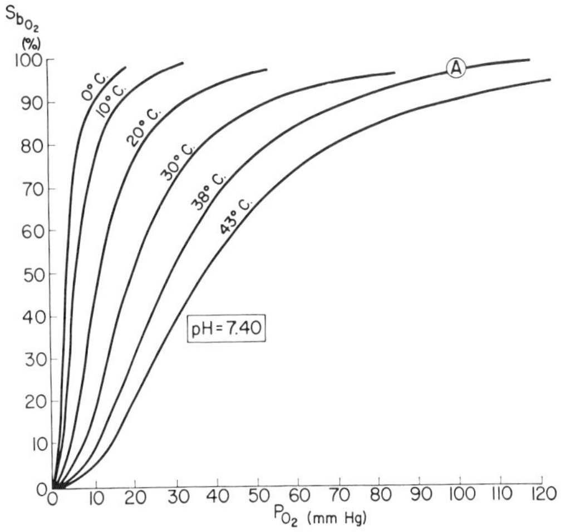

Fig. 7-5
Effect of temperature on the oxyhemoglobin dissociation curve.

ments. Oxygen delivery rate increases as oxyhemoglobin saturation decreases. Blood from one individual may differ significantly with respect to oxygen delivery rate from that of another.

Oxygen association in erythrocytes is a slower process than dissociation. Diffusion of O_2 through the erythrocyte membrane and interior of the erythrocyte requires ten times as long as does combination of dissolved hemoglobin with O_2. The increasing oxygen delivery rate of blood with decreasing oxyhemoglobin saturation is an intrinsic mechanism of blood itself that protects tissues against hypoxia. This intrinsic mechanism is in addition to other mechanisms such as those regulating regional blood flow.

CARBON DIOXIDE TRANSPORT

Each minute the metabolizing cells of the human body consume about 250 ml of O_2 and produce about 200 ml of CO_2 for a metabolic respiratory quotient of about 0.8. The transport of this CO_2 by the blood from tissues to lungs is the subject of this section.

Atmospheric air contains only traces (0.03%) of CO_2. Unless CO_2 is added to inspired gas, the CO_2 present in venous blood, alveolar gas, and arterial blood originates in metabolizing body cells. Carbon dioxide diffuses from these tissue cells into the systemic capillary blood and is carried in the veins, both in chemical combination and physical solution, to the lungs, where some of it diffuses into the alveolar gas to be eliminated in the exhalatory stream. The P_{CO_2} is greater in actively metabolizing cells than in blood flowing through the systemic capillaries; carbon dioxide therefore diffuses from these cells into the plasma.

Carbon dioxide is carried in the blood as (1) dissolved CO_2, (2) carbonic acid, or H_2CO_3, (3) bicarbonate ions, or HCO_3^-, (4) carbaminohemoglobin and other carbamino compounds, and (5) physiologically insignificant amounts of carbonate ion, or $CO_3^=$. When whole blood is chemically analyzed for total CO_2 content, all these molecular species are included. Since the CO_2 content of erythrocytes is considerably lower than that of plasma, it is essential to specify whether blood or plasma is being analyzed and to realize that the hematocrit is a variable affecting whole blood total CO_2 content.

Reactions, compounds, and consequences

In plasma. Of the CO_2 dissolved in plasma, a small amount reacts slowly with water to form carbonic acid; this H_2CO_3 dissociates into $H^+ + HCO_3^-$, and the resulting H^+ are buffered by plasma buffering systems.

Dissolved CO_2 in plasma also reacts with the free amino groups of various plasma proteins to form carbamino compounds. This rapid chemical reaction requires no catalyst:

$$R\text{—}NH_2 + CO_2 \rightleftharpoons R\text{—}NHCOO^- + H^+$$

In erythrocytes. However, most of the CO_2 that diffuses from tissue cells into the plasma enters the erythrocytes, where three events occur:

1. Some remains within the red blood cell as dissolved CO_2.

2. Some combines with hemoglobin to form carbamino compounds; the resulting H^+ are buffered by the hemoglobin molecule in a chemical process termed the *isohydric shift*. This process is facilitated by the simultaneous loss of O_2 from systemic capillary blood to the tissues because the conversion of oxyhemoglobin to reduced hemoglobin results in a weaker acid, which then takes up additional H^+ with little change of pH.

Carbon dioxide combines with hemoglobin (as well as other proteins) at the free amino ($-NH_2$) sites. In the hemoglobin molecule, combination takes place in the globin moiety in close proximity to the heme portion. The presence of O_2 on the heme portion appears to interfere somewhat with carbamino compound formation. Carbon dioxide does not combine at $-NH_3^+$ sites, which, however, are in equilibrium with $-NH_2$:

$$\begin{array}{ccc} Hb{-}NH_2 + CO_2 & \rightleftharpoons & Hb{-}NHCOOH \\ \upharpoonleft\downharpoonright & & \upharpoonleft\downharpoonright \\ Hb{-}NH_3^+ & & Hb{-}NHCOO^- + H^+ \end{array}$$

3. Some CO_2 combines with water to form H_2CO_3, which then dissociates to form H^+ and HCO_3^-. The conversion of CO_2 and H_2O into H_2CO_3 is very rapid because the enzyme, carbonic anhydrase, is concentrated within the erythrocyte. Carbonic anhydrase speeds the normally slow reaction, but as a catalyst does not change its equilibrium. In blood the hydration of CO_2 is an important and rapid reaction only within the erythrocyte.

$$CO_2 + H_2O \overset{\substack{\text{Carbonic} \\ \text{anhydrase} \\ \downarrow}}{\rightleftharpoons} H_2CO_3 \rightleftharpoons HCO_3^- + H^+$$

This reaction also results in the formation of H^+, which are buffered by functional groups of the hemoglobin molecule with minimal change in pH. Again, the simultaneous conversion of some oxyhemoglobin to reduced hemoglobin facilitates the buffering (isohydric shift).

The preceding events result in an accumulation of HCO_3^- within the red blood cell. Some HCO_3^- diffuse out into the plasma to reestablish HCO_3^- concentration equilibrium between erythrocyte and plasma. If this diffusion of bicarbonate anions were accompanied by the diffusion of an equal number of cations, electrical neutrality would be maintained within the erythrocyte. However, the erythrocyte membrane is not freely permeable to cations so that chloride anions from the plasma diffuse into the erythrocyte to preserve electrical neutrality. This movement is termed the *chloride shift*. Simultaneously, some water moves into the erythrocyte to maintain osmotic equilibrium, resulting in a slight swelling of the erythrocytes in venous blood.

As O_2 uptake and CO_2 unloading proceed in the pulmonary capillaries, the reverse reactions occur.

Although plasma contains much more of the metabolically produced CO_2 than do the erythrocytes, and although plasma *transports* more than 60% of the CO_2 entering systemic capillary blood, chemical reactions within the erythrocyte account for almost all the additional HCO_3^- transported in the plasma. If carbonic anhydrase is inhibited, as by acetazolamide administration, the uncatalyzed reaction $CO_2 + H_2O \rightleftharpoons H_2CO_3$ proceeds slowly and will not be completed in the systemic capillaries or even in transit from veins to heart. The reverse reaction, $H_2CO_3 \rightleftharpoons CO_2 + H_2O$, which normally takes place in the fraction of a second that mixed venous blood is in the pulmonary capillaries, is also slow and continues long after the blood has left the pulmonary capillaries and entered the systemic circulation. Therefore, if carbonic anhydrase is inhibited, P_{CO_2} decreases gradually in venous blood until it reaches the pulmonary capillaries, where some CO_2 is eliminated; however, P_{CO_2} rises as blood flows through the systemic arteries, and the unloading reaction slowly proceeds to completion; tissue P_{CO_2} rises as a result. An instantaneous method for measuring blood P_{CO_2} would be required to analyze the dynamics of this disturbance, but CO_2 retention under these conditions has been demonstrated.

Carbon dioxide dissociation curve

Just as the amount of O_2 in blood is a function of P_{O_2}, so the amount of CO_2 in blood is a function of P_{CO_2}. The solubility coefficient (C_s) for CO_2 in blood at 37° C is 0.063 vol %/mm Hg. Chemical reactions that form HCO_3^- and the combination of CO_2 with hemoglobin account for most of the CO_2 content of blood. The CO_2 dissociation curve, or blood buffer curve, describes the formation of HCO_3^- from CO_2, or from dissociation or ionization of H_2CO_3, as a function of P_{CO_2} (Fig. 7-6). This curve is an experimentally determined curve resulting from the analysis of HCO_3^- in blood equilibrated with gas of various CO_2 pressures. The relationship between CO_2 pressure and CO_2 content is nearly linear in the physiologic range. The curvature, or departure from linearity, reflects the chemical reactions of CO_2 with water and buffers. The curve may be lowered by increasing the P_{O_2} of the equilibrating gas mixture, or it may be raised by lowering its O_2 pressure. This effect of changing the level of the CO_2 dissociation curve by varying the P_{O_2} is called the *Haldane effect.* Because of this effect, arterial blood has a somewhat lower dissociation curve than venous blood. About 70% of this effect is because oxyhemoglobin has a reduced affinity for CO_2 due to formation of carbaminohemoglobin.

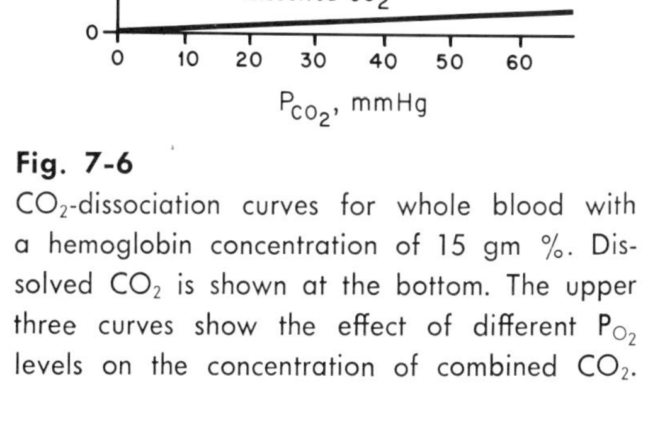

Fig. 7-6
CO_2-dissociation curves for whole blood with a hemoglobin concentration of 15 gm %. Dissolved CO_2 is shown at the bottom. The upper three curves show the effect of different P_{O_2} levels on the concentration of combined CO_2.

Body stores of carbon dioxide

Of the normal body gas stores, the CO_2 stores are the largest and the most complex. When pulmonary ventilation is eliminating CO_2 at precisely its production rate, CO_2 output equals metabolic CO_2 production, and a steady state exists. However, any change in alveolar ventilation produces an unsteady state, changing, in turn, the level of body CO_2 stores. If pulmonary ventilation is greater than that required to rid the body of current CO_2 production, the rather large body reservoirs of stored CO_2 are depleted. The body fluids, about 70% of body mass, normally hold 50 ml of CO_2 for each 100 ml of fluid (50 vol %); bone contains over 100 vol % of CO_2. Thus a 70 kg man contains about 35 L of stored CO_2. This equals the resting metabolic CO_2 production for a period of about 140 minutes. When alveolar ventilation is subnormal, metabolic CO_2 is stored and the CO_2 reservoirs fill.

If CO_2 production remains constant, the relationship between alveolar P_{CO_2} and alveolar ventilation is a rectangular hyperbola. If alveolar ventilation doubles, alveolar P_{CO_2} is halved; if ventilation is halved, P_{CO_2} is doubled. This relationship holds only after a new storage level is achieved and remains constant, that is, after a new

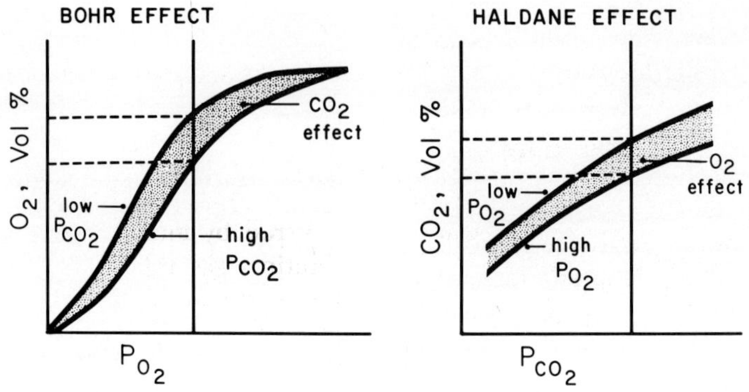

Fig. 7-7
Reciprocal interaction of O_2 and CO_2 on blood-gas transport. Increased P_{CO_2} decreases the affinity of hemoglobin for O_2 (Bohr shift), whereas decreased P_{O_2} increases CO_2 content (Haldane effect).

Table 6
Typical blood-gas and pH values for healthy man at rest*

	Inspired air	Alveolar gas	Arterial blood	Mixed venous blood	Arteriovenous difference
P_{H_2O} (mm Hg)	Varies	47			
P_{O_2} (mm Hg)	159†	104	100	42	58
S_{O_2} (%)			96	75	21
O_2 content (vol %)			18.97	14.71	4.26
O_2 combined with Hb (vol %)			18.67	14.59	4.08
O_2 in physical solution (vol %)			0.30	0.12	0.18
O_2 capacity of Hb (vol %)			19.45	19.45	0
P_{CO_2} (mm Hg)	0.3†	40	40	46	6
Total CO_2 (vol %)			48.5	52.2	3.7
content‡ (mM/L)			21.8	23.5	1.7
Total CO_2 (vol %)			58.3	62.1	3.8
content§ (mM/L)			26.2	27.9	1.7
Combined CO_2§ (vol %)			55.6	59.0	3.4
CO_2 in physical solution§ (vol %)			2.78	3.13	0.35
Combined CO_2 / dissolved CO_2§			20.0/1	18.8/1	1.2/1
Plasma pH			7.40	7.376	0.024

*Sea level: P_B = 760 mm Hg; assume Hb = 14.3 gm %.
†On basis of dry atmospheric air.
‡Whole blood.
§Plasma.

steady state is achieved. Once attained, however, the alveolar ventilation rate must remain at the new level or, if it changes, the level of CO_2 stores will follow it. The CO_2 stores of the body are readjusting almost continuously. The rate of adjustment of CO_2 stores during hyperventilation or hypoventilation with air is about one eighth as fast as that for O_2. Both processes are simple exponential functions with time.

Interrelation of O_2 and CO_2 transport mechanisms

Oxygen unloading and CO_2 loading in systemic capillaries are mutually helpful processes. A reciprocal relationship exists so that increased P_{CO_2} aids in unloading O_2 and decreased P_{O_2} aids in loading CO_2 in the tissues. The reverse occurs in the lung, where decreasing P_{CO_2} increases the affinity of hemoglobin for O_2 and increasing P_{O_2} reduces the affinity of hemoglobin for CO_2. These two effects, the *Haldane effect* on CO_2 loading and the *Bohr effect* on O_2 loading, result from the unique physicochemical properties of hemoglobin; they are contrasted in Fig. 7-7.

Since the oxyhemoglobin dissociation curve shifts to the right when P_{CO_2} increases, the affinity of hemoglobin for O_2 decreases; for a given P_{O_2} less hemoglobin is oxygenated. The O_2 released from hemoglobin as a result of increasing P_{CO_2} is available to the tissues.

Deoxygenation of hemoglobin increases affinity for CO_2; thus at a given P_{CO_2} more CO_2 combines with hemoglobin, adding to that carried as HCO_3^- and as dissolved CO_2. Total blood CO_2 content increases.

These two mechanisms, both dependent upon the characteristics of hemoglobin, facilitate the efficient exchange of respiratory gases in regions of high metabolic activity, where O_2 consumption and CO_2 production are increased. Table 6 shows typical blood-gas and pH values for healthy man at rest.

CHAPTER 8 Diffusion of gases in the lung

The continuous exchange of O_2 and CO_2 between blood and the atmosphere is accomplished by the simultaneous processes of pulmonary ventilation, pulmonary perfusion, and alveolocapillary diffusion. Diffusion (Chapter 2) is a critical step in respiratory gas exchange; indeed, some of what has been termed alveolar ventilation is actually diffusion of inspired gas in terminal airways.

In health, diffusion rapidly equalizes mixed venous gas pressures with alveolar gas pressures. At rest, blood traverses a pulmonary capillary in approximately 0.75 second, P_{O_2} equalizes in 0.3 to 0.4 second, and P_{CO_2} equalizes in about 0.1 second. If an alveolocapillary pressure difference increases so that more gas must move to equalize pressure, or if pulmonary capillary transit time for blood decreases through increase of cardiac output, or if diffusion is impaired, then equalization of gas pressures may not occur within the fraction of a second available. Alveolocapillary gas pressure difference may increase as a result of abnormal mixed venous gas pressure or abnormal alveolar gas pressure.

DETERMINANTS OF GAS TRANSFER

The *volume* of a gas that moves across the alveolocapillary membrane *per unit time* depends upon (1) the characteristics, or physicochemical properties, of that gas, (2) the characteristics of the lung, and (3) the pressure gradient across the alveolocapillary membrane.

Gas characteristics

Velocity of gas molecules. At a given pressure the product mv^2 is constant*; thus larger gas molecules move more slowly. Since the rate of diffusion of a gas is directly proportional to the velocity of its molecules, larger gas molecules diffuse more slowly whether in gas or liquid. Since the mass of a molecule m is reciprocally related to v^2, the relative rates of diffusion of two gases are inversely proportional to the square roots of their molecular weights, or densities (Graham's law). Thus, on the basis of molecular weight only, O_2 diffuses slightly faster than CO_2:

$$\frac{\sqrt{44}}{\sqrt{32}} = \frac{6.63}{5.66} = 1.17$$

Solubility coefficient. The rate of transfer of a gas across a biologic membrane depends upon the solubility coefficient, C_S, of that gas in the aqueous phase of the membrane. At 38° C, CO_2 is approximately twenty-one times as soluble as O_2 in the aqueous fluids of the body and diffuses much faster than O_2 across the alveolocapillary membrane. Impaired diffusion interferes with O_2 transfer long before CO_2 transfer is affected; indeed, outward diffusion of CO_2 is never a clinical problem except in patients whose diffusion is so

*The velocity of gas molecules is also a function of temperature; velocity increases as temperature increases. The rate of diffusion of a gas in a liquid is directly proportional to the square root of the absolute temperature.

severely impaired that life can be maintained only by administration of high P_{O_2} mixtures.

However, in body fluids the relative diffusion rates of O_2 and CO_2 depend on solubility *and* molecular weight. Thus, although somewhat heavier, the much more soluble CO_2 diffuses about twenty times faster than O_2 across the water-containing alveolocapillary membrane.

Lung characteristics

Membrane area. The total volume of gas that diffuses across the alveolocapillary membrane per unit time is limited by the area of membrane available for diffusion. Lung size as well as the distribution of alveolar ventilation and pulmonary capillary blood flow are important determinants of this gas-exchanging area. Thus the rate of diffusion is directly related to the functioning area of alveolocapillary membrane.

Diffusion distance. The rate of diffusion is inversely related to the length of the pathway between the alveolus and the hemoglobin molecule within the erythrocyte. The pathway involved in the diffusion process from alveolus to hemoglobin molecule can be divided into five steps: (1) the liquid alveolar lining layer; (2) the alveolocapillary membrane where diffusion depends upon the O_2 (or CO) pressure gradient from alveolar gas to pulmonary capillary plasma, tissue thickness and characteristics, and gas-exchanging surface area; (3) diffusion in plasma until the gas molecule meets the erythrocyte membrane; (4) diffusion across the erythrocyte membrane; and (5) random movement until contact and chemical combination with a hemoglobin molecule occurs.

The diffusion pathway across the alveolocapillary membrane varies normally from 0.1 to 0.5 μ, but in disease it may increase greatly; appreciable reduction of alveolocapillary membrane thickness by any circumstances appears unlikely. The sum of the distances in steps 3, 4, and 5, from membrane to hemoglobin molecule, is sometimes called intracapillary distance.

Liquid viscosity. ~~The rate of diffusion of a gas is inversely related to the viscosity of the liquid through which it diffuses.~~ Viscosity is essentially constant for the alveolar lining liquid, for the aqueous phase of the alveolocapillary membrane, and for the blood plasma in the pulmonary capillary.

Transmembrane pressure gradient

The volume of a gas that diffuses across the alveolocapillary membrane per unit time is directly related to the mean gas pressure difference between alveolus and pulmonary capillary. The greater the mean gas pressure difference the larger will be the volume of gas that diffuses across the alveolocapillary membrane. Three factors maintain the pressure differences that promote the transfer of O_2 and CO_2 across the alveolocapillary membrane.

Alveolar ventilation. As alveolar ventilation increases, the composition of alveolar gas approaches that of inspired air. Normal alveolar ventilation maintains a P_{O_2} of approximately 100 mm Hg and a P_{CO_2} of 40 mm Hg, creating a *source* of O_2 and a *sink* for CO_2 as these gases diffuse across the alveolocapillary membrane.

Pulmonary capillary blood flow. Pulmonary capillary blood flow keeps the mean P_{O_2} of capillary blood close to that of the mixed venous blood presented to the lung. It thereby maintains a suitable sink for O_2 and source of CO_2, facilitating continuous transfer of these two gases.

Chemical reactions. Hemoglobin is a sink for the stream of O_2 molecules that moves from alveolar gas into the erythrocyte. After combination with hemoglobin, O_2 exerts negligible backpressure, maintaining the alveolocapillary O_2 pressure difference as O_2 transfer proceeds.

The CO_2-buffering mechanism of blood, including carbaminohemoglobin, is a source of CO_2, favoring a CO_2 pressure difference, despite the stream of CO_2 molecules across the alveolocapillary membrane. The kinetics of the CO_2 reactions in blood favor the maintenance of a normal pressure difference. The velocity of the chemical reactions is sufficiently great to remove O_2 from solution and to supply CO_2 for diffusion from the erythrocyte.

All factors that affect the rate of gas diffusion across the alveolocapillary membrane are represented in the following equation:

$$\dot{V} \propto \frac{C_S \times T \times A \times dP}{\sqrt{MW \times L \times \eta}}$$

where $\dot{V}$ is the volumetric rate of gas transfer by diffusion, C_s is the solubility coefficient, T is the absolute temperature, A is the gas-exchanging membrane area, dP is the gas pressure gradient, MW is the molecular weight of the gas, L is the length of diffusion pathway, and η is the viscosity of the liquid. The pressure gradient, dP, in turn, is a function of alveolar ventilation, pulmonary capillary blood flow, and the velocity of the chemical reactions involved.

Pulmonary diffusing capacity

Pulmonary diffusing capacity (D_L), or lung transfer factor (T_L), is a measure of the lung *conductance* for a gas. This term quantitates the pulmonary transfer of a specific gas, including the effects of alveolar ventilation, pulmonary capillary blood flow, and the velocity of chemical reactions involved.

Gas transfer between alveoli and pulmonary capillary blood obeys the fundamental law of diffusion:

$$\frac{dV}{dt} = D(P_1 - P_2)$$

where $\frac{dV}{dt}$ is the rate of diffusion of a given gas in milliliters per minute across a given membrane, D is the diffusion constant for that gas in relation to the membrane in ml × min^{-1} × mm Hg^{-1}, and ($P_1 - P_2$) is the pressure difference for that gas in mm Hg between the two sides of the membrane. D is directly proportional to the solubility of that gas in the membrane under stated conditions and to the total membrane surface area available for diffusion, but D is inversely proportional to membrane thickness and to the square root of the molecular weight of the gas.

Another form of this equation, expressed in terms of D_L is as follows:

$$D_L\ [\text{ml (STPD)} \times \text{min}^{-1} \times \text{mm Hg}^{-1}] = \frac{\dot{V}}{P_A - P_{\bar{c}}}$$

Division of volume transferred per minute by the gas pressure difference normalizes pulmonary diffusing capacity, and thus facilitates comparison of the transfer rates of different gases across the lung. Changes in pulmonary diffusing capacity thus reflect changes in the lung.

D_L is a measure of the conductance across the lung, since it increases as the ease of gas transfer increases. The reciprocal of D_L is "resistance" to gas transfer. It consists of the resistance to transfer in the alveoli, across the alveolocapillary membrane, and in the blood. Series resistances are additive, so the reciprocals of the diffusing capacity of alveoli, the diffusing capacity of the membrane, and the diffusing capacity of the blood are additive:

$$\frac{1}{D_L} = \frac{1}{D_A} + \frac{1}{D_M} + \frac{1}{D_b}$$

D_A is negligible because of the small distance for diffusion within the alveolus. This should not be confused with diffusion within the airways; D_A refers only to diffusion from the center of the alveolus to the alveolocapillary membrane.

Diffusing capacity of the membrane accounts for half the total resistance to O_2 transfer. The resistance to diffusion in the blood, D_b, accounts for the other half.

This latter factor is affected by capillary blood volume, hemoglobin concentration, and the rate of chemical reaction of O_2 with hemoglobin.

The contribution of the alveolocapillary membrane to the alveoloerythrocyte diffusion impediment is expressed by the following equation:

$$\frac{\theta V_c}{D_L} - \frac{\theta V_c}{D_M} = 1$$

where θ is reaction rate, V_c is pulmonary capillary blood volume, normally about 100 ml, D_L is pulmonary diffusing capacity, and D_M is diffusing capacity of the alveolocapillary membrane.

Tests of pulmonary diffusing capacity

The pulmonary diffusing capacity of a gas is defined as the volume in ml (STPD) that diffuses across the alveolocapillary membrane per minute per mm Hg of mean pressure difference. In general, pulmonary diffusing capacity is calculated as follows:

$$D_L = \frac{\text{Rate of gas transfer}}{\text{Mean alveolar gas tension} - \text{Mean pulmonary capillary gas tension}}$$

Pulmonary diffusing capacity is the factor that limits the transfer of any gas, large volumes of which are transferred before transmembrane pressure difference decreases. Because of specific chemical reactions that occur in the blood this condition applies to three gases: CO_2, O_2, and CO. As indicated earlier, the high pulmonary diffusing capacity for CO_2, a result of its water solubility, implies that diffusion impairment must produce hypoxemia before it produces CO_2 retention and hypercapnic acidosis.

A test gas must be considerably more soluble in blood than in the alveolocapillary membrane. The diffusing capacity for O_2 and CO are affected by some of the same factors, since both gases combine with hemoglobin. Hemoglobin removes CO from solution very effectively, forming carboxyhemoglobin. The affinity of hemoglobin for CO is 210 times as great as that for O_2 (Haldane number). At equilibrium at sea level a P_{CO} of 1.46 mm Hg, or 0.065%, produces the same percent saturation of hemoglobin as does a P_{O_2} of 100 mm Hg, or 14.0% O_2. Thus P_{CO} back pressure is nearly zero when blood CO concentration is low.

The dynamics of CO uptake differ from that of O_2 uptake in the lungs because mixed venous blood has appreciable O_2 content and tension as it enters the pulmonary capillaries; the rate of diffusion of O_2, but not CO, depends upon a diminishing pressure gradient as blood traverses the pulmonary capillary. Thus CO transfer is not limited by the rate of pulmonary capillary blood flow; it is limited by the rate of diffusion across the alveolocapillary membrane and by diffusion across the erythrocyte membrane and the rate of the subsequent chemical combination with hemoglobin.

D_{LCO} can be calculated from measurements of the transfer rate and the mean alveolar P_{CO} during the time of measurement, assuming mean pulmonary capillary P_{CO} (back pressure) to be zero. It is difficult to calculate D_{LO_2} because *mean* pulmonary capillary P_{O_2} cannot be measured. Subjects who smoke cigarettes or have otherwise been exposed to CO may have appreciable carboxyhemoglobin levels in the blood, invalidating the test results.

Two methods are commonly used to determine pulmonary diffusing capacity for carbon monoxide (D_{LCO})—the breath-holding method and the steady state method; the breath-holding method is now used more widely. The subject inspires a gas mixture containing 0.4% CO and an inert insoluble gas, such as helium or neon, in air and holds a single breath in his lungs for 10 seconds. The volume of CO removed by the blood is calculated from the alveolar volume and the change in P_{CO} in the alveolar gas during the breath-holding period. In this method mean pulmonary capillary P_{CO} is neglected. D_{LCO} is then calculated as follows:

$$D_{L_{CO}}\ (\text{ml} \times \text{min}^{-1} \times \text{mm Hg}^{-1}) = \frac{60\ V_A}{t(P_B - 47)}\ \ln \left[\frac{F_{Init_{CO}}}{F_{Final_{CO}}}\right]$$

where V_A is alveolar volume, t is breath-holding time in seconds, $F_{Init_{CO}}$ is fractional concentration of CO in alveolar gas at the beginning of the breath-holding period, and $F_{Final_{CO}}$ is fractional concentration of CO in alveolar gas at the end of the breath-holding period. A disadvantage of this method is that very ill or dyspneic patients, or subjects who are exercising, may have difficulty in holding their breath for the required 10 seconds.

In such cases the steady state measurement can usually be made. This consists of breathing from a gas mixture containing 0.25% CO for a measured period of time, during which mixed expired gas is collected and an alveolar gas sample is taken. The rate of CO-uptake per minute is calculated, and the mean alveolar CO pressure is determined by analysis of the alveolar gas sample. For the most accurate measurement, blood samples should also be obtained for determination of P_{CO} to estimate the CO back pressure.

The combination of differing solubility and molecular weight result in the fact that D_{LO_2} is 1.23 times greater than D_{LCO}:

$$\frac{D_{O_2}}{D_{CO}} = \frac{O_2\ \text{solubility}}{CO\ \text{solubility}} \times \frac{\sqrt{MW\ CO}}{\sqrt{MW\ O_2}}$$

$$= \frac{0.024}{0.018} \times \frac{\sqrt{28}}{\sqrt{32}} = 1.23$$

Thus pulmonary diffusing capacity for CO is converted to that for O_2 by multiplying D_{LCO} by the factor 1.23. A similar calculation for CO_2 in relation to O_2 indicates that it must diffuse at about twenty times the rate of O_2 through an aqueous medium.

Factors that affect pulmonary diffusing capacity

Body position. Pulmonary diffusing capacity is greater in the recumbent position by 15% to 20% over that measured with the subject upright. Two factors are probably responsible for this finding: (1) pulmonary blood volume increases when a subject is recumbent; (2) pulmonary blood flow is distributed more evenly when a subject is recumbent, tending to match more closely the distribution of ventilation within the lung, thus providing a larger effective area for diffusion. Pulmonary diffusing capacity also increases with body size.

Physical exercise. The pulmonary diffusing capacity of healthy subjects increases by 25% to 35% during muscular exercise; most of the increase is achieved with moderate levels of physical activity. The increase probably results from several factors:

1. Increased ventilation of certain lung areas.
2. Increased lung perfusion, with improved distribution of $\dot{V}_A/\dot{Q}_c$ ratios, bringing the mean P_{CO} nearer to zero in the capillary blood.
3. During exercise hemoglobin concentration increases as a result of sympathoadrenal discharge, splenic contraction, and possibly other factors. Increased hemoglobin increases D_b slightly, partly due to the reduction of CO back pressure at any given rate of CO uptake.
4. During heavy exercise decreased mixed venous P_{O_2} may decrease competition for hemoglobin and, thereby, decrease the back pressure of CO (usually considered negligible but is, in fact, not quite zero).

Pulmonary disease. Diseases that decrease pulmonary diffusing capacity (D_L)

do so by reducing effective surface area and/or by increasing diffusion distance.

1. Reduced effective surface area.
   a. Loss of lung tissue by excision or destruction of lung decreases both alveolar gas volume and capillary blood volume.
   b. Alveolar closure or regional airway obstruction decreases alveolar volume.
   c. Capillary obstruction, pulmonary embolism, or regional vasoconstriction reduces capillary volume.
   d. Mismatching of ventilation with perfusion reduces the effective, or functioning, membrane area for gas transfer.
2. Increased diffusion distance (increased length of diffusion pathway, or alveolocapillary diffusion block).
   a. Thickened alveolocapillary membrane (e.g., fibrosis) increases diffusion distance and decreases pulmonary diffusing capacity (D_L). Such conditions probably also decrease D_L by impairing the distribution of ventilation, producing regions of decreased compliance and thus reducing the effective membrane area for diffusion.
   b. Accumulation of fluid in the lung decreases D_L. Fluid may accumulate within the alveolocapillary membrane itself (interstitial edema) or on the alveolar surface (intra-alveolar edema) due to increased permeability, increased intracapillary pressure, or increased surface tension as a result of surfactant deficiency.
   c. Increased intracapillary diffusion distance also affects D_L. Low hemoglobin concentration (anemia) increases intracapillary diffusion distance. It also diminishes the sink for CO and favors the development of CO back pressure.

The clinical syndrome of *alveolocapillary diffusion block* includes a variety of bronchopulmonary diseases that have in common the single feature of increased alveolocapillary diffusion pathway. The diseases that produce this pathophysiologic condition include pulmonary berylliosis, asbestosis, sarcoidosis, interstitial fibrosis, adenomatosis, alveolar proteinosis, and to some extent, mitral stenosis. The clinical picture includes hypoxemia and cyanosis, which are aggravated by exercise, alveolar hyperventilation, decreased arterial blood P_{CO_2}, and often essentially normal ventilatory capacity.

Tests of pulmonary diffusing capacity cannot distinguish between lengthened diffusion pathway, on the one hand, and decreased surface area, on the other; furthermore, diffusing capacity may decrease by a combination of the two. Attempts to relate pulmonary diffusing capacity to alveolar volume (D_L/V_A) can be misleading, since V_A does not reliably reflect *effective* area, although if V_A is reduced, D_L is predictably low. If $\dot{V}_A/\dot{Q}_c$ ratios (Chapter 9) are uniform throughout the lung, D_L/V_A helps to differentiate the cause of decreased pulmonary diffusing capacity; however, $\dot{V}_A/\dot{Q}_c$ ratios are often also abnormal in patients who have reduced pulmonary diffusing capacity.

GAS POCKETS

The absorption of gas from pockets within the body involves solubility, diffusion, and perfusion. Gas pockets in the body gradually decrease in size and disappear or, if the walls are rigid, develop a "negative" pressure. The rate of disappearance of a gas depends upon its composition, the metabolic rate, and physical activity. After its creation a closed, collapsible gas pocket quickly reaches a composition that is essentially independent of its initial composition; this composition and the resulting gas tension diffusion gradients are then maintained until absorption is complete. No matter what gases constitute the pocket initially, O_2, CO_2, and water vapor quickly become a part of it. As could be predicted, P_{CO_2} reaches its steady state value in the pocket more quickly than P_{O_2}. Absorption proceeds at a constant rate after steady state gas tension values, and therefore gradients, are achieved.

Values for tissue P_{O_2} and P_{CO_2} can be obtained from analysis of the equilibrated gas phase. Except in the intestine, gas pocket values for P_{CO_2} are from 40 to 50 mm Hg, whereas those for P_{O_2} are from 20 to 45 mm Hg. Gas pockets disappear because they are ultimately subject to the atmosphere and its pressure; the blood supply in their walls is essentially venous, and venous blood is incompletely saturated. Blood, in its passage through metabolizing tissues, may lose 60 mm Hg in P_{O_2} but gain only 5 mm Hg in P_{CO_2}. This uneven exchange leaves venous blood with a 55 mm Hg deficit in total gas pressure; however, the partial pressures of the various gases comprising a pocket add up to a value that is close to atmospheric pressure. After the rapid initial composition changes, during which any large gradients are minimized, there is, for each gas, a tension gradient from gas pocket to the blood leaving the vicinity of the pocket. Each gas present diffuses along this tension gradient into the blood, and the pocket is gradually absorbed. Although CO_2 is much more soluble than N_2 in body fluids, a pocket contains both as long as it lasts; complete loss of CO_2, which is not possible, would leave a reverse CO_2 tension gradient. The pace of CO_2 loss is set by the gas that diffuses from the pocket most slowly. The presence of N_2 in a gas pocket retards absorption greatly; it is clear that atmospheric nitrogen delays atelectasis of occluded alveoli and is thus of value for air-breathing animals.

Gas pockets occur within the body as a result of trauma, disease, obstruction of spaces such as the middle ear or paranasal sinuses, rapid decompression with aerobullosis,* or experimental production. Two such gas pockets in particular are well studied—pneumothorax and pneumoperitoneum. If the pocket is in the middle ear, where volume is fixed by bone structure, the gas loss is often replaced by a fluid transudate.

It is impossible completely to eliminate dissolved N_2 from body fluids by pure O_2 breathing as long as the skin is exposed to air; even though relatively insoluble, N_2 trickles across the skin barrier into the body. It was suggested in Chapter 1 that O_2 uptake by dry skin occurs but is not very important. However, skin has a layer of cornified epithelium, removal of which may decrease the diffusion barrier to gases. It may be that scrubbed, wet skin permits passage of more O_2 than is commonly supposed and is even more permeable to CO_2. Scholander found that the nitrogen:argon ratio in the swim bladder of deep-sea fish is similar to the ratio of these two gases in air, and he concluded that the swim bladder N_2 of those fish is not derived from metabolism but, rather, from gases dissolved in the water.

*See Glossary, hypobarogenous aerobullosis, p. 209.

CHAPTER 9 Distribution of inspired gas, distribution of pulmonary blood flow, and ventilation-perfusion ratio

Even under physiologic conditions inspired gas and pulmonary blood flow are unevenly distributed. Diffuse bronchopulmonary diseases often exaggerate this nonuniform distribution of ventilation and perfusion. Indeed, ventilation-perfusion ratio inequality is the commonest clinical cause of arterial hypoxemia.

NONUNIFORM DISTRIBUTION OF VENTILATION

Physiologic causes

1. During inspiration the shape of the thoracic cage and the movement of the ribs increase lung volume proportionately more at the base of the lung than at the apices. The volume of the upper part of the chest increases only two thirds as much per 100 gm of lung tissue as that of the lower chest because the upper ribs are less curved and the upper thoracic cage less mobile.

2. The descent of the hemidiaphragms expands the lower lobes of the lungs more than the upper lobes; downward movement of the lung above the hilum (upper lobes) must stretch the supporting trachea and is thus less than the downward movement of the lower lobes.

3. At any given level of the upright lung, inspiration expands the peripheral lung more than the deeper tissue. Thoracic expansion decreases intrapleural pressure; this expands the lung by "pulling" it out. The expansion of deeper lung tissue is also limited by its larger, stiffer supporting airways.

4. The distribution of a single inspiration within the lung is sequentially uneven. In the upright lung the weight of lung tissue (lung density is 0.2 that of water) and blood results in a more positive (less "negative") intrapleural pressure at the bottom of the thorax. Dependent (lower) lung regions are relatively less inflated because transpulmonary pressure is less in the lower lobes than in the upper lobes (Fig. 9-1). Because the compliance curve is sigmoid and transpulmonary pressure (P_l) is greater in the upper lobes, the first portion of an inspiration beginning at FRC level goes preferentially to the upper lobes, and the last portion is distributed more to the lower lobes. Fig. 9-1, illustrating this fact, assumes that the change in *transpulmonary* pressure during inspiration is evenly distributed; that is, transpulmonary pressure *change* is the same for upper and for lower lobes. The lung is most compliant in the middle of the pressure-volume curve; when inspiration begins at FRC,

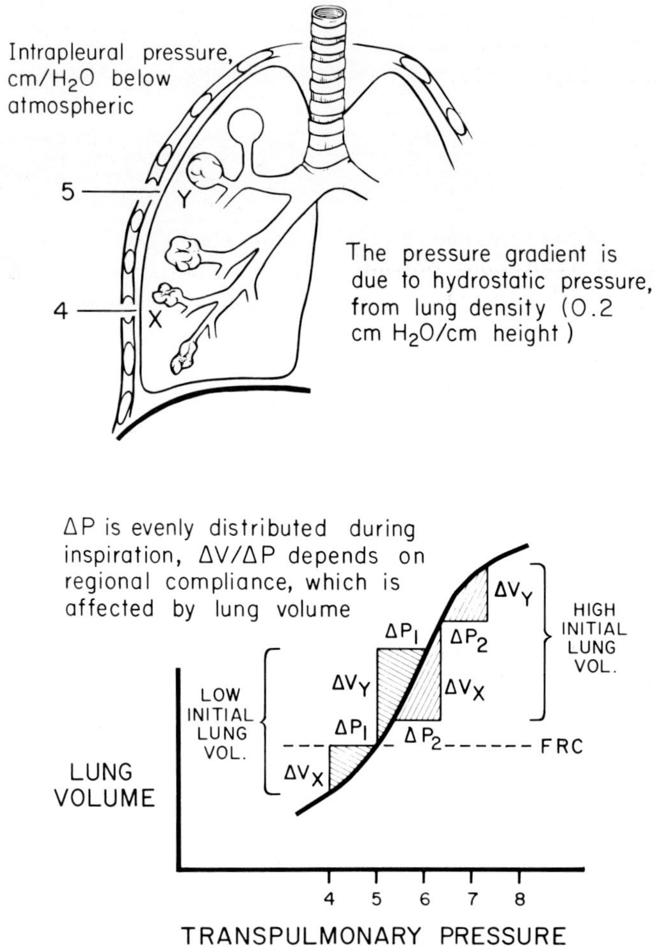

Fig. 9-1
Effect of hydrostatic pressure due to lung density on the distribution of inspired gas at low and high lung volumes.

a given pressure difference moves air into the upper lobes first; the lower lobes fill later.

Pathologic causes

Physiologic factors produce a certain degree of uneven distribution of inspired gas; pathologic changes of lung or airway exaggerate this uneven distribution of ventilation. Regional elasticity changes (e.g., pulmonary fibrosis) change lung compliance, and less compliant lung regions inflate less for a given transpulmonary pressure difference. Regional obstruction of airways (e.g., a check-valve mechanism in pulmonary disease or masses that compress the airways) increases resistance to air flow, and some lung regions are ventilated inadequately. Intrathoracic fluid accumulation may limit regional expansion, change compliance, and produce nonuniform distribution of inspired gas.

NONUNIFORM DISTRIBUTION OF PERFUSION

Physiologic causes

1. The weight of the column of blood in the pulmonary circulation produces a

vertical hydrostatic pressure gradient in the pulmonary blood vessels. Thus, although the arteriovenous pressure difference may be the same in all pulmonary vessels, hydrostatic pressure is greater in the dependent small vessels, dilating them. Poiseuille's law indicates the powerful effect of blood vessel diameter on blood flow; for the same arteriovenous pressure difference, blood flow is greater in the dependent vessels.

2. Because of the acute angle at which the right pulmonary artery branches from the main pulmonary artery, momentum carries relatively more blood into the left pulmonary artery. This difference increases with the velocity of blood flow as, for example, when cardiac output increases.

Blood flow decreases from the bottom to the top of the healthy upright human lung, reaching low values at the apex. This uneven distribution of blood flow, resulting from the hydrostatic pressure gradient within the pulmonary blood vessels, impairs pulmonary gas exchange to some extent. When healthy subjects are accelerated on a centrifuge, inequality of blood flow increases and may become severe. In the weightless state the distribution of pulmonary blood flow is more uniform, and the efficiency of the lung for gas exchange may be optimal.

Pathologic causes

Any alteration in the pulmonary circulation that produces a regional change in resistance to blood flow aggravates the uneven distribution of pulmonary perfusion. Kinking or compression of blood vessels due to intrathoracic masses, or embolic obstruction of pulmonary vessels contributes greatly to nonuniform distribution of pulmonary blood flow. A regional vasoconstriction, whether by direct action on blood vessels or mediated via the autonomic nervous system, also contributes to nonuniform pulmonary perfusion.

DISTRIBUTION OF VENTILATION-PERFUSION RATIOS

The gas-exchanging function of the lungs is achieved through interaction of the ventilatory gas stream with the blood perfusing the gas-exchange regions; hence, the ventilation-perfusion relationship, abbreviated $\dot{V}_A/\dot{Q}_c$ ratio, has great physiologic importance. Various terms have been used to describe the abnormalities related to the distribution of the $\dot{V}_A/\dot{Q}_c$ ratio; these include inequality, nonuniformity, unevenness, and inhomogeneity. Concern for the $\dot{V}_A/\dot{Q}_c$ ratio is directed toward its distribution within the lung. The overall (mean) ratio reflects the average resting alveolar ventilation (about 4 L [BTPS] /min) and the average normal pulmonary capillary blood flow (about 5 L/min). The overall (or mean) calculated $\dot{V}_A/\dot{Q}_c$ ratio is thus 0.8. However, ventilation and perfusion must be distributed to the same areas to accomplish gas exchange.

The importance of matching the distribution of ventilation with the distribution of perfusion is illustrated in a type of *reductio ad absurdum* as follows: Assume that total pulmonary ventilation and total pulmonary capillary blood flow are both normal so that the overall mean $\dot{V}_A/\dot{Q}_c$ ratio is 0.8. However, assume also that the entire ventilation goes to the right lung, whereas the entire perfusion goes to the left lung. The $\dot{V}_A/\dot{Q}_c$ ratio for the right lung is therefore infinity, whereas the $\dot{V}_A/\dot{Q}_c$ ratio for the left lung is zero. No gas exchange would occur in either lung, and the condition is obviously incompatible with life.

Fatal mismatching of ventilation with perfusion occurred in emphysema patients after unilateral lung transplantation; blood flow went preferentially to the new lung because of high vascular resistance in the old one, and inspired gas went primarily to the old, abnormally compliant lung.

As discussed earlier, there is normally

a nonuniform distribution of both ventilation and perfusion in the lung. Furthermore, there is a greater proportionate ventilation and a greater proportionate perfusion in the lower, or dependent, portions of the lung. However, the patterns of unevenness for ventilation do not precisely match those for perfusion, resulting in $\dot{V}_A/\dot{Q}_c$ variations throughout the lung.

MEASURING THE DISTRIBUTION OF $\dot{V}_A/\dot{Q}_c$ RATIOS

The degree of nonuniform distribution of inspired gas is commonly studied by means of the single-breath nitrogen test. This test has the virtue of being simple, rapid, and harmless. After a single deep inhalation of pure O_2, the subject expires forcefully while the N_2 concentration in the expired gas stream is recorded with a nitrogen analyzer. Analysis of the record of N_2 concentration versus the time thus obtained yields information regarding the uniformity of distribution of inspired gas.

A test for gross disturbance of the distribution of pulmonary blood flow involves the breathing of pure O_2 for 15 minutes, after which a sample of arterial blood is drawn and analyzed for O_2 saturation or tension. Failure to achieve either full saturation or an arterial P_{O_2} above about 550 mm Hg indicates venous-to-arterial shunting.

Another procedure for evaluating the distribution of pulmonary blood flow involves intravenous injection of macroaggregated radioiodinated serum albumin. The injected aggregates lodge in pulmonary capillaries where blood is flowing. The perfused areas of the lung are then mapped by external scanning to produce a lung scan.

In yet another method, Xe^{133} is dissolved in saline and injected intravenously. Scintillation counters placed on the chest wall record the distribution of pulmonary blood flow.

A simultaneous study of the distribution of ventilation and the distribution of blood flow involves the inhalation of an appropriate radioactive gas. A method for estimation of the uniformity of the distribution of $\dot{V}_A/\dot{Q}_c$ ratios is shown in Fig. 9-2. The subject inhales a gas mixture containing Xe^{133}, a radioactive gas emitting sufficient energy to be detected by scintil-

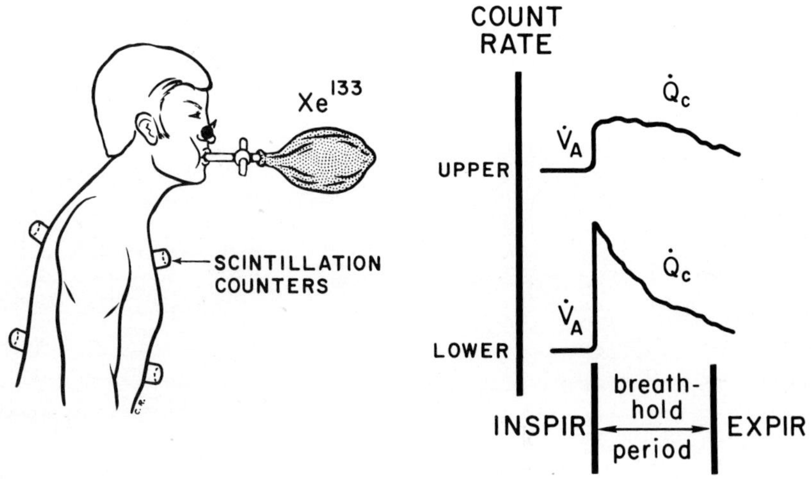

Fig. 9-2
A system using scintillation counters and radioactive xenon gas for simultaneous estimation of $\dot{V}_A$ and $\dot{Q}_c$ in an upright subject.

lation counters placed on the chest wall at different levels. The inspired gas is held in the lungs for 10 to 15 seconds, after which it is expired. Each scintillation counter detects a count rate that depends upon the amount of Xe^{133} distributed to the region of the lung beneath it. Fig. 9-2 shows that the increased count rate of the detectors placed low on the chest is much larger than that of the detectors placed high on the chest. This observation indicates that more of the inspired volume is distributed to the lower part of the lung than to the upper part under the conditions of this test.

The rate at which radioactivity decreases during the breath-holding period depends on the rate at which perfusion of the region under a scintillation counter removes the radioactive gas from the region. As Fig. 9-2 shows, because perfusion of the lower lobes is greater than that of the upper lobes the rate of decrease during the breath-holding period is much faster in the lower part of the lung. Information about the distribution of ventilation and the distribution of perfusion is thus derived from a single test.

CONSEQUENCES OF NONUNIFORM $\dot{V}_A/\dot{Q}_c$ RATIO DISTRIBUTION

Corrected to milliliters of ventilation per 100 gm of lung tissue, the upper lobes are ventilated approximately 65% but are perfused only about 10% as much as the lower lobes; blood flow is more disproportionate than ventilation between upper and lower lobes. The $\dot{V}_A/\dot{Q}_c$ ratio is much higher in the upper lobes (3.3) than in the lower lobes (0.55). There is thus a sixfold difference in the $\dot{V}_A/\dot{Q}_c$ ratio between upper and lower lobes. Because much of the ventilation and most of the blood flow go to the lower lobes their $\dot{V}_A/\dot{Q}_c$ ratio is closer to the overall mean value of 0.8.

Alveolar gas composition differs from region to region of the lung because ventilation and perfusion, which determine O_2 and CO_2 exchange, are nonuniformly distributed and imperfectly matched. Only if $\dot{V}_A/\dot{Q}_c$ ratios were evenly distributed throughout both lungs, would a sample of expired gas reflect the true mean gas pressures to which the pulmonary capillary blood was exposed. Hence, actual "alveolar gas" samples do not provide the data required for calculation of respiratory dead space, and anatomic dead space differs from physiologic dead space even in healthy subjects.

PHYSIOLOGIC ADJUSTMENTS TO NONUNIFORM $\dot{V}_A/\dot{Q}_c$ RATIO DISTRIBUTION

Regional lung responses improve the distribution of $\dot{V}_A/\dot{Q}_c$ ratios, restoring a more even pattern after alteration by various factors such as postural change or bronchopulmonary disease. Hyperperfused regions remove more O_2 from alveolar gas, decreasing alveolar P_{O_2}; this regional hypoxemia causes regional vasoconstriction, diverting blood to other lung regions. Even slight regional vasoconstriction strongly affects the distribution of perfusion; blood flow decreases in the region of vasoconstriction, and because total blood flow remains unchanged, perfusion of other regions increases.

In regions of relative hyperventilation and high $\dot{V}_A/\dot{Q}_c$ ratio, alveolar P_{CO_2} is low because of CO_2 washout. Regional hypocapnia produces local bronchoconstriction, redistributing ventilation, decreasing the $\dot{V}_A/\dot{Q}_c$ ratio in regions where it was high, and increasing the $\dot{V}_A/\dot{Q}_c$ ratio in regions where it was low. The regional responses affecting the distribution of $\dot{V}_A/\dot{Q}_c$ ratios within the lung are summarized in Table 7. These responses constitute a local homeostatic mechanism, favoring equalization of $\dot{V}_A/\dot{Q}_c$ ratio distribution.

Despite the surprising degree of non-

Table 7
Regional responses affecting distribution of $\dot{V}_A/\dot{Q}_c$ ratios within the lung

Regional abnormality	Effect	Reflex response	Result
Decreased Q or increased $\dot{V}$ (high $\dot{V}_A/\dot{Q}_c$ ratio)	Regional hypocapnia	Bronchoconstriction	Decreased regional $\dot{V}$ (reduced $\dot{V}_A/\dot{Q}_c$ ratio)
Decreased $\dot{V}$ or increased Q (low $\dot{V}_A/\dot{Q}_c$ ratio)	Regional hypoxemia	Vasoconstriction	Decreased regional $\dot{Q}$ (increased $\dot{V}_A/\dot{Q}_c$ ratio)

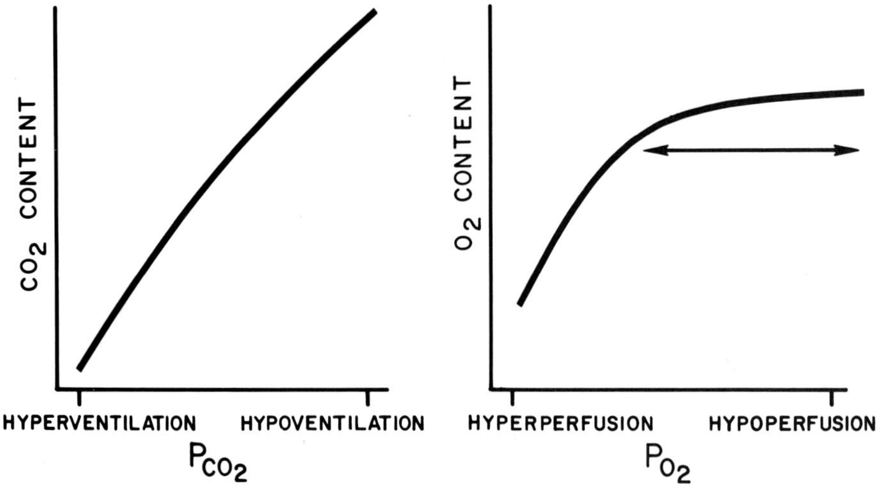

Fig. 9-3
Importance of CO_2-dissociation curve (left) and oxyhemoglobin dissociation curve (right) for gas exchange in areas of high or low $\dot{V}_A/\dot{Q}_c$.

uniformity of distribution and mismatching of ventilation and perfusion, the *efficiency* of gas exchange is 97% to 98% of the theoretic maximum value for both O_2 and CO_2. This calculation takes 100% as the maximum amount of each gas that would exchange if the normal total ventilation and total perfusion were perfectly distributed and matched throughout both lungs. The high efficiency of gas exchange despite striking variations of $\dot{V}_A/\dot{Q}_c$ ratio distribution is a result of the slopes of the dissociation curves for CO_2 and O_2 (Fig. 9-3). The CO_2 dissociation curve (P_{CO_2} versus CO_2 content) slopes appreciably in the physiologic range; CO_2 unloads efficiently in regions of hyperventilation and high $\dot{V}_A/\dot{Q}_c$ ratio despite low P_{CO_2}. In contrast, the oxyhemoglobin dissociation curve is relatively flat in the physiologic range; thus, even in regions of hyperperfusion (relative hypoventilation and low P_{O_2}) O_2 content decreases little and blood loads O_2 efficiently despite a low $\dot{V}_A/\dot{Q}_c$ ratio. As long as the overall mean $\dot{V}_A/\dot{Q}_c$ ratio is normal, the slopes of the two dissociation curves for O_2 and CO_2 tend to maintain efficient gas exchange despite regional variations of the distribution of ventilation and perfusion.

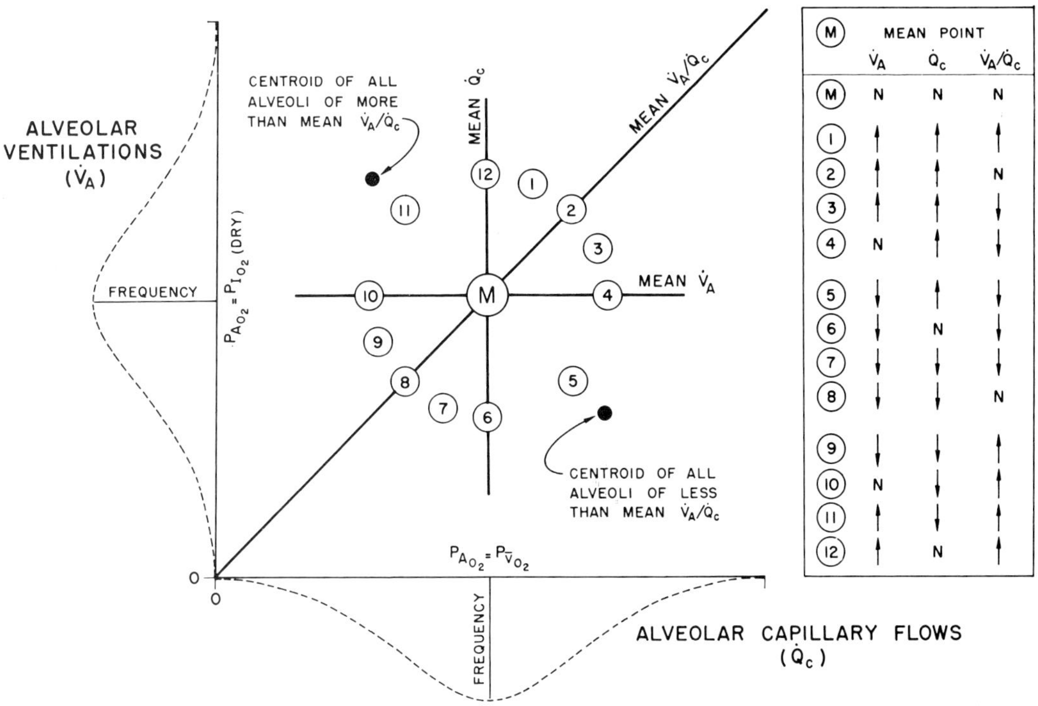

Fig. 9-4
Illustration of $\dot{V}_A/\dot{Q}_c$ ratios and classification of alveoli with respect to $\dot{V}_A/\dot{Q}_c$ relationships (schematic only; not based on actual data).

CONSEQUENCES OF PATHOLOGICALLY NONUNIFORM $\dot{V}_A/\dot{Q}_c$ RATIO DISTRIBUTION

If the overall mean $\dot{V}_A/\dot{Q}_c$ ratio is normal, a pathologically nonuniform distribution of $\dot{V}_A/\dot{Q}_c$ ratios produces hypoxemia but not CO_2 retention. When ventilation and perfusion are very nonuniformly distributed and mismatched, regions of marked hyperventilation coexist in the lung with regions of marked hypoventilation. Regions of hyperventilation, high $\dot{V}_A/\dot{Q}_c$ ratio, and low blood CO_2 content compensate for regions of hypoventilation, low $\dot{V}_A/\dot{Q}_c$ ratio, and high blood CO_2 content. If overall alveolar ventilation is essentially normal, *average* arterial blood CO_2 content is also normal.

Regions of low $\dot{V}_A/\dot{Q}_c$ ratio produce hypoxemic blood. In regions of hyperventilation and high $\dot{V}_A/\dot{Q}_c$ ratio, blood O_2 content cannot increase further because normal ventilation almost fully saturates hemoglobin. Thus, the mixture of blood from hyperventilating regions with that from hypoventilating regions is hypoxemic.

The population of alveoli with greater than average $\dot{V}_A/\dot{Q}_c$ ratios (Fig. 9-4) has higher than average P_{O_2} values and overcontributes this high P_{O_2} to the expired gas. Blood returning from this population of alveoli undercontributes its high P_{O_2} to pulmonary vein blood. The population of alveoli with less than average $\dot{V}_A/\dot{Q}_c$ ratios has lower than average P_{O_2} values and undercontributes this low P_{O_2} to expired gas. Blood flowing through this population overcontributes its low P_{O_2} to pulmonary vein blood. Even in the absence of an alveolar-arterial P_{O_2} gradient

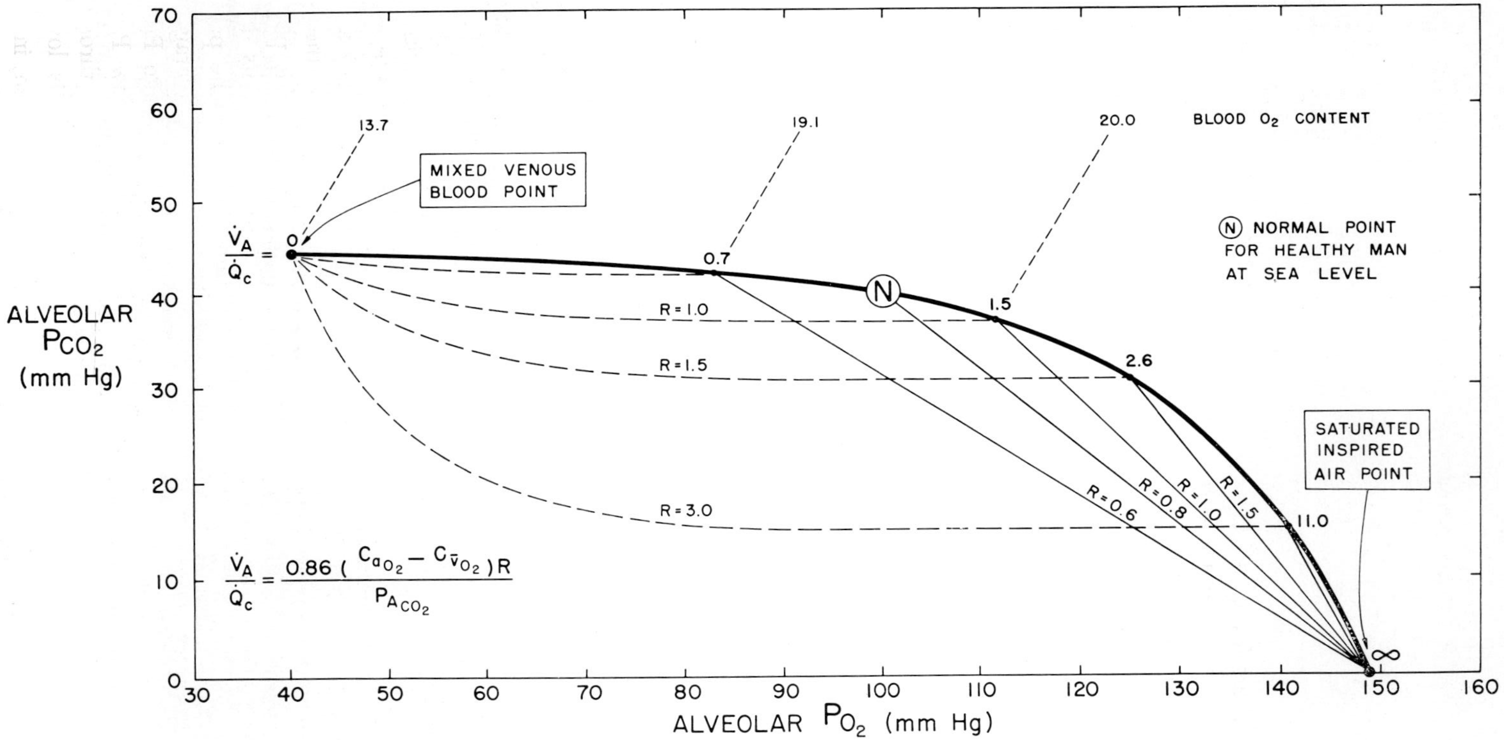

$$\frac{\dot{V}_A}{\dot{Q}_c} = \frac{0.86\,(C_{a_{O_2}} - C_{\bar{v}_{O_2}})\,R}{P_{A_{CO_2}}}$$

Fig. 9-5

O_2-CO_2 diagram. The heavy line indicates all possible combinations of O_2 and CO_2 tension that can theoretically exist in the alveoli and pulmonary capillary blood for the particular inspired gas and mixed venous blood tensions indicated by the two heavy dots. Every point on this ventilation-perfusion line is determined by a particular $\dot{V}_A/\dot{Q}_c$ ratio. (From Rahn, H., and Fenn, W. O.: A graphical analysis of the respiratory gas exchange, Washington, D. C., 1955, The American Physiological Society.)

for any single alveolus, this mismatching of ventilation and perfusion gives rise to an overall alveolar-arterial P_{O_2} gradient.

The alveolar gas concentrations at all possible $\dot{V}_A/\dot{Q}_c$ ratios can be plotted on an O_2-CO_2 diagram (Fig. 9-5). The limits of the heavy line are the inspired gas point where $\dot{V}_A/\dot{Q}_c = \infty$ and the mixed venous blood point where $\dot{V}_A/\dot{Q}_c = 0$.

The consequences of large variations in the distribution of $\dot{V}_A/\dot{Q}_c$ ratios are complex and interesting. For instance, in the healthy erect subject, because of relative hyperventilation of the upper lobes, much of the CO_2 is exchanged there. Because of the proportionately larger blood flow to the lower lobes more of the O_2 is taken up there. Thus the pattern of O_2 and CO_2 exchange differs from place to place within the lungs.

In chronic diffuse bronchopulmonary disease, maldistribution and mismatching of ventilation and perfusion commonly increase functional dead space and shunt-like effects, causing firstly hypoxemia and finally CO_2 retention. Alveolar P_{O_2} may be normal or even increased as a result of compensatory hyperventilation. However, ventilation-perfusion problems must be distinguished from alveolar hypoventilation, which decreases alveolar P_{O_2} and increases alveolar P_{CO_2}.

THE O_2-CO_2 DIAGRAM

Our understanding of alveolar gas, its composition, its changes, and its physiologic significance, is greatly facilitated by the O_2-CO_2 diagram. This diagram plots alveolar P_{CO_2} versus alveolar P_{O_2}, permitting simultaneous visual appreciation of the static and dynamic relationships of the two respiratory gases (Fig. 9-5). Oxygen tension, or P_{O_2}, is plotted on the horizontal axis, and CO_2 tension, or P_{CO_2}, on the vertical axis. In its simplest form the diagram shows the normal alveolar gas of healthy man at sea level rest (alveolar $P_{O_2} = 100$ mm Hg, alveolar $P_{CO_2} = 40$ mm Hg), the saturated inspired air point (inspired $P_{O_2} = 150$ mm Hg, inspired $P_{CO_2} = 0$), and a straight line joining these two points whose slope, R, is proportional to the respiratory exchange ratio.

If pure O_2 is breathed, the R line slope on the O_2-CO_2 diagram is no longer proportional to the steady state respiratory exchange ratio, R_S. Since no N_2 is present, the sums of P_{CO_2} and P_{O_2} must equal $P_B - 47$. A plot of this situation would show the inspired gas point (inspired $P_{O_2} = P_B - 47$, inspired $P_{CO_2} = 0$) and the alveolar gas point (alveolar $P_{O_2} = P_B - 47 - 40$, alveolar $P_{CO_2} = 40$). The R line slope is then –1; its slope is always –1 whenever pure O_2, or a mixture containing only O_2 and CO_2, is breathed, irrespective of the metabolic respiratory quotient, R_S.

If a resting sea level resident begins to hyperventilate with air, alveolar P_{O_2} is increased and alveolar P_{CO_2} is reduced (Fig. 14-2). Eventually, if a constant level of hyperventilation is maintained, the alveolar gas point comes to rest on the R line, the alveolar pathway during the intervening unsteady state having described a portion of a clockwise loop. Initially, alveolar P_{O_2} rises much more rapidly than alveolar P_{CO_2} drops.* With continued hyperventilation, however, alveolar P_{CO_2} gradually drops until the alveolar gas point reaches the R line and a steady state of hyperventilation is achieved—that is, there is no further change in the level of body CO_2 stores. Resumption of normal breathing is followed by alveolar gas value changes that complete the clockwise loop on the diagram; the alveolar gas values return to their original point on the R

*Large quantities of CO_2 are stored in the body, mostly as HCO_3^-. Substantial depletion of this stored CO_2 must occur before P_{CO_2} can fall appreciably. Since O_2 is not stored in appreciable quantities, alveolar P_{O_2} reacts more quickly to changes in pulmonary ventilation.

line. However, before this steady state is again achieved, alveolar P_{O_2} drops with more rapidity than alveolar P_{CO_2} rises, since it takes time to accumulate metabolically produced CO_2 and augment the body stores.

The closed hyperventilation-and-recovery loop on the O_2-CO_2 diagram graphically portrays the impact of unsteady states on alveolar gas composition and respiratory exchange ratio. When CO_2 output equals CO_2 produced, a steady state exists; when CO_2 output equals current metabolic CO_2 production plus CO_2 from stores, R_A (alveolar R) is larger than R_S. When only a fraction of current metabolic CO_2 production is expired and the balance is being stored, R_A is less than R_S. Summarizing:

$$\frac{\dot{V}_{CO_2}}{\dot{V}_{O_2}} = R_S \quad \text{(steady state)}$$

$$\frac{\dot{V}_{CO_2} + CO_2 \text{ from stores}}{\dot{V}_{O_2}} = \text{High } R_A \text{ (unsteady state)}$$

$$\frac{\dot{V}_{CO_2} - CO_2 \text{ being stored}}{V_{O_2}} = \text{Low } R_A \text{ (unsteady state)}$$

The R line slope on the O_2-CO_2 diagram is proportional to the respiratory exchange ratio, R_E, calculated from analysis of expired gas, except when pure O_2 is breathed. However, not one, but many R lines can be drawn. When $\dot{V}_{CO_2} = \dot{V}_{O_2}$, R_E is 1 and the R line slope is –1; an R line slope steeper than –1 indicates an R_E greater than 1. Early in hyperventilation the slope of a line connecting the alveolar gas point with the inspired air point is steeper than 1, indicating an R_E greater than 1, or a CO_2 output that is in excess of O_2 uptake. During recovery from hyperventilation R_E is low, the R

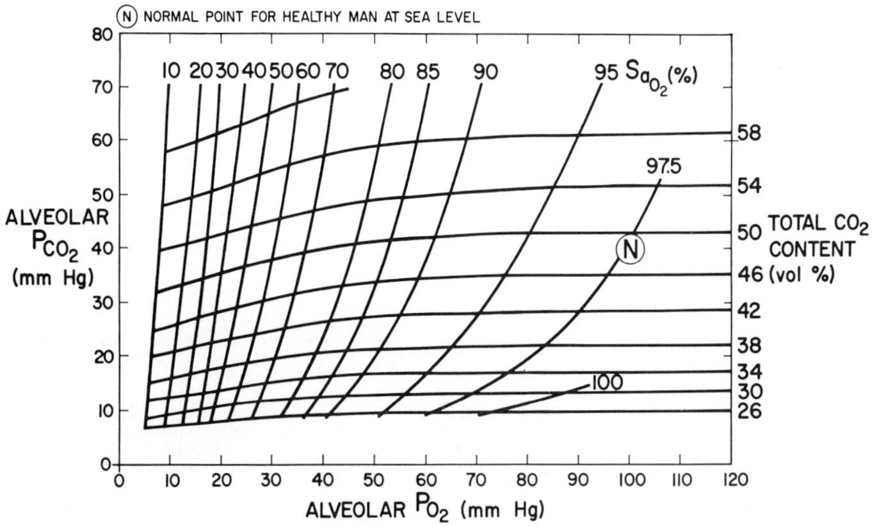

Fig. 9-6

O_2-CO_2 diagram. Isopleths for O_2 saturation and CO_2 content of whole blood. Oxyhemoglobin capacity is 20 vol %. Slope of O_2 isopleths represents the Bohr effect, and slope of CO_2 isopleths represents the Haldane effect. (From Rahn, H., and Fenn, W. O.: A graphical analysis of the respiratory gas exchange, Washington, D. C., 1955, The American Physiological Society.)

line slope on the O_2-CO_2 diagram is gradual and much of the current metabolic CO_2 production is being stored rather than blown off.

Hypoventilation and recovery also produce a clockwise loop on the O_2-CO_2 diagram. An example of such hypoventilation is respiration during anesthesia, which involves such a loop. Initially, the drop in alveolar P_{O_2} far exceeds the rise in alveolar P_{CO_2}. As CO_2 stores increase, alveolar P_{CO_2} rises until a steady state for that level of ventilation is reached at the R line. Recovery completes this clockwise loop but requires an extended period of many minutes, during which the R line slope is greater while excess CO_2 stores are blown off in the expired gas.

Values for O_2 content and oxyhemoglobin saturation can be taken from a family of oxyhemoglobin dissociation curves plotted on an O_2-CO_2 diagram. Each curve is associated with a given P_{CO_2}—that is, a different Bohr effect. Such a plot is shown in Fig. 9-6.

The versatility of the O_2-CO_2 diagram is illustrated by Fig. 14-1, p. 151, which shows the effects of departure from normal alveolar gas values. Hypoxia, CO_2 narcosis (not anesthesia at these P_{CO_2} values), hyperoxia, and hypocapnia surround the normal area. The rounded corners of these regions imply a synergism between adjacent effects.

CHAPTER 10 pH homeostasis

Free hydrogen ions (H^+) are rare in most body fluids, but their concentration is very important. The activity of enzymes and the solubility of salts are dependent upon H^+ concentration. At chemical neutrality there is only 1×10^{-7} (1/10,000,000) of a mole of H^+ per liter of solution. The concentration in arterial blood plasma is even less—about 4×10^{-8} (4/100,000,000) of a mole of H^+ per liter. However, gastric juice may contain a million times this concentration.

Chemically, any solution containing in excess of 1×10^{-7} mole of H^+ per liter is considered to be acidic, and any solution containing less than that concentration is alkaline or basic. Note that the chemically neutral H^+ concentration of 1×10^{-7} mole per liter is acid with respect to arterial blood plasma, which has a lower concentration.

What is an acid and what is a base?

Many years ago it was found that organic ash has an alkaline reaction. Since the most abundant cation in such ash is potassium (K^+), it was assumed that K^+ is a base. But K^+, in vitro, does not reduce H^+ concentration. Organic ash is alkaline because of the anion associated with K^+, and not because of K^+ itself. Older literature refers to potassium and sodium as bases, but this usage is giving way to more descriptive and accurate terminology. An acid is any substance that increases H^+ concentration or that is a proton donor. Conversely, a base is any substance that reduces H^+ concentration or that is a proton acceptor.

The hydrogen ion, or proton, does not exist free in aqueous solutions but, rather, exists combined with a molecule of water as the hydrated hydronium ion, H_3O^+. Although it is more accurate to speak of hydronium ions, we may use the terms proton or hydrogen ion (H^+) for simplicity without introducing errors into these considerations.

Carbon dioxide combines with water to form carbonic acid, which then dissociates into H^+ and HCO_3^-. Since CO_2 increases H^+ concentration, it may be called an acid.* Since ammonia (NH_3) can accept a proton to form the ammonium ion (NH_4^+), ammonia is a base.

What is pH?

The concentration of hydrogen ions in a solution is expressed as gram-ionic weights per liter. At 25° C water has a H^+ concentration of 10^{-7} as well as a OH^- concentration of 10^{-7} moles per liter. Thus the pH of water at 25° C is 7. A greater accuracy is obtained if one substitutes the thermodynamic *activity* of the H^+ for its *concentration.*

It is obviously inconvenient to refer to H^+ concentrations such as 1/10,000,000 of a mole per liter. To avoid this inconvenience, acidity is usually expressed in

*Actually, it is an acid *anhydride.*

terms of pH, which is defined as the logarithm of the reciprocal of the H^+ concentration. In other words, the pH of a solution is the negative logarithm of its H^+ concentration. Accordingly, a solution at chemical neutrality with 1/10,000,000 (or 1×10^{-7}) mole of H^+ per liter has a pH of 7.

Note that as H^+ concentration increases, pH decreases. Note further that the concentration of H^+ in a solution at pH 6 is ten times that in a solution at pH 7. Because of the logarithmic nature of the pH scale a decrease of 0.3 pH unit, although appearing small, actually represents a *doubling* of the H^+ concentration. The logarithmic nature of the pH scale must also be remembered when comparing pH differences and when making ratios involving pH.

pH homeostasis—concept and physiologic importance

Normal acidity within and around body cells is absolutely essential for maintenance of the dynamic, biochemical equilibrium that life processes involve. Cellular metabolism and function require that acidity be kept within very narrow limits. Normal acidity is maintained within the body by a sensitive, well-integrated mechanism involving pH-sensitive receptors, kidneys, lungs, and several buffer systems.

Enzymes are biologic catalysts and, as such, speed the achievement of chemical equilibria. The physiologic importance of pH homeostasis becomes clear when we realize that a multitude of biochemical processes in any biologic system are catalyzed by specific enzymes and that each enzyme is optimally active at a specific pH. We may imagine, then, the biochemical chaos that results when appreciable shifts of pH occur, affecting the multitude of enzymes, each to a different degree, and some actually in opposite directions. Accordingly, it is not surprising that the extreme range of plasma pH compatible with life in higher forms is from approximately 7.0 to 7.8. pH homeostasis is perhaps a better term than acid-base balance because it is indeed the maintenance of normal pH with which the homeostatic mechanisms are concerned.

The term *blood* pH always refers to *plasma* pH, which is higher than the intracellular pH of the erythrocyte. Note that *arterial* blood samples are required for clinical characterization of acid-base status and that blood temperature is an important variable.

BUFFER SYSTEMS AND THE HENDERSON-HASSELBALCH EQUATION

Strong acids, such as hydrochloric, sulfuric, and nitric acids, dissociate almost completely into H^+ and their associated anions. As there is little attraction in solution of chloride, sulfate, or nitrate ions for H^+, these anions are very weak bases. However, weak acids are weak because they do not yield their H^+ readily. When they do, the anions thus formed remain rather avid for the H^+ they have lost and are therefore rather strong bases.

In low pH solutions where H^+ are relatively abundant, a H^+ lost from a weak organic acid is almost immediately replaced, so that at any instant most weak organic acid molecules are undissociated. As the pH increases, however, replacement of dissociated H^+ is slower, so that at any given instant a larger fraction of the organic acid molecules are dissociated. For any organic acid there is a pH at which only half of the organic acid molecules are undissociated; the other half are dissociated into H^+ and their anions, or bases. The pH at this point is termed the pK for that particular acid. The pK is defined as the negative logarithm of the H^+ concentration at which half of the acid molecules are associated and half are dissociated.

The relationships among pH, strength of a weak acid, or pK, and the base-to-acid concentration ratio for any buffer system are given by a modified form of the law of mass action called the Henderson-Hasselbalch equation:

$$pH = pK + \log_{10} \frac{[base]}{[acid]}$$

where base is the anion (the acid molecule less its H^+). Some acids, such as carbonic, have 2 H^+, each of which may be lost. It is convenient, although not precisely accurate, to think of this as a stepwise process. In such a case each H^+, or step, has its own pK. Under physiologic conditions the dissociation of only the first H^+ of carbonic acid is important, and we refer to this dissociation as the pK_1.

Phosphoric acid is an example of an acid with 3 H^+, each with its own pK. Physiologically, one is concerned primarily with the second of these (pK_2), which at normal body temperature is about 6.8. The Henderson-Hasselbalch equation for dissociation of this second H^+ of phosphoric acid is as follows:

$$pH = 6.8 + \log_{10} \frac{[HPO_4^{=}]}{[H_2PO_4^{-}]}$$

At pH 6.8, $HPO_4^{=}$ and $H_2PO_4^{-}$ are present in equal concentration. At pH 7.8 there is ten times as much $HPO_4^{=}$ as $H_2PO_4^{-}$. At pH 5.8 there is ten times as much $H_2PO_4^{-}$ as $HPO_4^{=}$. A phosphate buffer in which equal quantities of these ions are used resists large changes in pH. If acid is added, the free H^+ combine with $HPO_4^{=}$ to form $H_2PO_4^{-}$, with relatively little change in pH. If alkali is added to this pH 6.8 buffer, the pH reduction is minimized by release of H^+ from $H_2PO_4^{-}$ as it becomes $HPO_4^{=}$.

The *buffer capacity* of a solution is the amount of H^+ that can be added to, or removed from, a solution for a change of 1 pH unit. Buffer capacity depends upon the concentration and nature of the buffer substances and upon the pH in relation to the pK of the buffer. The slope of a buffer dissociation or titration curve is greatest at the pK of the buffer. It follows that buffers are most effective in the pH range that centers on their pK. Buffer capacity may also be defined as d(V)/d(pH), or the slope of the acid-base titration curve. This definition, however, involving as it does the ratio of a number to a logarithm, does not permit ready comparison of buffer slopes in different pH ranges. If H^+ concentration were used to express buffer capacity instead, direct comparison would be possible. *Effective buffer capacity* refers to the in vivo capacity of organs to buffer perfusates and is more relevant to the physiologic behavior of intact living organisms.

Astrup suggested that the total surplus of acid or base in the *extracellular space* can be estimated by the following formula:

0.30 × Body weight (kg) × Base excess or deficit per liter of blood = Amount of $NaHCO_3$ or NH_4Cl required to restore standard plasma bicarbonate ion concentration to normal

However, more than half of the buffering capacity of the body is intracellular. It is therefore important to distinguish *blood* from *total body* acid-base balance. For example, after the experimental intravenous infusion of acid or base, acid-base changes in blood continue for hours, reflecting total body buffering capacity, metabolism, and compensating mechanisms.

The isohydric shift

In terms of buffer capacity, hemoglobin is the most important buffer in blood. This is true because blood contains about 15 gm of hemoglobin per 100 ml, and because the imidazole groups of globin histidine have a pK that it close to blood pH. Hemoglobin and oxyhemoglobin have different pK's, but each combines with H^+. Hemoglobin has a high pK, about 7.93; oxyhemoglobin has a much lower pK, about 6.68, and is the stronger acid. At an intracellular pH of 7.2 the ratio of $\frac{Hb^-}{HHb}$ is about $\frac{1}{5.4}$, whereas the ratio of $\frac{HbO_2^-}{HHbO_2}$ is $\frac{3.3}{1}$. As some oxyhemoglobin molecules are losing O_2 to the tissues and becoming reduced hemoglobin, there is a rapid influx of H^+, many of which are taken up by hemoglobin with no change in pH. This buffer effect is known as the *isohydric shift*. At pH 7.2 about 84% of the hemoglobin is in the form of HHb, whereas only about 23% of the oxyhemoglobin is $HHbO_2$. Of the total oxyhemoglobin that loses O_2 to become reduced hemoglobin, 23% was already combined with H^+, 16% will not combine with H^+, but 61% will take up H^+ from solution before a pH decrease occurs. Thus an important consequence of the isohydric shift in the systemic capillaries is that if 0.7 mM of CO_2 enters the blood for every 1.0 mM of oxyhemoglobin reduced (metabolic respiratory quotient = 0.7), all H^+ produced by this quantity of CO_2 are buffered (no blood pH decrease) by the reduced hemoglobin just formed without dependence on the other blood buffer systems. Over the physiologic range of pH, the titration curve of oxyhemoglobin is *almost* a straight line. This line has a slope of about 2.54 mM of H^+ per pH unit.

The most interesting buffer system for the respiratory physiologist is the carbonic acid–bicarbonate system (CO_2 system). Carbon dioxide combines with water to form carbonic acid, which then dissociates into bicarbonate ions and hydrogen ions:

$$CO_2 + H_2O \overset{\text{Carbonic anhydrase}}{\rightleftharpoons} H_2CO_3 \rightleftharpoons H^+ + HCO_3^-$$

This reaction is catalyzed by an enzyme, carbonic anhydrase, which is found in red blood cells, renal tubules, gastric mucosa, and the eye. This enzyme speeds the reversible reaction of CO_2 with H_2O to produce H_2CO_3 by a factor of approximately 7,500. Carbonic acid is a rare and transitory intermediate between CO_2 and HCO_3^-. Because of this fact, CO_2 itself is usually treated as if it were the proton donor. When this is done, the *apparent* pK_1, termed pK_1', is about 6.11 and the Henderson-Hasselbalch equation for plasma at 38° C is written* as follows:

$$pH = 6.11 + \log_{10} \frac{[HCO_3^-]}{[CO_2]}$$

This pK_1' is assumed constant because blood temperature, solute concentrations, and acid strength satisfy the necessary conditions. The $[CO_2]$ is expressed as mM/L so that it matches $[HCO_3^-]$ in mM or mEq/L. However, $[CO_2]$ in the denominator may also be expressed as the constant *a* times P_{CO_2}. The constant *a* is a proportionality constant relating CO_2 in mM/L to P_{CO_2} in mm Hg and is equal to 0.0301.

GRAPHIC REPRESENTATION OF ACID-BASE PATTERNS

As we have seen, a buffer system involves three variables, so that actual measurement of any two permits determination of the third. This determination can be made by arithmetic calculation, or it

*The pK_1 of H_2CO_3 is about 3.4. At pH 7.4 the ratio of $[HCO_3^-]$ to $[H_2CO_3]$ is about 10,000:1. Physiologically, however, CO_2 is a much more useful quantity, since it is about 500 times as abundant as H_2CO_3. If we pretend that it is CO_2 and not H_2CO_3 that dissociates yielding H^+, we can use the ratio of $[HCO_3^-]$ to $[CO_2]$, but we must correct the pK_1 by the equilibrium constant of 500. This *apparent* pK_1, the pK_1', which goes with the apparent ratio of $[HCO_3^-]$ to $[CO_2]$, has a value of about 6.1. Note that it is incorrect to use this pK_1' of 6.1 with the ratio of $[HCO_3^-]$ to $[H_2CO_3]$.

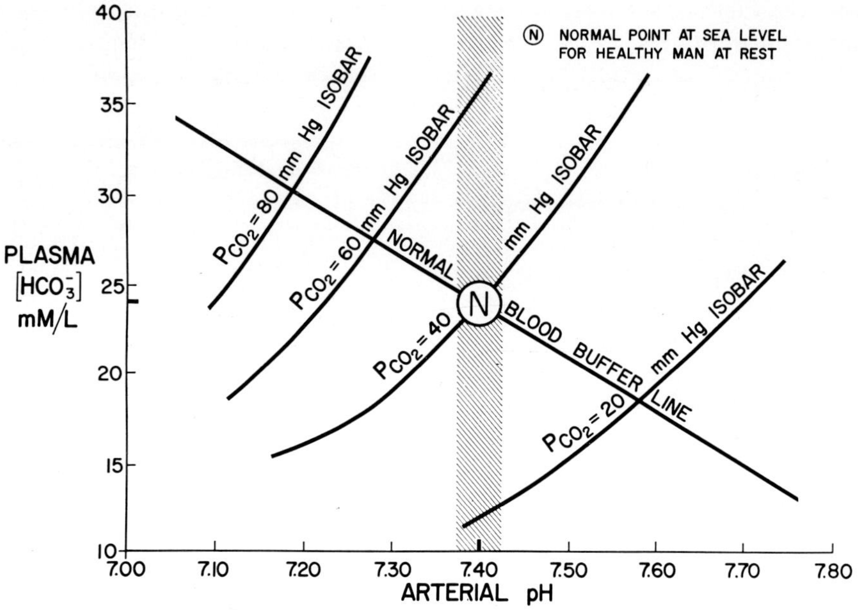

Fig. 10-1
The pH-bicarbonate diagram for analysis of acid-base status. (Modified from Davenport, H. W.: The ABC of acid-base chemistry, ed. 4, Chicago, 1958, The University of Chicago Press.)

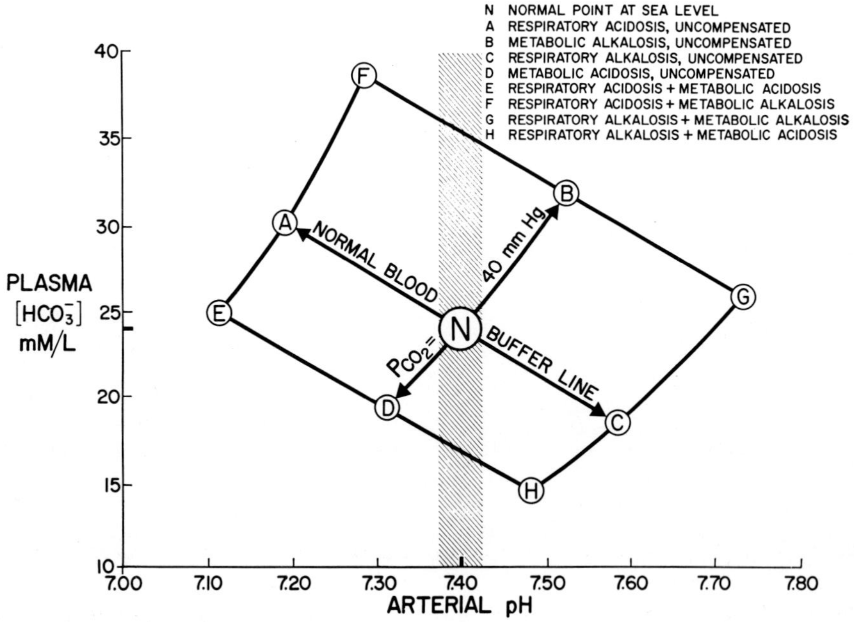

Fig. 10-2
Pathways of acid-base disturbance. (Redrawn from Davenport, H. W.: The ABC of acid-base chemistry, ed. 4, Chicago, 1958, The University of Chicago Press.)

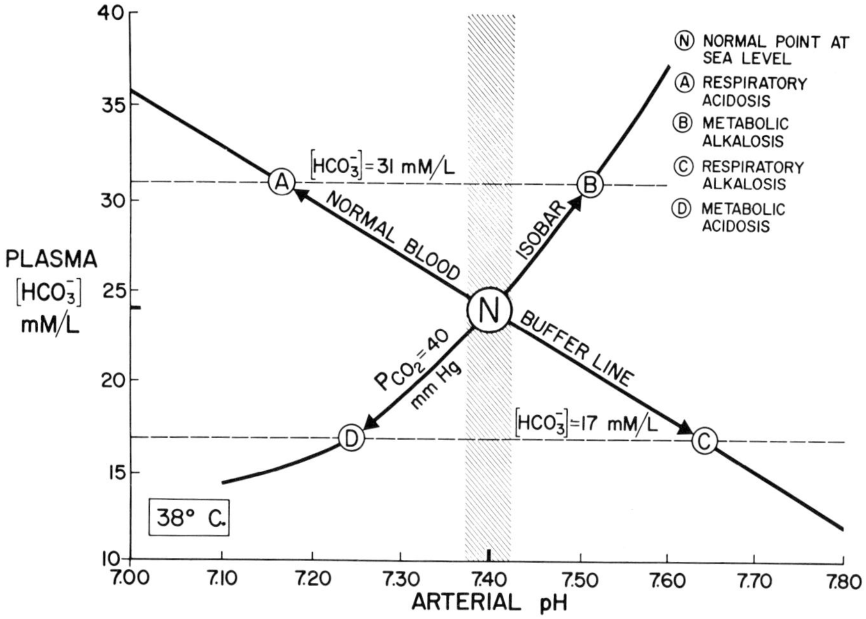

Fig. 10-3

A pH-bicarbonate diagram to illustrate the impossibility of distinguishing acidosis from alkalosis with only one kind of CO_2 content information. (Redrawn from Davenport, H. W.: The ABC of acid-base chemistry, ed. 4, Chicago, 1958, The University of Chicago Press.)

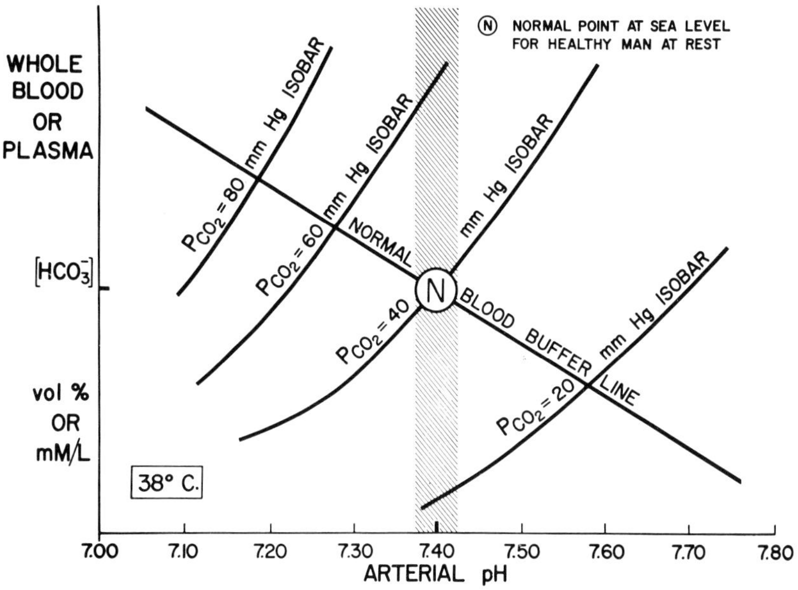

Fig. 10-4

Diagram for analysis of acid-base status. Whole blood or plasma values of bicarbonate ion concentration are plotted on the vertical axis. Expression in terms of mM/L is usually preferable. Whole blood analysis eliminates the problem of plasma separation but introduces hematocrit as a variable affecting the ordinate value. (Redrawn from Davenport, H. W.: The ABC of acid-base chemistry, ed. 4, Chicago, 1958, The University of Chicago Press.)

can be done graphically. In the following section we discuss three of the several possible ways of graphing the Henderson-Hasselbalch buffer equation and present two graphs that can be used at altitude as well as at sea level.

The Henderson-Hasselbalch equation for the carbonic acid–bicarbonate buffer system lends itself nicely to two-dimensional graphic representation and solution. Any pair of the three variables can be plotted on cartesian coordinates against one another, and the third variable then portrayed as a family of isovalue lines or curves. One of these representations plots HCO_3^- concentration as a function of pH, with P_{CO_2} appearing as a family of isobars (Figs. 10-1 to 10-5). As P_{CO_2} is increased or decreased, the values for pH and HCO_3^- concentration describe a nearly straight line, termed the *blood buffer line,* or *curve.* The shaded vertical bands in Figs. 10-1 to 10-5 indicate the approximate range of normal arterial pH and emphasize the basic fact that the various homeostatic mechanisms function to maintain normal pH. The points marked Ⓝ in all six acid-base diagrams indicate normal values for healthy, resting subjects acclimatized at sea level.

It is difficult to overestimate the significance of the basic algebraic fact that if any two variables in the Henderson-Hasselbalch equation are measured, the third can be calculated—but that *one alone* does not suffice. This point is illustrated in Fig. 10-3.

Technically speaking, the term *CO_2 content information* may include both HCO_3^- and total CO_2 concentrations. If both of these are known, the P_{CO_2} can be calculated from the equation

$$[HCO_3^-] = [\text{Total } CO_2] - aP_{CO_2}$$

and the acid-base status is determined. Furthermore, it should be emphasized that

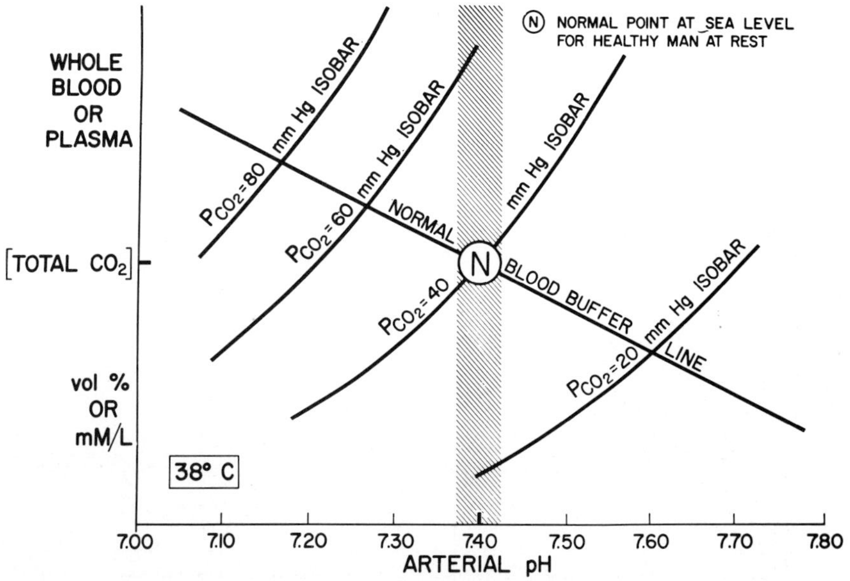

Fig. 10-5

Diagram for analysis of acid-base status. Whole blood or plasma values of total CO_2 concentration are plotted on the vertical axis. Expression in terms of mM/L is usually preferable. Whole blood analysis eliminates the problem of plasma separation but introduces hematocrit as a variable affecting the ordinate value.

if total CO_2 concentration instead of HCO_3^- concentration is plotted on the vertical axis, a different linear scale must be used, and that the P_{CO_2} isobars will then need to be recalculated.

Another graphic solution of the Henderson-Hasselbalch equation plots the ratio $\frac{[HCO_3^-]}{[CO_2]}$ (Fig. 10-6). When temperature and consequently pK_1' are constant, this ratio is the pH. The pH is about 7.4 when the ratio is 20:1, 40:2, 60:3, or 80:4. It is about 7.1 when the ratio is 10:1, 20:2, 30:3, or 40:4. These and other pH lines radiate from the origin of the graph. This representation is particularly useful for the respiratory physiologist because P_{CO_2}-$[HCO_3^-]$ dissociation curves can be superimposed upon the graphic solution of the Henderson-Hasselbalch equation. Ventilation can also be represented, since ventilation is inversely related to P_{CO_2}.

Hyperventilation does not shift the plasma values *directly* to the left on this graph—but rather downward and to the left—along the *CO_2 dissociation,* or *blood buffer, curve.* Underbreathing shifts the plasma values to the right and somewhat upward along the CO_2 dissociation curve. The HCO_3^- concentration changes with ventilation because alterations in P_{CO_2} shift the equilibrium of the equation:

$$CO_2 + H_2O \overset{\text{Carbonic anhydrase}}{\rightleftharpoons} H_2CO_3 \rightleftharpoons H^+ + HCO_3^-$$

During any second, many CO_2 molecules combine with water to form HCO_3^- and H^+. But during the same second, an equal number of HCO_3^- combine with H^+

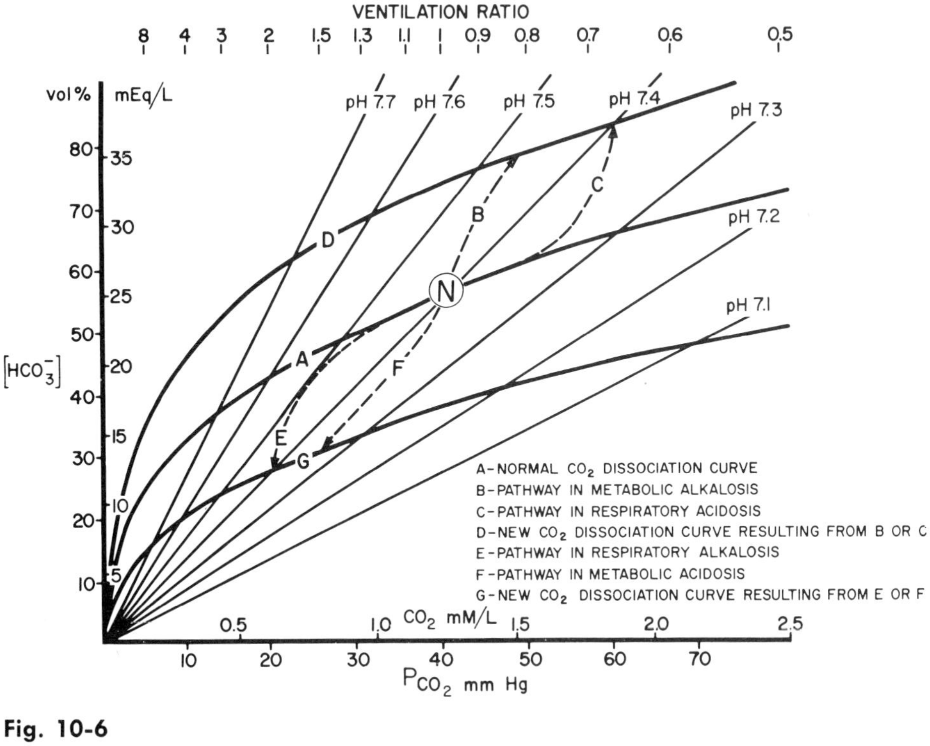

Fig. 10-6
Diagram for analysis of acid-base status, showing normal and abnormal true plasma CO_2 dissociation curves.

to form CO_2 and water. When CO_2 is removed from this system by overbreathing, fewer CO_2 molecules are available for combination with water to form HCO_3^-, but as many HCO_3^- and H^+ move to form CO_2 as before. Hence, overbreathing not only reduces CO_2 but also reduces the populations of HCO_3^- and H^+. This illustrates the chemical principle of driving an equilibrium reaction to one side by removing one of the reactants (CO_2) from that side. The diagram shows this not only by the slope of the CO_2 dissociation curve but also by departure from the pH 7.40 line in the direction of a higher pH. This is alkalosis. Since it is generated by a change in respiration, it is *respiratory* alkalosis.

Underbreathing out of proportion to CO_2 production produces effects that are opposite to those of overbreathing. Carbon dioxide accumulates, more CO_2 is available to form HCO_3^- and H^+, and the populations of both of these ions increase. In the diagram this corresponds to a rightward movement along the CO_2 dissociation curve, involving an increase in HCO_3^- and a lower pH. This is acidosis—in this case, *respiratory* acidosis.

The quantitative aspects of respiratory acidosis and alkalosis are more fully appreciated if there is some notion of the relative abundance of the molecular species involved. When metabolizing tissue cells produce CO_2, some of this CO_2 moves into red blood cells, where carbonic anhydrase converts most of it to HCO_3^- and H^+. The H^+ thus produced are largely removed from solution by combination with hemoglobin, oxyhemoglobin, intracellular and plasma proteins, polypeptides, and amino acids. Thus, when CO_2 is stored in body fluids as HCO_3^-, most of the H^+ produced with the HCO_3^- are buffered and eventually excreted in the urine. When mixed venous blood encounters the lower P_{CO_2} in the lungs, dissolved CO_2 quickly leaves the blood, forcing combination of HCO_3^- with H^+ to produce more dissolved CO_2; but most of the H^+ that enter into this union did not exist as free H^+, having come from blood buffers.

If arterial plasma has a pH of 7.40 and contains 24 mEq/L of HCO_3^-, the following approximate populations exist:

$$\begin{array}{ccccccc} CO_2 + H_2O & \xrightarrow[]{\text{Carbonic anhydrase}} \!\!\!\rightleftharpoons & H_2CO_3 & \rightleftharpoons & H^+ & + & HCO_3^- \\ 120{,}000 & & 240 & & 4 & & 2{,}400{,}000 \end{array}$$

(each × 10^{-8} mole/L)

Any shift in equilibrium, to either left or right, has a much greater proportionate effect upon H^+ than it does upon HCO_3^-. But the availability of buffers, where H^+ may be either stored or retrieved, changes this picture. Even though the H^+ concentration is only 4×10^{-8} mole/L, H^+ are replaced as soon as they combine with HCO_3^-.

The *Siggaard-Andersen curve nomogram* is another graphic representation of the Henderson-Hasselbalch equation. It is widely used in the clinic with the Astrup micromethod for blood-gas and pH analysis. It involves the following definitions:

Acidosis and *alkalosis* are defined in terms of pH. Blood pH is *plasma* pH. *Respiratory* acidosis is the result of increased arterial P_{CO_2}, whereas *respiratory* alkalosis is the result of decreased P_{CO_2}. *Metabolic* (nonrespiratory) acidosis is an acidosis that is reflected in a decrease of standard bicarbonate, whereas *metabolic* alkalosis is an alkalosis that is reflected in an increase of standard bicarbonate. *Total CO_2 content* is the total content of CO_2 in plasma separated from the cells at the actual P_{CO_2}. *CO_2 combining power* is the total content of CO_2 in plasma separated from cells at the actual P_{CO_2} and then equilibrated to a P_{CO_2} of 40 mm Hg before analysis. *Standard bicarbonate* is the *plasma* bicarbonate ion concentration measured under the standard conditions of 38° C, P_{CO_2} = 40 mm Hg and full oxygenation of the hemoglobin. It thus expresses the *metabolic* aspect of acid-base balance only and is normally 24 mEq/L. Standard bicarbonate is estimated on the Siggaard-Andersen curve nomogram by intersection of the P_{CO_2} = 40 mm Hg line with the pH-log P_{CO_2}, or blood buffer, line. The term *buffer base* is used as defined in 1948 by Singer and Hastings as the sum of the cations corresponding to the buffer anions, including the cations corresponding to the hemoglobin anions. Thus an anemic patient can have an abnormal buffer base value without *any* actual abnormality of acid-base chemistry. The value of the buffer base concept has accordingly been questioned.

The pH-versus-log P_{CO_2} plot, or blood buffer line, is *linear* in the physiologic region. This line is determined by equilibrating aliquots of a blood sample at two different P_{CO_2}'s and then measuring the two resulting pH values. It is usual clinical practice to determine this line by means of only two points. The exact values of P_{CO_2} to which the two aliquots are equilibrated are not critical, but they must be precisely known and equilibration must be complete. The actual pH of the blood sample is also determined, and its P_{CO_2} is then estimated from the blood buffer line. Blood buffer capacity, or the slope* of the pH-log P_{CO_2} line, is largely a function of hemoglobin concentration. However, it is only *approximately* proportional to hemoglobin concentration because blood contains other buffers. NBB on the curve nomogram means *normal buffer base*. The pK of reduced hemoglobin is 7.93, whereas the pK of oxyhemoglobin is 6.68. Oxygenation of hemoglobin is thus an important variable. If a blood sample is 100% saturated, as assumed in the Siggaard-Andersen curve nomogram, then this method will easily predict hemoglobin concentration within the stated ± 3 gm % range. Siggaard-Andersen and Engel determined the base excess curve empirically by adding known amounts of acid or base to various blood samples.

As the fundamental relationship of acid-base chemistry, the Henderson-Hasselbalch equation is used in many ways—in tables, nomograms, slide rules, and computers, as well as in each of the three possible two-dimensional cartesian graphs just described.

*Δ log P_{CO_2}/Δ pH.

Although these devices generate data, they are neither intellectually satisfying nor especially successful in providing the conceptual model necessary for comprehension and analysis of acid-base information. The Acid-Base Surface model* is a three-dimensional plot of the Henderson-Hasselbalch equation. The three continuous variables—pH, P_{CO_2}, and $[HCO_3^-]$—are represented on a triaxial rectangular cartesian coordinate system with scales and ranges so chosen that the three-dimensional surface is inscribed within the physiologically relevant acid-base cube. The Acid-Base Surface is thus a unifying synthesis of the three two-dimensional representations of this equation, all of which are in current use. Although a three-dimensional surface is inherently no more *accurate* than the projection of that surface onto a two-dimensional coordinate system, such a projection results in a complex distortion of the three-variable relationship and is absolutely incapable of showing the true *continuous* nature of the third variable. Three-dimensional visual presentation of a three-variable problem thus yields a complete model that is conceptually simpler.

Clinically, acid-base status is usually well characterized by plotting an arterial point on a graph such as Fig. 10-1. However, it is sometimes also necessary to measure blood electrolyte concentrations and the pH of other body fluids. In actual practice the clinical diagnosis of acid-base disturbances is usually also based upon the history, physical examination, and clinical laboratory data. However, in uncertain or serious cases the principle illustrated in Fig. 10-3 may be of utmost importance.

CARBON DIOXIDE TENSION AND THE RENAL EXCRETION OF BICARBONATE

The kidney is the key to compensation for initial respiratory changes. It is now

*The Acid-Base Surface model is available from Acid-Base, Inc., 2045 Franklin St., Denver, Colo. 80205.

known that renal HCO_3^- retention or excretion depends not upon HCO_3^- concentration, nor upon pH, but rather, upon the P_{CO_2}. Bicarbonate ion concentration is high in both metabolic alkalosis and uncompensated respiratory acidosis. In the latter situation HCO_3^- is retained by the kidney; in the former it is not. Bicarbonate ion concentration is low in both metabolic acidosis and uncompensated respiratory alkalosis. In the latter HCO_3^- is excreted by the kidney, taking the concentration still lower; in the former it is not.

It is the cells of the distal convoluted tubule of the kidney that excrete or retain HCO_3^- in relation to the P_{CO_2}. These cells are rich in the enzyme carbonic anhydrase. When P_{CO_2} is normal, HCO_3^- and H^+ are rapidly formed. The filtrate at this level contains not only Na^+ but also HCO_3^-, in the same concentration as plasma. The cell walls lining this tubule appear to have a cation exchange mechanism, or pump, on the tubular side that exchanges H^+ and K^+ within the cells for Na^+ in the lumen of the tubule. When H^+ reach the tubule by this route, they are free to combine with HCO_3^- in the tubule to form CO_2 and water. The HCO_3^- formed within the cells by the action of carbonic anhydrase moves, along with Na^+, across the opposite wall of the cell and into the capillary.

Why do H^+ and HCO_3^- combine freely to form CO_2 and water in the renal filtrate whereas the enzymatic action of carbonic anhydrase is necessary in the renal tubular cells and red blood cells? There are two possible answers: Either the reaction proceeds slowly without catalysis, but the filtrate remains in the tubule for some time, or red blood cells are being continually destroyed, their contents entering the circulation, and the smaller molecules passing through the glomerulus. Small amounts of carbonic anhydrase may pass through the glomerulus and be present in the filtrate at the level of the distal tubule.

What happens to the CO_2 produced from union of H^+ and HCO_3^- in the filtrate? Carbon dioxide diffuses readily through cell walls. If a CO_2 gradient is established from the lumen of the tubule to the renal cells and blood, CO_2 diffuses toward the region of lower concentration.

Why does the high P_{CO_2} of respiratory acidosis "save" HCO_3^-? There is a P_{CO_2} concentration gradient from plasma to renal tubular cells. As a result of this gradient, CO_2 moves quickly into these cells and shifts the reaction

$$CO_2 + H_2O \overset{\text{Carbonic anhydrase}}{\rightleftharpoons} H_2CO_3 \rightleftharpoons H^+ + HCO_3^-$$

to the right, producing more H^+, which exchange with more Na^+ and combine with more tubular HCO_3^-, preventing this latter ion from being excreted.

Why does the kidney excrete HCO_3^- when P_{CO_2} is low, as it is in respiratory alkalosis? Carbon dioxide moves from the cells, including renal tubular cells, into the blood. The preceding reaction is shifted to the left, depleting the H^+ population of these cells. Fewer H^+ exchange with Na^+; therefore, fewer H^+ are available to combine with HCO_3^- in the filtrate, and more HCO_3^- is excreted.

What is the effect of renal retention or excretion of HCO_3^- on the acid-base picture? If respiratory acidosis persists, the high P_{CO_2} will cause the kidney to retain HCO_3^-. This HCO_3^- retention results in an upward shift (Fig. 10-6) away from the CO_2 dissociation curve and in the direction of normal pH. If the condition persists, there will be complete *compensation* to pH 7.40. If respiratory alkalosis persists, the low P_{CO_2} will force renal excretion of HCO_3^-, moving the plasma values down from the normal CO_2 dissociation curve until pH is again 7.40. In either case a new CO_2 dissociation curve applies. Any further respiratory change will move the plasma values along that new curve.

What makes the kidney stop manipulating HCO_3^- once normal pH has been reestablished? In compensated respiratory acidosis the high P_{CO_2} continues to force H^+ into the filtrate; but the concentration of filtered HCO_3^- is high due to the high plasma level. With this high HCO_3^- level in the filtrate, some escapes combination with H^+ and is excreted in the urine. In compensated respiratory alkalosis the level of filtered HCO_3^- is so low that little of it escapes the tubular H^+, even though their level is also low.

Infusion of acid into the blood quickly drives the reaction

$$CO_2 + H_2O \underset{\text{anhydrase}}{\overset{\text{Carbonic}}{\rightleftharpoons}} H_2CO_3 \rightleftharpoons H^+ + HCO_3^-$$

to the left, depleting HCO_3^- and stimulating the peripheral chemoreceptors to increase breathing. The CO_2 thus produced is quickly blown off by the acid-induced hyperventilation. This sudden drop in HCO_3^- concentration is seen in Fig. 10-6 as an abrupt downward departure from the normal CO_2 dissociation curve to lower HCO_3^- and pH levels. But in contradistinction to renal compensation, respiratory compensation is rapid. Hyperventilation accompanies downward departure from the normal CO_2 dissociation curve. This reduces P_{CO_2} so that the direction (Fig. 10-6) is downward and to the left at the same time. In contrast to renal compensation, respiratory compensation is *incomplete*. Excess H^+ produce increased breathing. If compensation to pH 7.40 were complete, there would be no excess H^+, and thus no drive for hyperventilation.

Removal of acid (as by vomiting or aspiration of stomach contents) or addition of base (such as HCO_3^-) is seen as abrupt upward departure from the normal CO_2 dissociation curve to higher HCO_3^- levels and higher pH values. This is metabolic alkalosis. Except by renal removal of excess HCO_3^-, compensation for metabolic alkalosis is the poorest of those for any of the four primary acid-base disturbances; it succeeds in restoring the afflicted subject's plasma only about one third of the distance back toward normal pH. Compensation is by hypoventilation, which elevates P_{CO_2}. This compensation is poor because only a small fraction of normal ventilatory drive is due to H^+ in the blood. Reduction or even removal of this small stimulus does not reduce breathing drive very much. Because breathing is not reduced very much P_{CO_2} does not rise very much.

Changes in pulmonary ventilation change P_{CO_2} and shift plasma values along the CO_2 dissociation curve (Fig. 10-6). Whenever such changes are transient (measured in minutes), the normal CO_2 dissociation curve continues to apply. However, when ventilatory changes persist for longer periods of time (hours or days), the kidney retains or excretes HCO_3^- and a new CO_2 dissociation curve applies. If HCO_3^- has been retained, this new dissociation curve is higher than the old one. If HCO_3^- has been excreted, the new curve is below the old one. When a HCO_3^- shift establishes a new CO_2 dissociation curve, subsequent changes in ventilation will then move the plasma values along that new curve. When renal compensation is complete, the new curve intersects the pH 7.4 line at whatever resting arterial P_{CO_2} level the ventilation has set.

How do we know whether the CO_2 dissociation curve has been shifted up or down? We equilibrate a *blood* sample with a gas mixture that has the composition of resting, sea level, alveolar gas (P_{CO_2} = 40 mm Hg, P_{O_2} = 100 mm Hg)* and analyze the *plasma* for its bicarbonate content; this is the *standard bicarbonate*. A high value indicates a high CO_2 dissociation curve; a low value indi-

*If the P_{O_2} of this equilibration gas mixture is high or low, the Haldane effect will produce a different CO_2 dissociation curve.

cates a low CO_2 dissociation curve. A primary metabolic disturbance shifts the CO_2 dissociation curve up or down immediately. Ventilatory changes shift plasma values along the CO_2 dissociation curve.

It is sometimes helpful in understanding acid-base disturbances to consider the ratio of $[HCO_3^-]$ to $[aP_{CO_2}]$. If the primary disturbance is in the numerator, it is metabolic. If HCO_3^- concentration increases, there is metabolic alkalosis. If HCO_3^- concentration decreases, there is metabolic acidosis. If the primary change is in the denominator, the disturbance is respiratory. In respiratory acidosis an increased P_{CO_2} decreases the ratio and lowers the pH. If the P_{CO_2} decreases, thus increasing the ratio, the primary disturbance is respiratory alkalosis.

ACID-BASE PATTERNS IN VARIOUS PHYSIOLOGIC STATES

Metabolic acidosis almost always produces hyperventilation. The H^+ stimulus increases ventilation as the acidosis develops, so that partial compensation for the primary disturbance is present almost from the start. However, exercise severe enough to incur a sizable O_2 debt produces a metabolic acidosis (due to lactic acid accumulation in muscle and blood) that is uncompensated. Despite large increases in CO_2 production, arterial P_{CO_2} remains essentially normal. Compensation would require that the arterial P_{CO_2} decrease. Without such compensation the accumulation of a given quantity of lactic acid during exercise produces a greater drop in pH than would the same quantity of lactic acid infused at rest.

Gastric mucosa has the capacity to concentrate H^+ 1 million times. The production of HCl in quantity depletes the blood and the rest of the body of H^+. This depletion, which follows the ingestion of large meals, is reflected in the *alkaline tide,* a blood pH shift to the alkaline side, or temporary metabolic alkalosis. Pancreatic juice is highly alkaline, containing bicarbonate and phosphates. It neutralizes acid stomach contents, which pass into the small intestine. The intestinal reabsorption of gastric contents restores blood pH to normal. Loss of gastric contents through vomiting or gastric aspiration produces metabolic alkalosis.

During sleep metabolic rate decreases. There is also reduced sensitivity to CO_2. Accordingly, arterial P_{CO_2} increases slightly, producing slight respiratory acidosis. Overnight renal compensation for this respiratory acidosis is, presumably, incomplete. Patients with chronic, diffuse, obstructive bronchopulmonary disease may accumulate considerable CO_2.

Acid-base disturbance and compensation

Biochemical correction of acid-base disturbances should never be undertaken without thorough knowledge of the acid-base status, as well as knowledge of the significance of existing compensatory changes.

Metabolic acidosis occurs physiologically during exercise but is also observed during periods of low cardiac output, such as during surgical procedures involving cardiac bypass by means of a pump-oxygenator or resuscitation after cardiac arrest. Uncontrolled diabetes mellitus is a common clinical cause of ketosis and metabolic acidosis. Metabolic acidosis is also an aspect of the clinical syndrome *uremia,* which occurs when failure supervenes in the course of chronic, diffuse renal disease. Ammonium chloride tablets are often used to produce metabolic acidosis for clinical purposes.

Chronic, diffuse bronchopulmonary disease is an increasingly common clinical cause of respiratory acidosis. The sequence of events as pulmonary failure supervenes is invariably hypoxemia, CO_2 retention, and finally frank respiratory acidosis. What are critical acute changes in pH, P_{O_2}, and P_{CO_2} in respiratory failure? Although no rigid criteria can be defined, an arterial blood pH less than 7.25, a P_{CO_2} greater than 60 mm Hg, and a P_{O_2} less than 50 mm Hg are considered urgent indications for treatment.

Hypokalemic metabolic alkalosis

Potassium depletion and alkalosis generally result from renal, adrenal, or gastrointestinal causes. Significant deficit of total body K^+ and alkalosis can also occur in patients with chronic, diffuse bronchopulmonary disease and cor pulmonale. The occurrence of metabolic alkalosis due to hypokalemia and/or hypochloremia is so frequent in such patients as to require special emphasis. The mechanism probably includes hyperaldosteronism secondary to cardiac insufficiency, reduced dietary intake of K^+, and the kaliuretic effects of diuretic or glucocorticosteroid medications. Depletion of body K^+ and alkalosis may exist despite the fact that serum K^+ levels are within normal limits. Although K^+ depletion is associated with an extracellular alkalosis, an intracellular acidosis is simultaneously present.

Potassium depletion and alkalosis in patients with chronic, diffuse bronchopulmonary disease and CO_2 retention may exert a very deleterious effect. Alkalosis itself reduces ventilatory drive, thus aggravating hypoxemia and CO_2 retention. These changes, in turn, further increase the pulmonary arterial pressure and work of the right ventricle. Alkalosis also shifts the oxyhemoglobin dissociation curve to the left, thereby diminishing the O_2 dumping effect that normally occurs in the tissues. Adequate replacement with potassium chloride is the treatment of choice. Replacement by nonchloride potassium preparations is often inadequate.

Diuretics and metabolic alkalosis

In general, intermittency in the administration of diuretics is a clinical point of considerable value, enhancing therapeutic efficiency, while minimizing the possibility of overtreatment.

Various potent diuretics have the capacity to produce serious electrolyte and pH disturbances, especially in patients with impaired pulmonary or renal function. Sometimes the combination of low-sodium diet and potent diuretics results in severe hyponatremia and the *low-salt syndrome.* Thiazide diuretics, as well as glucocorticosteroids, produce metabolic alkalosis. Uncompensated alkalosis in patients with chronic, diffuse bronchopulmonary disease reduces ventilatory drive, aggravating both hypoxemia and hypercapnia.

Acetazolamide (Diamox) is an inhibitor of the enzyme carbonic anhydrase. One important effect of acetazolamide is to decrease renal reabsorption of HCO_3^-, producing metabolic acidosis; another, through its action in erythrocytes, is to cause CO_2 retention and respiratory acidosis. Large doses of acetazolamide increase brain tissue P_{CO_2}.

The prototype thiazide compound, chlorothiazide (Diuril), was introduced in 1958 as a result of the search for improved diuretic agents similar in structure to the sulfonamide carbonic anhydrase inhibitor, acetazolamide. Chlorothiazides are commonly used in the treatment of cardiac insufficiency, including that associated with cor pulmonale. They act by increasing urinary excretion of water, Na^+, Cl^-, and, to a lesser degree, K^+ and HCO_3^-. Consequently, hyponatremia, hypokalemia, and hypochloremic alkalosis may occur. Patients already liable to hypokalemia or those receiving concomitant glucocorticosteroids or digitalis must be watched closely during thiazide therapy. Daily ingestion of foods high in K^+, such as orange juice, or supplemental KCl should be considered.

Tromethamine

Tromethamine, or tris(hydroxymethyl) aminomethane, is a white, crystalline, water-soluble, organic alcohol amine of empiric formula $NH_2C(CH_2OH)_3$. It was first used to postpone the death of fish in transport, which die as a result of CO_2 accumulation and acidosis. It is an interesting experimental agent and has occasional clinical use in the therapy of respiratory acidosis.

Tromethamine is a weak base, or proton acceptor, which after injection (usually intravenous) into the circulation becomes a component of a buffer system. A 0.3 molar solution contains 36 gm/L, is iso-osmotic with plasma, and has a pH of 10.2 at 38° C. After tromethamine has reacted with H^+ it forms salts with the associated anions, which are then excreted by the kidney. Tromethamine is an osmotic diuretic, increasing both urine flow and urine pH. At pH 7.40 tromethamine is 30% un-ionized. The un-ionized form can diffuse from its extracellular location into the cells, where it combines with the anions of intracellular fluids. The reaction of tromethamine with acids may be represented as follows:

$$(CH_2OH)_3CNH_2 + HA \rightleftharpoons (CH_2OH)_3CNH_3^+ + A^-$$

Alkalinizing agents, such as bicarbonates and tromethamine, are occasionally useful in treatment of the acid-base disturbance of respiratory failure. Their use is limited to cases in which arterial pH remains less than 7.25 after partial or complete restoration of arterial P_{CO_2} to normal, or cases in which arterial P_{CO_2} remains high despite vigorous treatment of airway obstruction, hypercapnia, and hypoxemia.

Tromethamine overdosage* depresses respiration by reducing P_{CO_2} and increasing pH, an unusual example of respiratory alkalosis. Hyperventilation is the fundamental cause of respiratory alkalosis, a term that refers to the acid-base picture after excessive CO_2 has been ventilated away or otherwise removed. Emotional stress is the commonest cause of hyperventilation. Acetylsalicylic acid and other salicylates increase ventilation out of proportion to metabolic rate, causing respiratory alkalosis; however, in large doses they produce metabolic acidosis as a result of interference with carbohydrate metabolism.

*Large doses have been reported to cause hypoglycemia.

CHAPTER 11 Neurogenesis of breathing

The breathing cycle involves successive, rhythmic contraction and relaxation of the inspiratory muscles. Active expiration, when it occurs, involves rhythmic contraction and relaxation of the expiratory muscles. The breathing muscles, which include the internal and external intercostal muscles and diaphragm, have two functions: they make the movements of breathing and they contribute to the maintenance of posture, resisting the effects of gravity on the chest. The fluctuations of breathing are therefore superimposed upon the postural tonus of the respiratory muscles. The act of breathing is coordinated in the brainstem; however, the mechanism is not fully understood.

As inspiration begins, inspiratory neurons fire faster—from 5 to 10 per second to 30 to 40 per second. Simultaneously, expiratory muscle tone is inhibited. As inspiration proceeds, additional inspiratory neurons are recruited. Toward the end of inspiration the frequency of inspiratory impulses diminishes. During quiet breathing, inspiratory neuron activity continues into the expiratory phase of the breathing cycle, smoothing the transition from inspiration to expiration. A sudden interruption of all inspiratory effort would allow the thorax to fall abruptly, producing a transient, significant rise of intrapleural pressure. Such a spasmodic breathing cycle would impede venous return to the heart, as well as increase resistance to air flow with every expiration.

METHODS FOR STUDY OF THE RESPIRATORY CENTERS

A respiratory center is a region of the central nervous system where neuronal activity coincides with the breathing cycle, or a region where stimulation of neurons produces responses that are primarily related to breathing. Various technics have been used to localize the respiratory centers of the central nervous system and to study their function. Technics have improved greatly since the early observations of the effects of ablation or transection of central nervous system tracts. Recent studies using electrolysis or local temperature block bear little resemblance to the crude surgical technics of early investigators.

Both electric stimulation and chemical injection of selected regions have yielded information about the respiratory centers. Such studies may mislead as well as fail to yield information about *normal* respiratory center activity; it is not known whether fiber tracts or nerve cell bodies are being stimulated, and electric current may affect adjacent areas of the brain. Thus the response of a region to an electric current does not guarantee its involvement in the genesis of normal breathing.

The action potentials of specific regions correlate with inspiration or expiration. In general, the recording of spontaneous electric activity is more relevant than observing the response to artificial stimula-

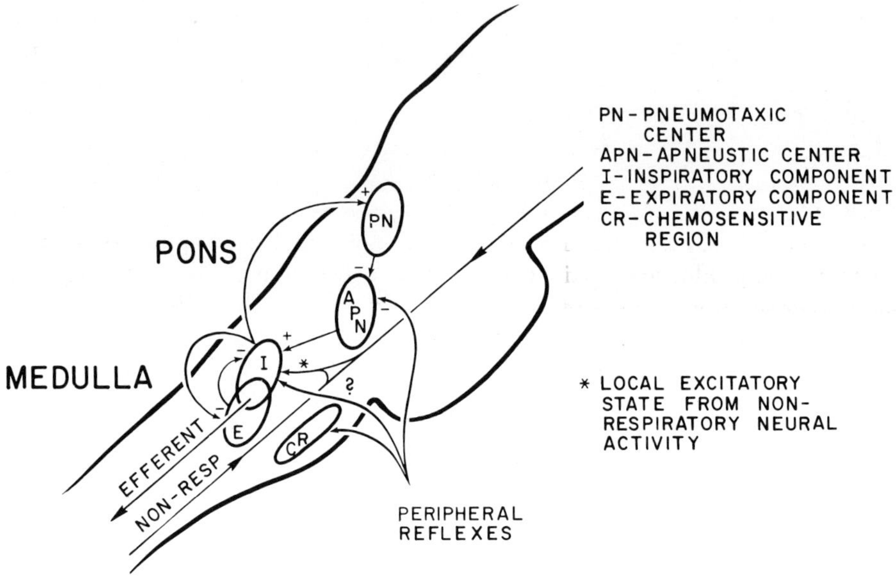

Fig. 11-1
Location and interaction of central nervous system respiratory centers.

tion; however, movement artifacts associated with breathing and with the blood pressure pulse may complicate interpretation.

Application of the foregoing technics and definitions has led to a general concept of the identity, location, and function of the central respiratory centers. Although there is general agreement on the identity and location of these centers, their function in the genesis of normal breathing and in the regulation of pulmonary ventilation remains in dispute. We will present our concept (Fig. 11-1), recognizing the possible validity of other conclusions.

MEDULLARY RESPIRATORY CENTERS

A primary respiratory center is located in the reticular formation of the medulla; functionally, it consists of inspiratory and expiratory components. Anatomically, these are two poorly delineated groups of neurons whose activities are synchronous with the inspiratory and expiratory phases of breathing, respectively.

The inherent rhythmicity of the medullary center results from the interaction between its inspiratory and expiratory components. Transection of the spinal cord and section of the cranial nerves in a decerebrate animal do not abolish this rhythmicity. Some believe that the pontine center periodically interrupts the tonic activity of the inspiratory component. However, experimental evidence suggests that the medullary respiratory centers can inherently produce *ataxic* (irregular) breathing.

The inspiratory component of the medullary center dominates the expiratory component. Stimulation of the inspiratory component produces an inspiratory effort that lasts as long as stimulation continues. Stimulation of the expiratory component causes only temporary expiratory effort as well as a temporary inhibition of inspiration; thus ventilation will resume despite continued stimulation. The inspiratory and expiratory components inhibit each other reciprocally; this reciprocal inhibition, together with other less well-defined influences, generates and maintains respiratory center rhythmicity.

Without a "local excitatory state" the rhythmicity of the medullary center would fade and finally fail. This essential state is produced and maintained by impingement of subthreshold stimuli from nonrespiratory neurons on the respiratory neurons. The respiratory stimulation produced by pain, cold, and certain other sensory inputs is probably a nonspecific neural effect on the threshold for reciprocal inhibition between inspiratory and expiratory components. The spanking of infants at birth is a well-known example of such nonspecific ventilatory stimulation; it is probably more theatrical than scientific unless central nervous system depression is severe. Digital stimulation of the anal canal and rectum is also used to initiate breathing in the newborn. Photic stimulation of the retina increases breathing, a response that is readily appreciated during retinoscopy. A sudden dousing with cold water evokes an inspiratory gasp. Pinching the skin and other painful stimulation elicit breaths in animals that have respiratory depression.

PONTINE RESPIRATORY CENTERS

Two centers in the pons, just anterior to the medulla, significantly affect the activity of the medullary center—the *apneustic* center, located at the level of the *area vestibularis,* and the *pneumotaxic* center, located in the anterior pons. These centers are less well defined and less active than the medullary center in producing action potentials synchronous with breathing. Their role in the neurogenesis of breathing and their effect on the rhythmicity of the medullary center have been studied with the technics of action potential recording, stimulation, and transection.

Apneustic center

Sectioning vagal afferents and transecting the brainstem between the apneustic and pneumotaxic centers produces a ventilatory pattern that consists of inspiratory spasms interrupted irregularly by transient expiratory efforts. This *apneustic breathing* is usually accompanied by decerebrate rigidity; indeed, some believe that the apneustic center is simply a part of the reticular facilitory system. With intact vagal afferents the same pontine section does not cause apneustic breathing. The apneustic center is believed to be inspirostimulatory and can be inhibited by vagal afferents or by the pneumotaxic center.

Pneumotaxic center

The pneumotaxic center, located in the anterior pons, inhibits the inspiratory activity of subordinate centers. It probably achieves this effect by inhibiting the apneustic center, although some believe that it directly inhibits the inspiratory component of the medullary center. The input of the pneumotaxic center is unknown, but it has been proposed that the inspiratory component of the medullary center facilitates pneumotaxic center activity. The pneumotaxic center is undoubtedly involved in the thermoregulatory breathing pattern of those animals that pant in response to hyperthermia.

The relationship between the medullary and pontine respiratory centers is shown in Fig. 11-2. Effects on the breathing pattern of brainstem transections that isolate central nervous system centers, with and without vagal influence, are predictable, if the following are true:

1. The medullary center is inherently rhythmic
2. The apneustic center stimulates the inspiratory component of the medullary center
3. The pneumotaxic center is stimulated by inspiratory component activity
4. The pneumotaxic center and the vagus nerve can inhibit the activity of the apneustic center
5. The vagus nerve affects the expiratory component of the medullary

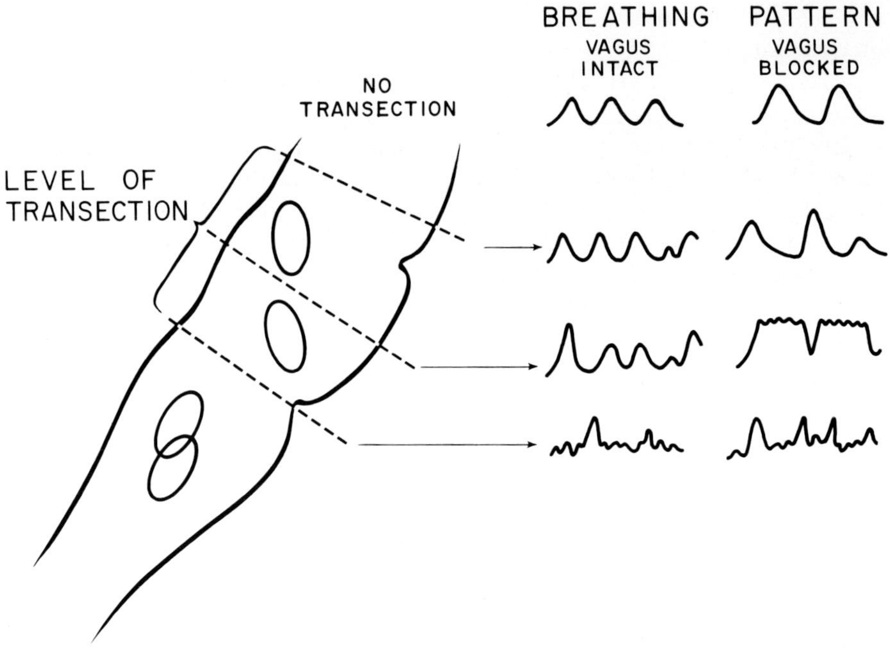

Fig. 11-2
Effect of midbrain transection at three different levels on the breathing pattern with vagus nerves intact and vagus nerves blocked.

center via the apneustic center rather than affecting it directly

MODIFICATION OF BREATHING BY HIGHER CENTRAL NERVOUS SYSTEM CENTERS

The breathing pattern can be modified by conscious control originating in the cerebral cortex—for example, voluntary hyperventilation or breath-holding. However, the ability of the cerebral cortex to override the basic rhythmicity of the medullary centers is limited, and most healthy subjects cannot hold their breath to the point of unconsciousness. We alter our breathing pattern voluntarily to speak or to sniff. We are less conscious of some cortically produced modifications such as breath-holding during a brief stint of vigorous physical activity (e.g., sprinting). We also modify our breathing pattern, and may even hold our breath, during the isometric muscular work of supporting heavy objects or straining at stool. Electric stimulation of certain areas of the cerebral cortex modifies the breathing pattern. Most of these areas also subserve other functions such as emotion (crying, laughing, sobbing), the autonomic nervous system (fright, thermoregulation), special senses (olfaction), or acts that directly control breathing (vocalization, swallowing, etc.).

CHAPTER 12 Regulation of pulmonary ventilation

In the previous chapter we discussed the genesis of the breathing cycle and described the central respiratory centers. Here we will present what little is known about the regulation of pulmonary ventilation. Endowed with inherent rhythmicity, the medullary respiratory center is a component of the complex system that regulates pulmonary ventilation. This regulatory system involves two feedback mechanisms.

1. The proprioceptive reflexes, originating in the lungs and chest wall, respond to mechanical changes in the lung-chest system, influencing the respiratory centers, and thereby increase the efficiency of breathing. Most of the afferent limbs of these reflexes are in the vagus nerves.

2. A humoral feedback system involving chemical factors (P_{O_2}, P_{CO_2}, and H^+) also influences the activity of the respiratory centers. In this system alveolar ventilation is a partial determinant of P_{O_2}, P_{CO_2}, and H^+, whereas these chemical factors, in turn, influence pulmonary ventilation. Although we will present each component separately, it is their coordinated systematic interaction (respiratory centers, proprioceptive reflexes, and humoral mechanisms) that regulates pulmonary ventilation, optimizing the breathing pattern for any metabolic level. Fig. 12-1 summarizes this concept.

PROPRIOCEPTIVE REFLEXES

The lungs and chest wall contain the receptors of a number of proprioceptive reflexes that affect breathing. At least eight kinds of receptors have been identified on the basis of structure, location, and afferent nerve type. The afferent, or sensory, pathways of most of the pulmonary reflexes are in the vagus nerves. We will describe only three of these pulmonary reflexes but do not wish to imply that other reflexes are unimportant for the breathing pattern.

Hering-Breuer inspiratory reflex

Perhaps the most familiar of the pulmonary reflexes is the Hering-Breuer reflex, which affects the depth of inspiration. Lung inflation stimulates pulmonary stretch receptors, which, in turn, influence medullary respiratory center activity. It remains unclear whether the receptors influence the medullary centers directly or act indirectly via pontine centers.

Hering and Breuer, in 1868, demonstrated that breathing can be interrupted by increased intratracheal pressure or by tracheal occlusion at the end of a normal inspiration (blocking expiration); both prolong the expiratory phase of the medullary center. Increased intratracheal pressure distends the airways and increases transpulmonary pressure. Airways distention is the apparent stimulus of the Hering-Breuer reflex, which originates in slowly adapting receptors located in the bronchi and bronchioles. Bilateral vagotomy abolishes this reflex.

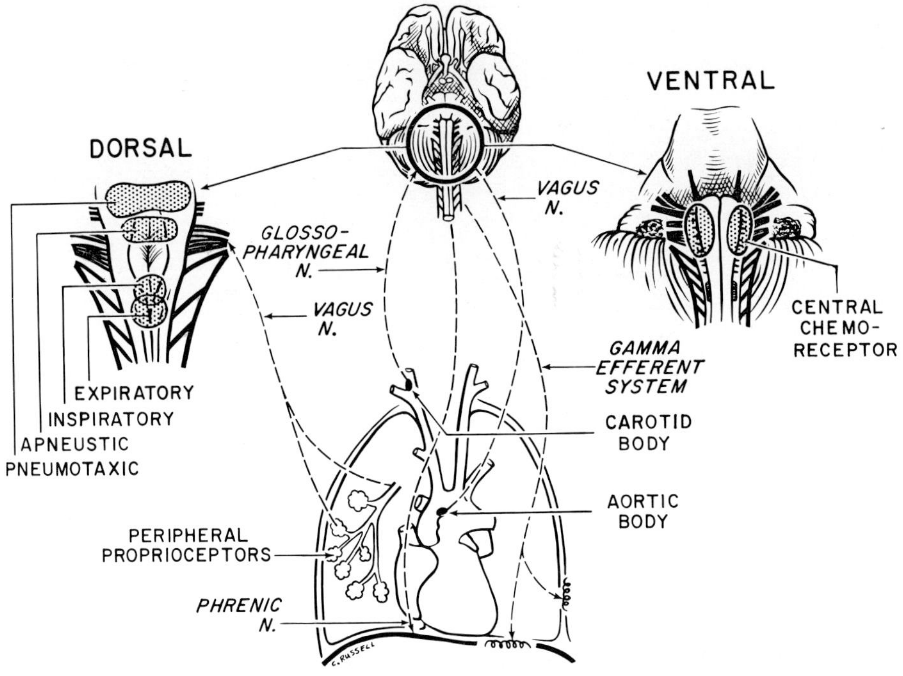

Fig. 12-1
The system that regulates pulmonary ventilation and generates the breathing pattern.

After discovery of the inspiro-inhibitory Hering-Breuer reflex, it was proposed that tidal volume is controlled on a breath-by-breath basis. This concept prevailed for more than 70 years, although rhythmic breathing was observed to resume despite continued vagal stimulation. Vagal tone probably affects the activity of the pontine apneustic center, which, in turn, influences the medullary respiratory center. After transection of the brainstem between the apneustic center and the medullary center, neither vagal section nor vagal stimulation affects medullary rhythmicity. On the other hand, after transecting the pons between the apneustic and pneumotaxic centers, intermittent vagal stimulation can produce rhythmic breathing movements. After the same transection with vagi sectioned but unstimulated, apneustic breathing occurs.

Hering-Breuer receptors adapt slowly—impulses continue for a relatively long time if intratracheal pressure remains increased. Because changes of the mechanics of the lung-chest system affect the sensitivity of this reflex, factors that decrease lung compliance or increase airway resistance sensitize these receptors. Veratrum alkaloids also increase the sensitivity of the Hering-Breuer reflex, probably by direct action on the receptors.

Species vary in the sensitivity of their Hering-Breuer reflexes; some physiologists have suggested that man has lost this reflex. However, in the study of this reflex the importance of lung geometry has been underestimated. Most studies have considered the relationship between intratracheal pressure and the ratio of breath-holding time to the breathing cycle interval. What would the *relative* species sensitivity be if pressure/unit lung volume or pressure/unit cross-sectional area of the airway were plotted against the number of suppressed breathing cycles?

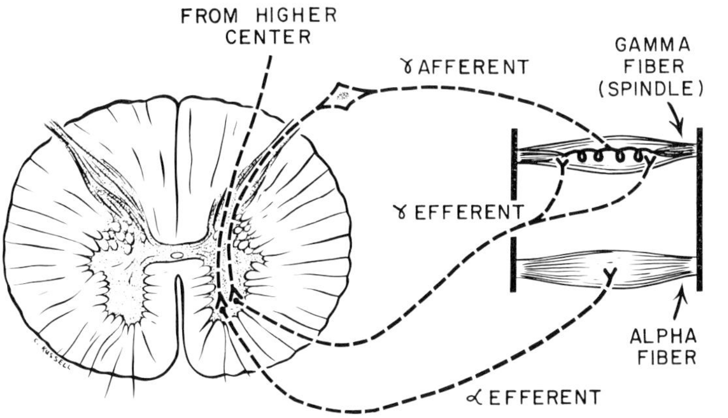

Fig. 12-2
The extravagal gamma-efferent system is a feedback system that modifies the breathing pattern.

Paradoxical reflex of Head

If the Hering-Breuer reflex is blocked by cooling the vagus nerve to 8° C, hyperinflation of the lungs causes an additional inspiratory effort that tends to inflate the lungs further. This inspirostimulatory reflex is the opposite of the inspiro-inhibitory Hering-Breuer reflex. The receptors for this reflex are in the lung parenchyma. They adapt rapidly, which means that they are mainly stimulated by rapid volume changes; they cease firing promptly after a volume change occurs. The reflex of Head may help to maintain hyperventilation that involves a large tidal volume, as, for example, during exercise, or it may be involved in gasping. The sensitivity of this reflex in man is not known. Sectioning the vagus nerves abolishes this reflex.

Deflation reflex

A third reflex, the deflation reflex, increases the force and frequency of inspiratory effort as the lungs are deflated by "negative" pressure or during lung collapse. This phenomenon is not the simple absence of the inspiro-inhibitory Hering-Breuer reflex. The receptors for the deflation reflex, located in bronchi and bronchioles, function below 8° C, unlike those for the Hering-Breuer reflex. Vagotomy abolishes this reflex. The deflation reflex may be involved in the hyperpnea of chest compression as well as pneumothorax. The role of the vagi in producing hyperventilation during pneumothorax remains undefined. The deflation reflex is basically nociceptive (receiving injury) and is not involved in the normal process of breathing.

Other types of receptors cause a ventilatory response to pulmonary emboli, to drugs such as serotonin and antihistamines, to mechanical stimulation of the upper airway, to chemical irritation of the lower airway, and to fluctuations of pulmonary blood pressure.

GAMMA-EFFERENT SYSTEM

Distinct from the vagal reflexes that modify the breathing pattern is the gamma-efferent, or muscle spindle, system. This feedback system detects and responds to changes of pulmonary compliance as well as resistance even after vagotomy. We do not fully understand this extravagal system that provides information about the relationship between inspiratory volume change and inspiratory effort (efficiency of inspiration). A conception of the gamma-efferent system is shown in Fig. 12-2.

Muscle spindles, or stretch receptors, are in parallel with alpha muscle fibers. Muscle fibers in series with stretch receptors alter the degree of parallel muscle fiber elongation required to stimulate stretch receptors. This system, which senses the force of and simultaneously detects the response to inspiratory effort, may be located in the diaphragm and intercostal muscles. Information about the response of inspiratory muscles to a given level of motor activity is integrated in the central nervous system; when a given level of motor activity fails to produce appropriate shortening of inspiratory muscles, the inspiratory effort is suspended and expiration results.

In restrictive lung disease, increased effort is required to inflate the lungs. The force of inspiratory muscle contraction increases. Because appropriate shortening of inspiratory muscles does not occur, inspiratory effort stops prematurely and tidal volume is small. These changes are detected and relayed to the central nervous system, which determines the optimal relationship between tidal volume and breathing frequency. Breathing frequency is increased to maintain alveolar ventilation. Fig. 12-3 shows the relation of breathing frequency to O_2 cost of breathing at constant alveolar ventilation in healthy subjects and in patients who have bronchopulmonary disease. Compared to healthy subjects, patients with restrictive lung disease breathe rapidly and have a small tidal volume; patients with obstructive lung disease breathe slowly and have a large tidal volume.

OTHER FACTORS AFFECTING VENTILATION

Blood pressure

An increase in systemic arterial blood pressure causes hypoventilation, and a decrease produces hyperventilation. This reflex originates in the aortic and carotid sinus baroreceptors. At normal arterial blood pressure, tonic baroreceptor activity inhibits ventilation. Baroreceptors in the walls of the atria and great veins, sensing increased blood pressure, may stimulate respiration, an action opposite to that of the systemic (aortic and carotid) baroreceptors. The physiologic importance for

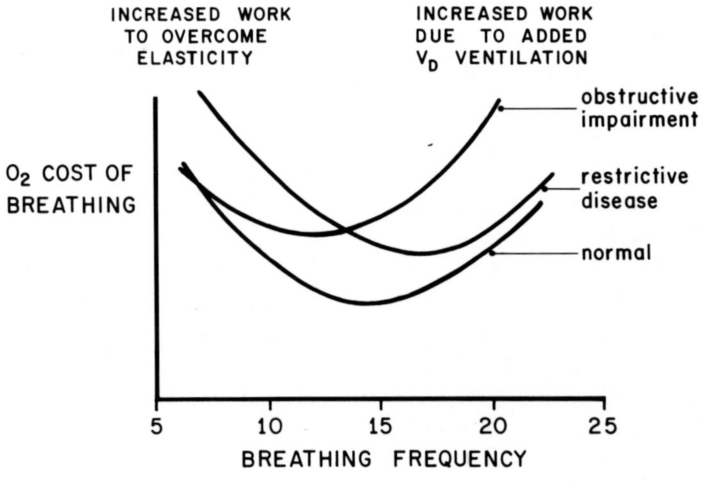

Fig. 12-3
The effect of breathing frequency on the O_2 cost of breathing in healthy subjects, patients with obstructive impairment, and patients with restrictive disease. The curves are not from actual data.

respiration of the atrial baroreceptors remains unclear.

Hormones

Certain physiologic states affect respiration; some of these, such as pregnancy, involve hormonal mechanisms. Characteristic respiratory changes occur during pregnancy. Progesterone stimulates ventilation and is probably responsible for the hyperventilation associated with pregnancy. As a result of chronic hyperventilation, pregnant women have a respiratory alkalosis (arterial P_{CO_2} decreases 6 to 8 mm Hg) that is compensated for by HCO_3^- excretion and metabolic acidosis. Indeed, the lowest arterial P_{CO_2} values in healthy, resting individuals are found in pregnant women at high altitude. Respiratory changes also occur during the menstrual cycle. Arterial P_{CO_2} decreases 3 to 4 mm Hg by the time of ovulation, a change that is also due to progesterone. This hormone also produces hyperventilation in healthy men, causing P_{CO_2} decreases that are comparable to those observed in women.

CHEMICAL FACTORS AFFECTING VENTILATION

There are situations in which ventilatory drive is purely chemical; however, waking ventilation, at rest or during exercise, is almost certainly driven to some extent by nonchemical factors. Certain patterns of ventilation have no positive chemical component. Indeed, some such as maximal voluntary ventilation have a negative chemical component (hypocapnic alkalosis).

Metabolic changes produce changes in CO_2 production, in O_2 consumption, and in the pH of body fluids. Chemical inputs affecting pulmonary ventilation are integrated with other inputs in the central nervous system. Because breathing is a vital function responsive to a variety of changing internal and external conditions, we are not surprised to find a complex interaction of driving factors and a complex integration of their inputs.

After artificial hyperventilation to reduce P_{CO_2} and elevate P_{O_2}, anesthetized animals undergo a period of apnea during which CO_2 rises and O_2 falls. Following voluntary hyperventilation, conscious physiologists* may wait to feel subjectively a certain level of stimulus before they resume breathing and, by so doing, demonstrate the apnea they have observed in anesthetized animals. However, conscious human subjects who do not know the purpose of this experiment resume breathing immediately without a period of apnea. Following hyperventilation, conscious human subjects exhibit a token breathing pattern of normal rhythm and frequency but ineffectual depth. Whether one does or does not experience apnea following hyperventilation probably depends upon his level of excitation. Psychogenic ventilatory drive readily supercedes chemical drive in most individuals who are awake and aware.

It has long been known that both hypercapnia and hypoxia are respiratory stimulants; hypercapnia is more potent than hypoxia. In 1911 Winterstein proposed a unified concept involving the final common path of increased H^+ concentration in the cells; metabolic acids and respiratory acidosis (due to CO_2 retention) produce H^+, whereas hypoxia favors accumulation of acids due to anaerobic metabolism. The discovery by Heymans in 1927 that hypoxia acts through peripheral chemoreceptors required revision of this theory, since it was known that CO_2 acts directly on the central nervous system. Additional information necessitated yet other changes in the theory. We still do not know whether molecular CO_2 acts independently and di-

*We have observed a tendency in our respiratory physiologist friends to use themselves as "healthy, objective subjects" in respiratory experiments when they are actually neither healthy nor objective.

rectly or whether its effect is mediated via pH.

In his *multiple factor theory* of the chemical regulation of pulmonary ventilation, Gray analyzed and quantified the chemical input to the brainstem. He added the ventilatory drives from CO_2, O_2, and H^+ algebraically to obtain the total chemical drive for pulmonary ventilation. In this scheme hypoxic drive may assume prominence, depressing P_{CO_2} by hyperventilation; however, CO_2 drive is not abolished and continues to exert a partial effect upon ventilation.

Carbon dioxide

Increased arterial P_{CO_2} is the most potent naturally occurring stimulus to ventilation. Fig. 12-4 shows a plot of ventilation as a function of inspired CO_2 concentration. Ventilation increases gradually up to a CO_2 concentration of 8% to 10%, after which it remains relatively constant, flattening slightly near the peak of the response and falling off at about 20% CO_2. The relationship between alveolar ventilation and arterial blood P_{CO_2} is more linear in the ascending portion of the curve. The sensitivity of the ventilatory response to hypercapnia is so great that a mere 2 to 3 mm Hg change in arterial P_{CO_2} produces a measurable effect.

Central chemoreceptor response to CO_2. In dogs and cats chemoreceptors for hypercapnia are located on the ventrolateral surfaces of the medulla near the exit of the ninth and tenth cranial nerves; these are presumed to be present also in man. Local application of H^+, CO_2, acetylcholine, or nicotine stimulates breathing within a few seconds. As an uncharged molecule, CO_2 diffuses freely from the blood across the blood-brain barrier into the cerebrospinal fluid (CSF), where it reacts with H_2O to form HCO_3^- and H^+. The H^+ thus produced stimulate the central chemoreceptors, which in turn affect the medullary respiratory center, increasing pulmonary ventilation. This ventilatory response is characterized more initially by tidal volume increase and later by progressively larger contributions from breathing frequency increase.

The blood-brain barrier is relatively impermeable to H^+ and HCO_3^-. As a result, a local respiratory acidosis in the central chemoreceptors is not quickly compensated and the CSF remains acidic until blood P_{CO_2} falls. Since blood P_{CO_2} is in equilibrium with CSF P_{CO_2}, increased alveolar

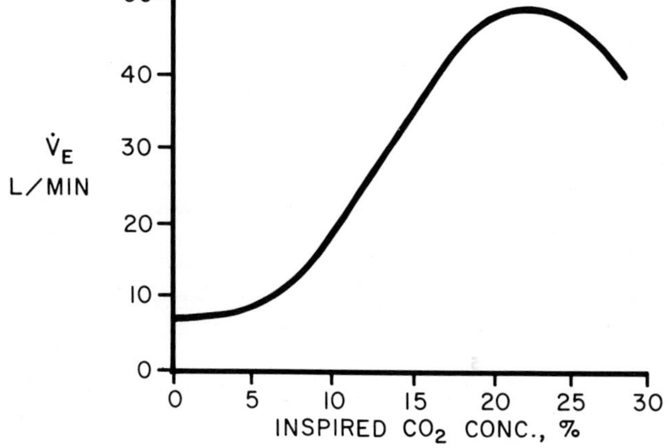

Fig. 12-4
Ventilatory response to CO_2 concentration in inspired gas.

ventilation reduces P_{CO_2} in both, returning CSF pH to normal. When *prolonged* hyperventilation lowers blood P_{CO_2}, CO_2 leaves the area of the central chemoreceptors, reducing H^+ concentration and producing a local respiratory alkalosis of the CSF. Chemoreceptor drive decreases until HCO_3^- can trickle through the blood-brain barrier from the CSF into the blood, compensating the local respiratory alkalosis of the central chemoreceptors.

Cerebrospinal fluid pH may explain the hyperventilation or hypoventilation of patients when arterial blood analysis does not. Furthermore, the adverse effects of excessively rapid therapeutic correction of acid-base disturbance can sometimes be understood in terms of central chemoreceptor physiology.

Cerebrospinal fluid has a lower buffer capacity than blood. The buffer capacity of blood is due largely to its protein content, especially hemoglobin. Because CSF is low in protein, its pH changes considerably more for a given P_{CO_2} change than does blood pH. Cerebrospinal fluid contains little, if any, carbonic anhydrase. Therefore, the reactions involving CO_2, carbonic acid, HCO_3^-, and H^+ proceed slowly; there may be a considerable delay before incoming CO_2 produces appreciable quantities of H^+. Is CSF a homogeneous fluid of identical chemical composition everywhere—even at the various sites of formation?

The physiology of the medullary chemoreceptors determines the low threshold and high sensitivity of pulmonary ventilation to P_{CO_2}. Regulated pulmonary ventilation is essential for the maintenance of a proper CO_2 and pH environment for the brain. Thus for the respiratory system, CSF is the essence of the milieu interieur.

Peripheral chemoreceptor response to CO_2. Arterial chemoreceptors in the angle of the bifurcation of the common carotid arteries and at the level of the aortic arch respond to hypercapnia. Carbon dioxide stimulates the chemoreceptors when the perfusing blood has a P_{CO_2} greater than 30 mm Hg. As P_{CO_2} rises, the frequency of nerve impulses increases. Because the sensitivity of the central mechanism is greater, peripheral chemoreceptors probably play only a minor role in the response to hypercapnia. Perfusion of the brain with hypercapnic blood produces a greater ventilatory response than such perfusion of the peripheral chemoreceptors. The sensitivity of the peripheral chemoreceptors for CO_2 increases during hypoxemia. Peripheral chemoreceptor response to hypoxemia is likewise affected by arterial blood P_{CO_2}. Indeed, this may be the most important physiologic effect of CO_2 on the peripheral chemoreceptors.

Hydrogen ions

Rapid intravenous injection of an acidic solution causes hyperventilation, whereas injection of dilute NaOH solution causes hypoventilation or even apnea. Hyperventilation occurs in metabolic acidosis even with the decreased arterial P_{CO_2} that partly compensates for the acidosis. Thus increased H^+ concentration directly stimulates pulmonary ventilation.

Ventilation is considerably less sensitive to pH change than it is to P_{CO_2} change. pH must decrease by 0.05 to 0.1 unit before ventilation responds significantly. However, if arterial P_{CO_2} is held constant by adjusting inspired CO_2 concentration to prevent the hypocapnia of acid-induced hyperventilation, a greater ventilatory response is observed for a given pH change.

The relative sensitivity of ventilation to P_{CO_2} versus H^+ is shown in Fig. 12-5. The steep rise of ventilation due to hypercapnia is a combination of the CO_2 stimulus acting primarily on central chemoreceptors and the H^+ stimulus acting primarily on peripheral chemoreceptors. The middle curve is recorded during an acidosis in which the P_{CO_2} is kept constant by adjusting inspired P_{CO_2}, and it is thus due

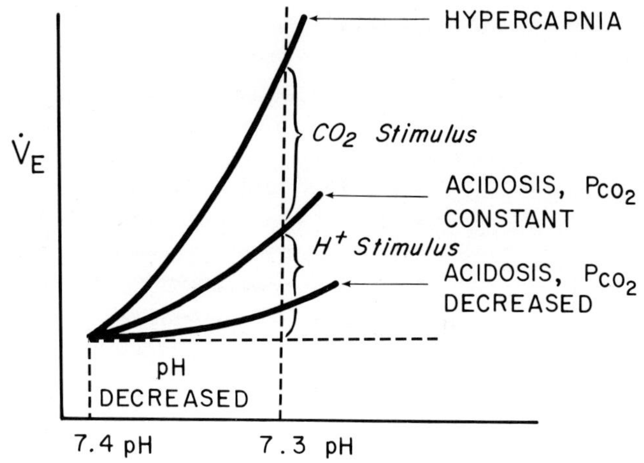

Fig. 12-5
Ventilatory response to hypercapnia and acidosis. The highest curve shows the effect of hypercapnia (increased P_{CO_2} and decreased pH). The lowest curve shows the effect of acidosis (low P_{CO_2} as a result of hyperventilation). The middle curve shows the response to acidosis alone (P_{CO_2} was kept constant by adjusting the CO_2 content of inspired gas).

only to the stimulus of H^+. The lower curve represents acidosis in which the induced hyperventilation is allowed to decrease P_{CO_2}. Concomitant hypocapnia inhibits much of the response to H^+.

In an animal with denervated peripheral chemoreceptors the injection of an acidic solution increases ventilation; thus acidosis stimulates ventilation through some other mechanism. Since blood pH change does not easily affect the cerebrospinal fluid surrounding the central chemoreceptors, one must consider some other mechanism such as a nonspecific excitatory state or a specific effect on medullary respiratory center activity. Thus acidosis probably stimulates central respiratory centers.

Oxygen

Although hypoxia stimulates pulmonary ventilation, the threshold for this effect is high and unpredictable. Decreasing inspired O_2 does not reliably stimulate ventilation until O_2 concentration falls to 12%, arterial P_{O_2} falls to 50 or 60 mm Hg, and oxyhemoglobin saturation falls to about 80%. The normoxic levels of healthy resting subjects acclimatized at sea level are probably not directly involved in the physiologic regulation of pulmonary ventilation.

The hyperventilation induced by hypoxia is a direct effect of decreased arterial blood P_{O_2} and only indirectly a function of decreased arterial blood O_2 content. This fact is supported by two observations: (1) at altitude, where P_{O_2} is low, hyperventilation occurs despite the normal blood O_2 content resulting from increased hemoglobin concentration; and (2) during carbon monoxide intoxication, ventilation does not increase.

If P_{CO_2} is held constant by adjusting inspired CO_2 concentration, hypoxia produces a larger ventilatory response than occurs with spontaneous air breathing. This is because hypoxia-induced hyperventilation with air reduces P_{CO_2}, which in turn inhibits the ventilatory response to hypoxia.

In contrast to CO_2, which acts at several sites, hypoxia stimulates breathing only through the peripheral chemoreceptors. However, hypoxia also has a central depressant effect that tends to reduce sensitivity to itself. Thus hypoxia stimulates ventilation if the peripheral chemorecep-

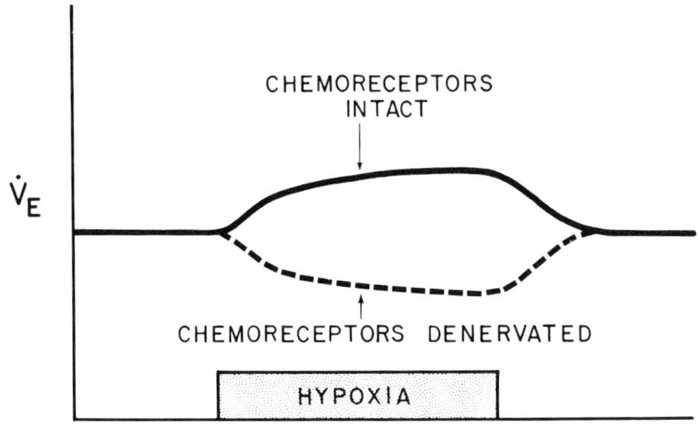

Fig. 12-6
Effect of chemoreceptor denervation on the ventilatory response to hypoxia.

tors are intact, but it depresses ventilation if they are denervated (Fig. 12-6).

There is a tonic level of peripheral chemoreceptor discharge during normal spontaneous air breathing. The large P_{O_2} decrease required to raise the level of chemoreceptor discharge significantly suggests that either there are two kinds of receptors or that other factors, central or peripheral, affect the response to hypoxia. The potent CO_2 effect on ventilation complicates the interpretation of studies of hypoxia. If healthy resting subjects acclimatized at sea level breathe pure O_2, ventilation usually decreases slightly and transiently, but as P_{CO_2} increases, ventilation rises slightly above the pre-oxygen control level.

INTERACTION OF CHEMICAL FACTORS AFFECTING VENTILATION

In the course of chronic diffuse bronchopulmonary disease, arterial hypoxemia always precedes hypercapnia. Thus hypoxemia occurs without concomitant hypercapnia, but the reverse is true only in patients with CO_2 retention who are receiving O_2 therapy. Alveolar ventilation is the most important determinant and prime regulator of arterial P_{CO_2}, whereas pulmonary blood flow is the major determinant of arterial P_{O_2}. It follows that arterial P_{CO_2} reflects the adequacy of alveolar ventilation with more fidelity than does arterial P_{O_2}.

It may be confusing to discover that P_{CO_2} and alveolar ventilation are *directly* related in some situations but *reciprocally* related in others. However, the paradox is only apparent. Carbon dioxide is only one of several ventilatory drivers. If another drive increases alveolar ventilation, expelling CO_2 more rapidly than it is produced, arterial P_{CO_2} falls. The withdrawal of CO_2 as a ventilatory stimulus diminishes the net response to the other drive. This situation is shown in Fig. 12-5, where the non-CO_2 ventilatory driver is acidosis.

The relationship between hypercapnia and hypoxia as ventilatory drivers is complex. Some interesting observations can be made by studying Fig. 12-7, which is an idealized set of curves constructed from published data. The greater sensitivity of ventilation to CO_2 than to O_2 is evident from the fact that equivalent distances along the horizontal axis represent a 4 mm Hg change of P_{O_2} but only a 1 mm Hg change of P_{CO_2}.

The relationships of pulmonary ventilation to both CO_2 and O_2 are nonlinear. A P_{O_2} isopleth (line of constant P_{O_2}) indicating CO_2 effect on ventilation reveals that when P_{CO_2} falls below the level of 35 to

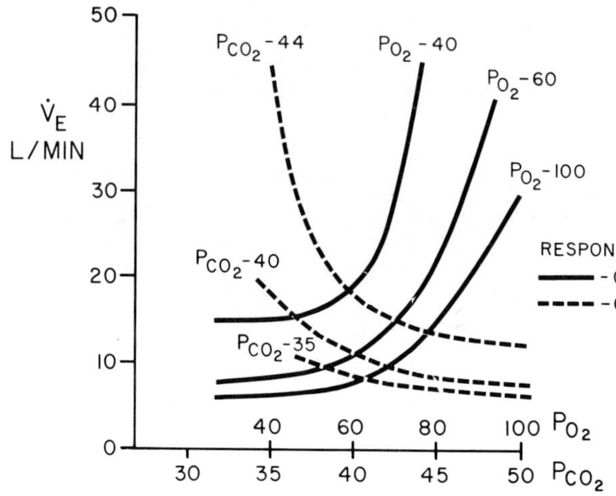

Fig. 12-7
Set of curves illustrating the ventilatory response to hypercapnia and hypoxia. The curves were constructed from published data. The solid lines represent the ventilatory response to P_{CO_2} at constant P_{O_2}. The broken lines represent the response to P_{O_2} at constant P_{CO_2}.

38 mm Hg, it no longer affects ventilation. Above that level pulmonary ventilation increases as P_{CO_2} increases. As P_{O_2} falls, CO_2 threshold decreases and CO_2 sensitivity increases. Thus hypoxia shifts the curve for P_{CO_2} upward and to the left.

The relationship of ventilation to P_{O_2} is also nonlinear. A P_{O_2} decrease from 60 to 40 mm Hg has a greater effect on the response to P_{CO_2} than a P_{O_2} decrease from 100 to 60 mm Hg. Cross-circulation and chemoreceptor denervation studies suggest that the effect of P_{O_2} on the sensitivity of ventilation to P_{CO_2} is probably mediated through the peripheral chemoreceptors.

The ventilatory response to hypoxia when P_{CO_2} is held constant is also nonlinear (see P_{CO_2} isopleth). Again, a strong interaction between P_{CO_2} and P_{O_2} is evident, since hypercapnia decreases the hypoxia threshold and increases the sensitivity to hypoxia. Since hypoxia depresses ventilation after denervation of the peripheral chemoreceptors, it is likely that the CO_2 effect is mediated primarily through them.

In summary, the important *interaction* between hypercapnia and hypoxia in the regulation of pulmonary ventilation should not be underestimated. During air breathing, for which the regulatory system evolved, hypercapnia is always preceded by hypoxemia. Therefore, as P_{CO_2} increases, the actual ventilatory response curve shifts up and to the left to isopleths of progressively greater hypoxia. This suggests that hypoxia plays an important role in the physiologic regulation of ventilation, and because it affects the response to CO_2, hypoxia may also play an important role in the regulation of ventilation in patients with pulmonary insufficiency.

Breath-holding and rebreathing

Breath-holding is voluntary apnea that persists until ventilatory drive exceeds the cortical inhibition a subject will or can exert. The length of time that the breath can be held depends upon P_{CO_2}, P_{O_2}, pH, lung volume, level of physical activity, prior hyperventilation, level of CO_2 acclimatization (tolerance), motivation, and self-discipline.

The study of breath-holding and rebreathing throws some light on the regula-

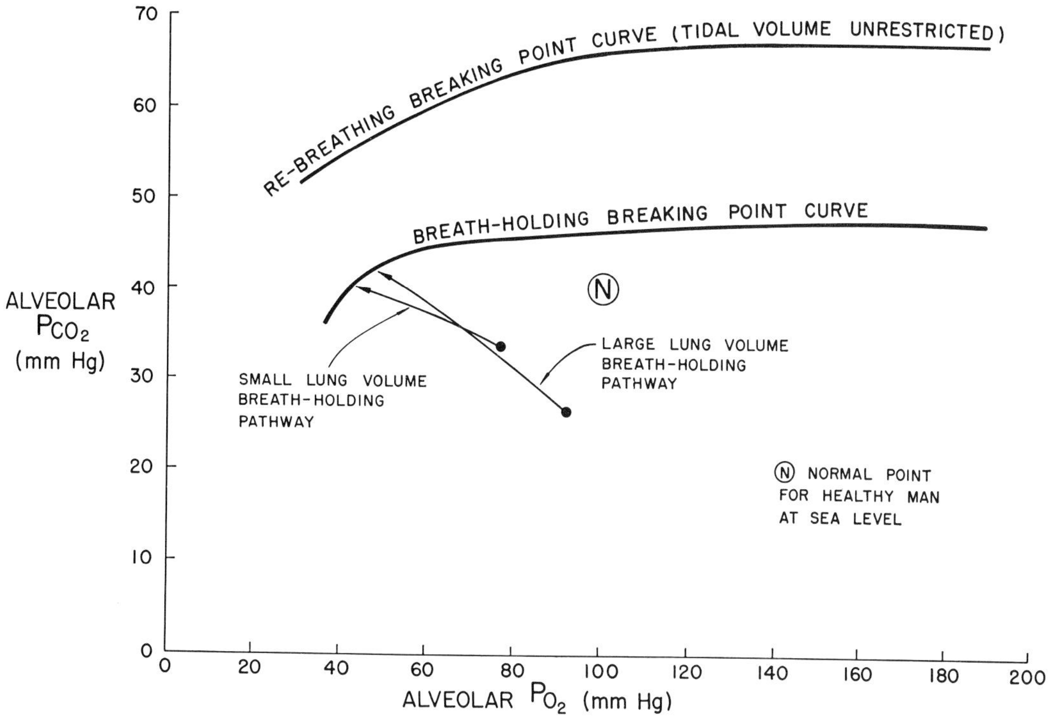

Fig. 12-8
O_2-CO_2 diagram, showing breath-holding as opposed to rebreathing of healthy man acclimatized at an altitude of 1,600 meters.

tion of pulmonary ventilation. Everyone who holds his breath experiences a desire to breathe. This sensation of air hunger, having both intensity and quality, is the cortical appreciation of several factors, including the brainstem excitation that results from chemical factor input. Resumption of breathing provides prompt and total relief from this distress.

If at the breaking point of breath-holding, a subject blows the gas then present in his lungs down a long tube, the gas trapped in the proximal end of this tube is alveolar gas (Haldane-Priestley alveolar gas sample). This forced expiratory alveolar gas sample is analyzed for its content of O_2 and CO_2. If a practiced breath-holder repeatedly holds his breath under the same conditions, his alveolar P_{CO_2} and P_{O_2} values are remarkably consistent at the breaking point. The values of alveolar P_{O_2} and P_{CO_2} thus obtained at the breaking point are plotted on an O_2-CO_2 diagram for graphic display and analysis (Fig. 12-8). If the subject was breathing a gas other than air, the values of P_{O_2} and P_{CO_2}, as well as their relationship, may be different at the breath-holding breaking point. If we obtain a subject's breaking-point values for each of an array of different gas mixtures, we can construct a breath-holding, breaking-point curve by joining the breaking points plotted for each mixture. When the O_2 content of the inspired gas mixture is initially high, hypoxia exerts little influence upon the breaking point and the influence of CO_2 is dominant. However, when breath-holding lowers P_{O_2} to severely hypoxic levels, the role of CO_2 in terminating breath-holding is less important. The breath-holding, breaking-point curve demonstrates a smooth transition from the extreme of almost pure hypoxia effect as the major chemical factor, ranging through synergism of hypoxia with

CO_2, to the extreme of almost pure CO_2 effect as the overwhelming chemical influence upon the breaking point.

During breath-holding, molecules of O_2 move from lungs to blood at a relatively constant rate that is a function of cardiac output. Lung volume decreases, passively increasing the fractional concentrations of the remaining lung gases (N_2 and CO_2). Thus alveolar P_{CO_2} would increase even if no CO_2 were to enter the lungs from the blood.

The rate of O_2 uptake from the lungs is constant when metabolic rate is constant. If initial lung volume is low, a constant rate of O_2 uptake rapidly changes the proportion of gases remaining in the lungs, the breaking-point curve is rapidly approached, and breath-holding time is relatively short. When metabolic rate is high, the rate of O_2 uptake and CO_2 production is also high. A combination of low initial lung volume and high metabolic rate results in an even more rapid rise of alveolar P_{CO_2} and fall of alveolar P_{O_2}; the breaking-point curve is even more rapidly approached, and breath-holding time is even shorter. Prolonged breath-holding requires a combination of large initial lung volume and low metabolic rate.

Is it more comfortable to hold one's breath at a volume somewhat less than full inspiration or at the volume of maximum inspiration? If a breath-holder relaxes against a closed glottis at full inspiration, the high relaxation pressure impedes venous return to the right heart, decreasing cardiac output and cerebral blood flow. An inspiratory effort against the closed glottis facilitates venous return, increasing cardiac output and cerebral blood flow.

Brief periods of intense hyperventilation lower alveolar and arterial P_{CO_2} but only slightly affect body stores of CO_2. However, moderate hyperventilation for several minutes significantly reduces body CO_2 stores, lowering the level of the CO_2 reservoir in which metabolically produced CO_2 can accumulate during subsequent breath-holding. If a subject hyperventilates breathing O_2, immediately prior to breath-holding his initial alveolar gas concentrations are remote from the breath-holding, breaking-point curve, and breath-holding time is correspondingly long.

Blood leaving the pulmonary capillaries returns to the left heart and traverses a segment of the systemic arterial circulation before the peripheral chemoreceptors can sense its composition. This delay is usually about 5 seconds but varies slightly. In addition a subject requires about a second to exhale an adequate alveolar gas sample into a Haldane sampling tube when the breath-holding breaking point is reached. Consequently, the composition of the alveolar gas analyzed for a breath-holding, breaking-point curve reflects a longer breath-holding time than the arterial blood chemical factors that are actually involved in producing a breaking point. One reason that breath-holding during exercise penetrates the resting breath-holding, breaking-point curve is that, despite decreased systemic arterial transit time, alveolar gas composition changes more rapidly. During exercise, breath-holding time may be decreased by incompletely adapted pulmonary stretch receptors.

Breath-holding breaking points are protective. Most subjects are unable to lose consciousness during either breath-holding or rebreathing; for them it is physiologically impossible and psychologically intolerable to penetrate the breaking-point curve. However, individuals who are acclimatized to high CO_2 or who have unusually powerful cortical inhibition (self-discipline or volition) can achieve unconsciousness as a result of simple breath-holding.

During tantrums small children sometimes hold their breath to unconsciousness, the cyanosis of lips and nails suggesting that hypoxemia is involved. Hypoxic unconsciousness can also cause drowning accidents among overly enthusiastic underwater swimmers. After extreme hyperventilation to suppress CO_2 drive, a breath-holding Valsalva maneuver, together with an increased rate of O_2 consumption, produces unconsciousness from cerebral hypoxia before CO_2 accumulates sufficiently to penetrate the breaking-point curve. Such loss of consciousness differs from that due to simple breath-holding in that it involves hypocapnia and an increased metabolic rate.

Holding a musical note to endurance while singing involves a breaking point. Sometimes this occurs because the singer has completely exhaled, but low-intensity note-holding when initial lung volume is high may last long enough to produce discomfort of chemical and other origin, particularly if the singer is also dancing or otherwise physically active.

Rebreathing is significantly different from breath-holding. If one rebreathes gas from a closed system, he reaches a breaking point at which further breathing from the system becomes intolerable, and he rips the apparatus from his face. If before he gasps for fresh air, the subject can be persuaded to exhale into an alveolar sampling tube, the gas can be analyzed and the results plotted on an O_2-CO_2 diagram. When rebreathing and breath-holding, breaking-point curves for the same subject are plotted on the same diagram, it is seen that rebreathing penetrates the breath-holding, breaking-point curve at all points (Fig. 12-8). Rebreathing renews vagal inhibition with each breath, whereas in breath-holding the slowly adapting pulmonary stretch receptors have adapted for many seconds and have little or no inhibition left to contribute.

Rebreathing from systems of varying volume dramatically demonstrates the effect of breath size on the inhibition deriving from pulmonary stretch receptors. As we decrease the lung volume a subject is permitted to attain, the rebreathing breaking-point curve shifts down and to the right until, if the subject is forced to breathe only in his expiratory reserve volume, alveolar P_{O_2} and P_{CO_2} at the breaking point are very little higher and to the left than the starting point.

If a person takes half-sized breaths for a minute or two from an open system in which CO_2 does not accumulate, he feels a sensation that may be termed air hunger and becomes very uncomfortable. However, if he inspires deeply, activating the slowly adapting stretch receptors, even though the inspired gas be pure nitrogen, he is suddenly and dramatically relieved.

HYPERPNEA OF EXERCISE

The hyperpnea of exercise has fascinated generations of physiologists. It was once thought that this hyperpnea is due to elevated blood P_{CO_2}, since exercise generates large amounts of CO_2. We know that this hyperpnea keeps arterial P_{CO_2} at a precisely constant level over a wide range of metabolic rates. However, this linear relationship between metabolic rate and pulmonary ventilation* fails at both ends of the metabolic spectrum (Fig. 12-9). During rest and very mild exercise, pulmonary ventilation is greater than that predicted by the central linear relationship because of psychogenic ventilation. During exhausting exercise, ventilation outstrips the metabolic rate and may under these conditions actually exceed the maximal voluntary ventilation!† Note that the disproportionate increase of pulmonary ventilation with respect to O_2 uptake begins at 2,500 ml (STPD)/min. This is about 62.5% of peak O_2 uptake or slightly less than the value (70%) above which an exercising

*A linear relationship also holds for metabolic rate versus heart rate.

†This apparent contradiction results from physiologic airway dilatation during exhausting physical work. The administration of bronchodilator drugs to healthy, resting subjects also produces some airway dilatation.

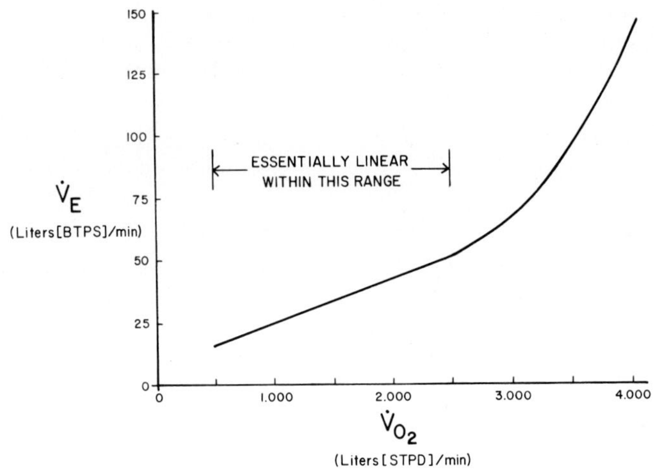

Fig. 12-9
Expiratory minute volume as a function of metabolic rate during physical exercise. Curve is constructed from published data.

subject cannot achieve a steady physiologic state.

The precise matching of pulmonary ventilation with O_2 uptake and CO_2 production has led some to postulate the existence of hypoxia or CO_2 receptors upstream from the alveoli in the pulmonary artery, right heart, or great veins. Such receptors would detect venous or mixed venous P_{CO_2} and "tell" some respiratory center how much pulmonary ventilation is necessary for homeostasis. Although postulated, such P_{CO_2} receptors have not been identified, and perfusion of upstream areas with CO_2-enriched blood does not increase pulmonary ventilation.

The precision of the relationship between metabolic rate and pulmonary ventilation also led to the notion that something senses metabolic rate and regulates ventilation to match it. Crossed perfusion experiments during which a thyromimetric drug was given indicated that ventilation responds to metabolic rate increase even when the only connection between central nervous system and the region of increased metabolic rate is neural. Muscle perfusion with CO_2-enriched blood does not stimulate the "metaboreceptors"; apparently CO_2 per se is not the stimulus. There is some evidence to suggest the existence of metaboreceptors in muscle; however, such receptors have not been identified either, and other evidence is contradictory.

Passive moment of the limbs causes hyperventilation. The magnitude of this response correlates well with the number of limbs (or joints) involved and with the frequency of joint movements. Joint denervation abolishes this effect. As discussed in Chapter 11, certain nonrespiratory inputs increase pulmonary ventilation by altering the "local excitatory state" of the central respiratory centers. However, joint receptor activity produces a larger ventilatory response than would be expected as a nonspecific effect. Evidence suggests that joint receptors specifically stimulate pulmonary ventilation and that this effect contributes to the ventilatory response of the exercising intact animal.

Pending further evidence, it is attractive to attribute the hyperpnea of exercise to the additive effects of several inputs, including metabolic rate, limb movement, and central nervous system threshold changes; but, in truth, the regulation of pulmonary ventilation during muscular exercise remains a mystery.

EMOTIONS AND RESPIRATION

Asleep as well as awake man's respiration reflects his emotional state. If something absorbs his interest, his breathing reflects his excitement. The anticipation of physical or sexual activity greatly increases ventilation *before* such activity begins. When he walks, runs, or climbs, his breaths synchronize with steps. That various intense emotions affect respiration is a common observation. Indeed, the respiratory system is a major mode of expression for a variety of feelings. The breath-holding of temper tantrums or anger; the singing, humming, or whistling of happiness; the sighing of passion; and the sobbing and crying of sorrow or grief are only a few examples. On occasion, cough is a symptom of psychogenic origin.

At any given time the emotional state of an individual is a mixture, blend, or "paint-pot" of various feelings. Correlations with respiration are accordingly difficult. Occasionally, however, certain feelings intensify and predominate to such an extent that their relationship to respiration becomes obvious; for example, panic-level anxiety produces hyperventilation.

Depression, which usually involves guilt, grief, and self-hatred, produces hypoventilation. Anger produces respiratory irregularities, including hyperventilation and breath-holding. Intense grief produces sighing respirations and a sensation of throat tightness or choking. Crying is a complex emotional expression, involving especially the expiratory phase of breathing.

Anxiety produces hyperventilation and increased cardiac output with a relatively slight increase of O_2 uptake. Hyperventilation is of practical importance for the performance of demanding tasks; the hypocapnia and respiratory alkalosis it produces are associated with a series of physiologic responses—decreased systemic arterial blood pressure, cerebral vasoconstriction, dizziness, numbness and tingling, increased susceptibility to fainting, impaired psychomotor function, tetany, and carpopedal spasm that produce a performance decrement. The hyperventilation of aircraft pilots to the point of psychomotor impairment is well documented. The spirographic sign of emotional stress pattern (p. 182) involves hyperventilation and appreciable moment-to-moment variation of rate, depth, and respiratory level. Such hyperventilation is less regular than that of nonemotional origin. Hysterical hyperventilation is a syndrome of extreme hyperventilation of sudden onset and incapacitating degree that is associated with episodes of intense panic-level anxiety. Air hunger occurs in psychogenic hyperventilation despite slight hyperoxia and appreciable hypocapnic alkalosis.

The emotional factors in asthma are a much-discussed example of psychogenic factors in respiratory disease. There is no doubt that emotionally induced hyperventilation aggravates the symptoms of any obstructive airway problem. In addition to this mechanism airway constriction, hypersecretion, and edema may be of emotional origin in certain patients; and as if this were not sufficiently complex, intense emotion can trigger allergic phenomena, for example, hives at a funeral.

ABNORMAL BREATHING PATTERNS

A variety of abnormal breathing patterns are related to central nervous system changes or malfunctions that interfere with the neurogenesis of normal breathing or with the interrelationships among regions that control or affect breathing.

Vagal breathing is the slow, deep pattern observed in anesthetized animals after section of both vagus nerves. It is due to interruption of proprioceptor afferents in the lungs and chest wall, modifying the activity of the pontine apneustic center. This breathing pattern is sometimes presented as the result of interference with the Hering-Breuer reflex, but this is probably an oversimplification since the vagi contain the afferents of many receptors. Furthermore, the concept that the Hering-Breuer reflex exerts a breath-by-breath effect on the breathing pattern is no longer widely accepted.

Apneustic breathing is characterized by sustained, cramplike, inspiratory efforts relieved irregularly by brief expirations. As previously described, this pattern is believed to be due to a loss of the normal inhibition of the pontine apneustic center, allowing its inspirostimulatory effect to be manifest. Apneusis is thus inspiratory apnea.

Biot's breathing is characterized by irregular periods of apnea alternating with periods in which four or five breaths of identical depth are taken. It is seen in patients who have increased intracranial pressure and is sometimes associated with midbrain lesions. A more specific description of its origin and significance is usually not attempted.

Coupled breathing, or *grouped breathing*, is a pattern in which breaths appear in pairs or triads separated by periods of apnea that last for several seconds. This pattern occurs in situations where the CO_2 level differs from the normal CO_2 threshold. Newcomers to high altitude frequently experience this pattern, accompanied by a dyspnea that is relieved only after the second deep breath. In healthy man at high altitude, breathing pure O_2 abolishes this pattern. Coupled breathing occurs spontaneously in anesthetized dogs, where anesthesia has raised the CO_2 threshold. The stimulus for this pattern of breathing is probably chemical, but the changes in sensitivity or the central changes that result in the prominence of the chemical drive are not understood.

Cheyne-Stokes breathing is a form of periodic breathing characterized by cycles of gradually increasing frequency and increasing tidal volume, followed by a gradual decrease in both frequency and depth of breathing—a *crescendo-decrescendo* pattern. It is usually seen in patients who have brain damage or who are terminally ill. It is also seen in infants and in some healthy people during sleep, particularly at high altitude. It occurs in patients who have increased circulation time between lungs and carotid chemoreceptors (and brain), for instance, those with cardiac insufficiency. The mechanism is related to the delay between hyperventilation-induced hypocapnia and decreased central nervous system drive to ventilation, as well as between hypoventilation-induced hypoxia and the ventilatory response mediated by the peripheral chemoreceptors. It is commonly seen after peripheral chemoreceptor denervation when the negative feedback system consists only of CO_2 acting through the central mechanism, which has a longer feedback delay than the peripheral chemoreceptors. When circulation time is normal and there is no apparent chemoreceptor impairment, Cheyne-Stokes breathing may result from midbrain lesions.

CHAPTER 13 Respiratory physiology of the newborn

One of the most fascinating achievements of the biologic world was the evolutionary transition of animal life from an aquatic to a terrestrial environment. The amphibia, able to survive in either environment, gradually became less dependent upon the aquatic environment and simultaneously more dependent upon the gaseous atmosphere.

In contrast to phylogenetic development, when a baby is born, the environmental change is sudden and dramatic. The fetus, comfortably surrounded by, and physiologically adapted to, the liquid amniotic fluid, must begin to breathe air, exchanging O_2 and CO_2 with the environment. Ordinarily, no amphibious period intervenes during which placental and pulmonary gas exchange overlap. Rather, with the onset of effective airbreathing placental function normally ceases, the transition between the two conditions occurring within seconds.

We will present the important factors involved in the respiration of the newborn: the physiologic and anatomic development of the fetus that accommodates it to intrauterine life and favors the transition to airbreathing; the mechanical factors concerned with the inception of airbreathing; the role of the nervous system in establishing and maintaining breathing; and the chemical and reflex factors that regulate respiration in the newborn.

RESPIRATORY PIGMENTS

Joseph Barcroft, who studied fetal physiology for nearly 40 years, demonstrated that fetal hemoglobin has an increased affinity for O_2 and that this increase is accompanied by a decreased O_2 affinity of maternal hemoglobin. The leftward shift of the fetal oxyhemoglobin dissociation curve is due to hemoglobin F, described in Chapter 7. The rightward shift of the maternal oxyhemoglobin curve probably reflects metabolic acidosis.

We must examine the *slope* of the oxyhemoglobin dissociation curve in the physiologically relevant range to understand how this affects the supply of O_2 to the fetus. Although umbilical arterial and venous P_{O_2} are both comparatively low, the dissociation curves in Fig. 13-1. show that both arterial and venous fetal blood contain more O_2 than maternal blood at the same P_{O_2}. Although more saturated with O_2 in the placenta, fetal hemoglobin releases less O_2 to the fetal tissues (change of percent saturation) as a result of the shift of the oxyhemoglogin dissociation curve. Furthermore, increased oxyhemoglobin saturation in both arterial and venous blood reduces the amount of CO_2 transported as carbaminohemoglobin, favoring fetal acidosis. Thus, although an interesting physiologic phenomenon, the oxyhemoglobin dissociation curve shift during fetal life is less important than once thought

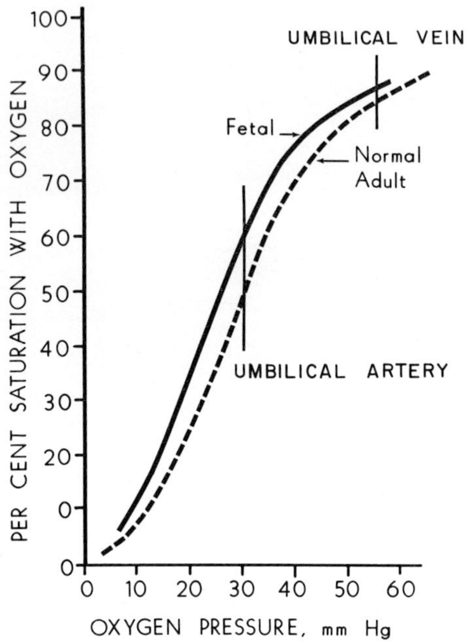

Fig. 13-1
Oxyhemoglobin dissociation curves for fetal hemoglobin (solid line) and adult hemoglobin (broken line). The curves show that fetal hemoglobin holds more O_2 but releases less to the tissues.

and, indeed, may actually work against the fetus.

The following considerations further support this de-emphasis of the importance of the shift of the oxyhemoglobin dissociation curve: The amount of material that moves across a membrane (e.g., O_2 moving across a placenta) depends upon the rate of supply of fresh material brought to the membrane (flow dependence) as well as upon the ease with which the material moves across the membrane (diffusion coefficient). Although transplacental P_{O_2} difference is comparatively large, suggesting an appreciable diffusion barrier to O_2 transfer, both maternal and fetal blood flow rates are high enough to ensure the fetus an adequate O_2 supply, even though oxyhemoglobin saturation is low by adult standards. The O_2 consumption of the fetal lamb does not rise when its oxyhemoglobin saturation is increased by administration of O_2 to the mother. It is of further interest that if temperature remains constant, O_2 consumption does not change after birth, despite increased P_{O_2}.

Since CO_2 diffuses easily in the tissues, transplacental P_{CO_2} and pH differences are likely to be small, and the fetus is usually neither hypercapnic nor acidotic unless the mother is. Normal acid-base values and P_{CO_2} measurements have been found in the fetal arterial blood of animals and in that of human infants during intrauterine exchange transfusions.

PRENATAL RESPIRATORY EFFORTS

Since Vesalius, who first described rhythmic breathing movements of the fetus, further observation has revealed that the normal fetus, at least near term, rarely makes respiratory movements unless subjected to asphyxia. The rapidity of such movements (40 to 80 per minute) when they do occur probably precludes much fluid movement through the small airways. Due to the relatively solid lung and soft chest wall, diaphragmatic gasps would suck little fluid into the lung but would, instead, probably collapse the chest. However, the fact that suspensions of radiopaque thorium oxide or india ink injected into the amniotic sac gain access to the fetal lung indicates that aspiration can occur.

Consideration of prenatal lung movements brings to mind the presence of fluid in the air spaces, its source during fetal life, and its fate at birth: How does the presence of this fluid affect the expansion of the lungs at birth and the ease with which the lungs can begin their gas-exchange function? Early work suggested that the lung fluid derived from aspirated amniotic fluid and that its occurrence was a dangerous complication of birth. However, recent work indicates that the presence of this fluid is a normal condition and that the lung itself is the source of the fluid during the last half of gestation. For example, analysis of blood, tracheal fluid, and amniotic fluid after injection of radioisotopes into fetal blood, suggests that the lung fluid comes from the fetus, not from the amniotic sac. Tracheal fluid with its higher Cl^- and H^+ concentrations, but lower protein and CO_2 levels than amniotic fluid, probably does not originate from the fluid surrounding the fetus. Rather, the lung fluid is an ultrafiltrate of blood plasma modified by subsequent selective reabsorption of some materials.

Surfactants are secreted into the liquid-filled alveolar spaces in utero. Normal surface tension has been reported in lungs of fetuses as small as 200 grams. Animal studies indicate that the rate of phospholipid synthesis increases with gestational age and that full development of biosynthetic pathways is achieved sometime during the third trimester of pregnancy. With the onset of air-breathing at birth, the rate of surfactant secretion increases further. As air-breathing begins, air displaces the liquid filling the alveolar spaces, and surfactants enter the rapidly formed alveolar lining layer.

THE START OF BREATHING

With proper obstetric management most healthy infants begin to breathe within seconds after birth, even before separation from the placenta. This was not the case when heavy maternal sedation and general anesthesia were widely used, causing serious depression of the infant and often requiring vigorous stimulation to start breathing.

The chest wall recoils elastically as the infant emerges from the birth canal, drawing 10 to 40 cc of air into the lungs to replace the fluid squeezed from the air passages during delivery. The glossopharyngeal musculature of some infants forces 5 to 10 cc of air into the trachea by means of "frog-breathing." Neither action is essential for the first breath, however, since babies delivered by cesarean section or those in whom a pharyngeal airway is inserted at birth expand their airways uneventfully.

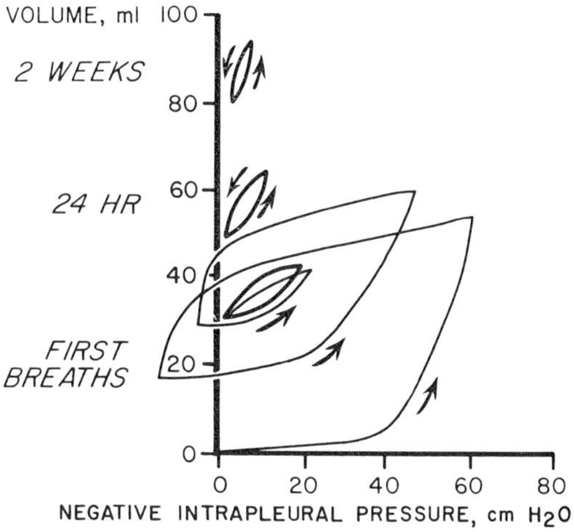

Fig. 13-2
Pressure-volume curves for the initial breaths of a newborn infant. Functional residual capacity and compliance change during the first weeks of life.

We will introduce our discussion of the mechanical factors associated with the initiation of breathing with a description of the relationship between pressure change and volume change in the thorax, as shown in Fig. 13-2. Intrapleural pressure is atmospheric before the first breath inflates the lungs. This fact, of considerable functional significance, indicates that the chest does not recoil outward until after birth. If the fetal chest recoiled outward, as it does in extrauterine life, one of two conditions would result:

1. The opposing recoil of the fluid-filled fetal lung would be small due to the lack of surface tension normally provided by an air-liquid interface. The two sets of opposing forces would balance at a large lung volume, and the lungs would then contain a larger fluid volume at birth (particularly with cesarean section) and rapid initiation of effective breathing would require a different mechanism.

2. If the lung did not follow the chest wall, intrapleural pressure would decrease

and liquid would fill the pleural space. This would interfere with expansion of the lungs at birth.

The mechanism of the permanent increase of chest volume that results from the first breath is not understood. It is described as a "plasticlike" phenomenon. Whatever its cause, this expansion sets up the opposing forces between lung and chest wall that produce and maintain a "negative" intrapleural pressure after breathing starts.

During the first breath (Fig. 13-2), intrapleural pressure falls to about – 40 cm H_2O with little volume change during the first 0.5 second or so; the subsequent sudden inflow of air is associated with very little further change of pressure. During expiration, pressure first decreases considerably, after which there is a rather sudden terminal volume decrease. The lungs do not empty completely during this expiration, thus establishing about one half of the neonatal residual volume with the first breath. Subsequent breaths stabilize a rather constant volume-pressure relationship over the next several hours at a compliance (ease of filling) of four to five times that at birth and at a flow resistance of one half to one quarter that of the first few breaths. Airway resistance decreases due to clearance of fluid from the airways and to the progressively more "negative" end-expiratory intrathoracic pressure. As functional residual capacity increases, small airways expand.

Since resistance to gas flow through the airways depends on radius, length, and the number of passages, airway resistance is predictably greater for infants than for adults. If lung dimensions were strictly proportional to body mass, the radius of infant airways would be one twentieth that of adults; the resulting extreme airway resistance would throttle pulmonary ventilation, since resistance to laminar flow varies inversely as the fourth power of tube radius. It is estimated that the radius of infant alveoli is about one half that of adults and that the terminal bronchioles are about three fourths of adult size. Infant airway resistance is about 25 to 30 cm $H_2O \times liter^{-1} \times second^{-1}$ as compared with about 2 cm $H_2O \times liter^{-1} \times second^{-1}$ for healthy adults. Total pulmonary ventilation of infants is about 560 cc/min, as compared with 8 L/min for adults. Thus total ventilation is fourteenfold greater in the adult, whereas airway resistance is about one fourteenth. However, the relationship between airway resistance and pulmonary ventilation is similar for adults and infants after the first few breaths.

During the first breath, movement of fluid in the airways creates a viscous resistance that contributes considerably to the pressure required to expand the lungs. For example, the viscous resistance to the movement of amniotic fluid in the airways of a guinea pig was 58 cm H_2O at a flow rate of 0.7 cc/sec.

Surface tension forces of the alveolar lining fluid are of great physiologic importance. Pulmonary surfactant affects the ease of breathing, the evenness of ventilation, and the efficiency of gas exchange. These concepts were described in detail in Chapter 5. Because of their importance for neonatal physiology the reader may wish to review them in connection with this chapter.

PERINATAL CIRCULATION

Normal fetal development depends on the placenta as the organ for gas exchange, a function that is transferred to the lungs at birth. The dramatic circulatory changes that occur at birth are matched at no other time in life. Contrary to earlier belief, the transition from fetal to adult circulation is gradual rather than abrupt, requiring a period of hours to days.

The pattern of circulation through the fetal heart is shown in Fig. 13-3. The most oxygenated stream of blood in the fetal circulation comes from the placenta and

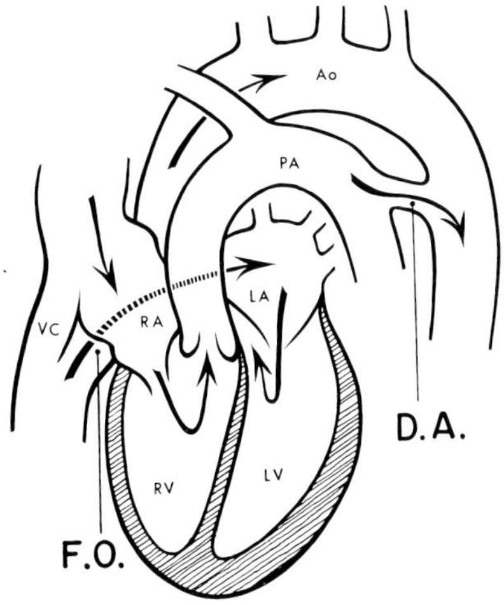

Fig. 13-3
Pattern of circulation in the fetal heart, showing the preferential shunting of blood from the placenta through the foramen ovale **(F.O.)** and the shunting of blood through the ductus arteriosus **(D.A.)**, bypassing the pulmonary circulation.

lower part of the body. This comprises about 75% of the venous return. About 85% of the total venous return shunts preferentially through the foramen ovale into the left atrium. The concept of a streaming pattern of blood flow through the right atrium derives from comparison of the O_2 content of blood in the carotid artery with that in the descending aorta; blood in the carotid artery has the composition of left ventricular blood (62% saturated with O_2), whereas that in the descending aorta (58% saturated with O_2) is a mixture of blood from the left ventricle with that shunted through the ductus arteriosus from the right ventricle. This circulatory pattern preferentially perfuses the brain, heart, and liver with blood of the highest systemic O_2 content.

At birth, blood ceases to flow through the placenta, a large peripheral vascular bed that had received more than one half of the cardiac output, and arterial pressure increases. High left ventricular pressure increases left atrial pressure. Simultaneous lung inflation reduces pulmonary vascular resistance, decreasing right ventricular pressure and, secondarily, right atrial pressure. The left-right atrial pressure difference closes the foramen ovale in the interatrial septum. Since this pressure difference is small, some right-to-left shunt may persist for 24 hours or longer.

At birth, pulmonary arterial pressure almost equals systemic arterial pressure and decreases only gradually. We are not surprised at this; a sudden fall in pulmonary vascular resistance would reverse the flow of blood through the ductus arteriosus before its lumen closes, resulting in a great imbalance of outputs from right and left ventricles.

Closure of the ductus arteriosus eliminates the circulatory shunt that bypasses the pulmonary circulation from pulmonary artery to aorta; hence, all venous blood flows through the lungs after birth. The ductus arteriosus is constricted by increased P_{O_2} and by catecholamines. Hypoxemia dilates the ductus, while constricting pulmonary arteries, and for some time after birth can reestablish a fetal pattern of circulation. This difference in reactivity of the ductus arteriosus and pulmonary arteries assists the hypoxic fetus by increasing effective cardiac output, but this difference is a liability to the hypoxic newborn infant because it increases ductal right-to-left shunt and further decreases O_2 uptake.

REGULATION OF RESPIRATION IN THE INFANT

Near term the fetal animal responds poorly to the chemical stimuli of acidosis, hypercapnia, and hypoxemia; however, younger fetuses respond to hypoxia with intrauterine gasps. Functional carotid chemoreceptors are present in the fetus, but for unknown reasons they are not generally active. However, it has been shown repeatedly that infants are responsive to chemical respiratory stimulants immediately after birth. Tonic chemoreceptor activity in infants is temporarily decreased by administration of pure O_2, and a ventilatory response to hypoxia is seen even during the first day of life. Measurement of the infant response to hypoxia is complicated by the influence of other variables, such as temperature, tactile stimuli, and perhaps other sensory inputs.

There is increasing reason to believe that the sensitivity of the newborn infant to CO_2 is comparable to that of the adult, but it is difficult to compare the ventilatory responses meaningfully. Is it more valid to compare the ventilatory response of infants with that of adults in terms of body weight or on the basis of body surface area? Apparent differences may result from such a choice.

As in the adult, decreased arterial blood pH in the infant is a stimulus to pulmonary ventilation that is independent of CO_2. Thus metabolic acidosis increases ventilation even in the presence of decreased arterial P_{CO_2}. Temperature also has an important effect on the pulmonary ventilation of infants; ventilation increases in response to modest cooling. More importantly, the sensitivity to hypercapnia decreases greatly during mild hypothermia.

The few studies that have been done with human infants indicate that neurogenic reflexes are active in the newborn. The neural pattern is presumed to be the same as that of adults (Fig. 11-1). Pulmonary stretch receptors are responsive in the fetus; the afferent impulses travel in the vagus nerve. These receptors inhibit the inspiratory activity of a medullary center (Hering-Breuer reflex), modifying the tonic effect of pontine centers on the medulla.

The paradoxical reflex of Head is an inspiratory gasp in response to a sudden increase of intratracheal pressure that distends the airway or inflates the lung; it is observed in the adult as well as in the newborn human infant. The afferent pathway of this reflex is in the vagus nerve. Except during "frog-breathing" and vigorous crying, the functional significance of this reflex in the infant is unknown.

Subthreshold stimuli establish a "local excitatory state" in the medullary center that is a prerequisite for rhythmic breathing. Both higher and lower nonrespiratory central nervous system mechanisms are involved. Skin temperature changes and tactile stimuli are not only important in the initiation of breathing at birth but also for the continuation of breathing throughout life. We are just beginning to appreciate the importance of the activity of nonrespiratory systems in establishing and maintaining respiration.

RESPIRATORY DISTRESS SYNDROME OF THE NEWBORN

Respiratory distress syndrome (RDS) is a multifactorial syndrome and the most frequent pulmonary complication of newborn infants. It usually contains elements of anatomic immaturity, hypoxia, and acidosis, as well as surfactant deficiency. The condition is more common in premature infants, in infants of mothers who have abnormalities of lipid metabolism (e.g., diabetes mellitus), and in infants who have experienced asphyxia during birth.

Normally, surfactant first appears in the lung at 24 to 28 weeks of fetal life; initially low, fetal pulmonary compliance increases during development. In RDS of the newborn a surfactant deficiency prevents the alveolar lining fluid from decreasing its surface tension as alveolar area decreases. Fig. 13-4 shows an idealized comparison of an extract from normal lung with the lung extract from a patient who died of RDS. Surface tension decreases only slightly as area is reduced in the abnormal lung extract.

The signs and symptoms of RDS appear to relate to a lack of change of alveolar surface tension during lung excursion. These include the following:

1. *Labored breathing.* Since alveolar sur-

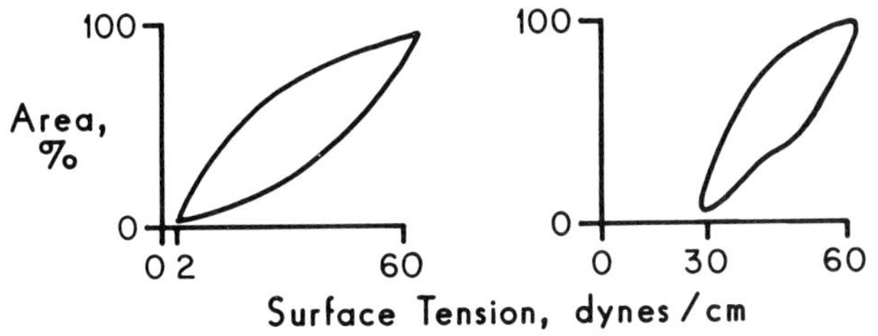

Fig. 13-4
Surface tension as a function of area for surfactant-containing lung extract (left) and surfactant-deficient lung extract (right).

face tension in RDS remains high, a greater transpulmonary pressure is required to increase alveolar volume during inflation (decreased compliance). Lung inflation thus requires more work. This increased work of breathing leads to hypoventilation, acidosis, exhaustion, and finally, collapse of the infant.

2. *Atelectasis.* In RDS an uneven atelectasis occurs with large patches of closed alveoli. The surface tension of small alveoli does not decrease sufficiently for them to remain open at the transpulmonary pressure required to maintain larger alveoli and they collapse. As a result, some blood passes from the pulmonary artery to the pulmonary veins without exposure to lung areas of gas exchange; this right-to-left shunt results in hypoxemia, CO_2 retention, and respiratory acidosis.

3. *Hyaline membrane.* The small radius of unopened alveoli and the increased surface tension due to surfactant deficiency unbalance the equilibrium forces that normally govern fluid movement across the alveolocapillary membrane. The high surface tension of the alveolar lining fluid increases the net force that drives fluid into alveoli and an ultrafiltrate of plasma moves into alveoli from the pulmonary capillaries, interfering further with gas exchange. This ultrafiltrate appears a glassy pale blue after the lung is processed and stained for microscopic examination; hence, *hyaline membrane.* The hyaline membrane was originally believed to consist of aspirated amniotic fluid and to cause the syndrome previously termed *hyaline membrane disease.* The "membrane" is now known to result from the syndrome whose fundamental cause appears to be a surfactant deficiency in the alveolar lining fluid of the newborn infant.

CHAPTER 14 Respiratory responses to unusual environments and special atmospheres

HYPOVENTILATION AND ASPHYXIA

Mammals evolved from forms that lived at sea level. Survival included the avoidance of asphyxia. These animals survived, in part, because they developed chemoreceptors which, when excited, increased breathing. Increased CO_2 and decreased O_2 usually occur together and elicit the same qualitative, but not necessarily the same quantitative, responses (Fig. 14-1). Both increase pulmonary ventilation and cerebral blood flow, but CO_2 is more effective. Both increase coronary blood flow, although hypoxia is more potent in this regard. Both cause airway constriction, and both lower body temperature.

Asphyxia can be produced in various degrees by breath-holding, rebreathing from a closed system or in a closed space, breathing through a tube that artificially increases dead space, chest-binding or otherwise limiting breath size, interposing obstruction to breathing, creating a large pneumothorax, opening the chest cavity so that breathing efforts are ineffective, or paralyzing the respiratory neuromuscular apparatus.

Asphyxia, or suffocation, still occurs today in certain situations—infants in their beds or with plastic films over the face that act as one-way respiratory valves, children closed in empty refrigerators, men trapped in ditch cave-ins or avalanches, and strangulation due to aspiration of food or to criminal assault.

Hypoxia

The term *anoxia* means no oxygen; *hypoxia* means less than normal oxygen pressure. Anoxia has frequently been used to describe situations that are hypoxic, not anoxic. Hypoxia may occur from a variety of causes operating at any of various transport levels, which Luft* has classified as shown in Table 8.

Hypoxia may be defined as either insufficient P_{O_2} or insufficient concentration of free O_2 molecules to meet the requirements of aerobic metabolism. *Histohypoxia* means a reduced P_{O_2} at the cellular level. The function of intracellular enzymes can be impaired in the presence of normal P_{O_2}, or such impairment may even be the result of excessive P_{O_2}, as shown by studies of hyperbaric oxygenation. Thus a term is needed to indicate all conditions involving impairment of aerobic metabolism. Strughold has suggested the term *hypoxidosis* for this purpose. Hypoxidosis includes (1)

*We are indebted to Dr. Ulrich C. Luft for his discussion of the problems involved in the classification of hypoxia.

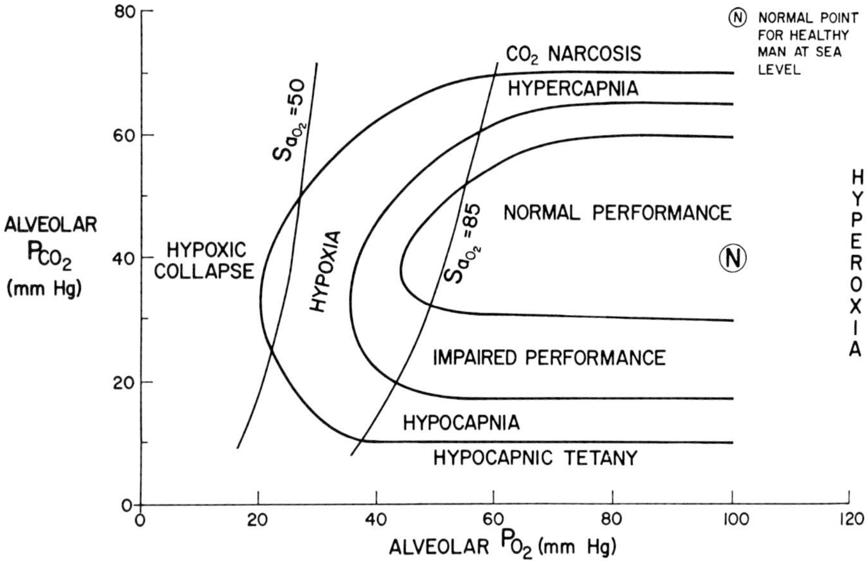

Fig. 14-1

O_2-CO_2 diagram, showing alveolar patterns of respiratory gas disturbance. (From Rahn, H., and Fenn, W. O.: A graphical analysis of the respiratory gas exchange, Washington, D. C., 1955, The American Physiological Society.)

hypoxia, (2) lack or dysfunction of intracellular enzymes, (3) lack of energy sources or substrate, and (4) excessive accumulation of metabolites.

Aerobic metabolism may be slowed in response to reduced energy requirements, although transport and utilization potentials for O_2 are normal. This type of hypometabolism is termed *hypoxidation* and includes the following: (1) hypothermia, (2) hibernation. (3) the effects of depressant drugs or anesthetics, and (4) hypothyroidism.

Increased tissue O_2 consumption does not produce histohypoxia unless capillary blood flow to the metabolizing tissue fails to match the increased requirements. When this happens, the primary site of hypoxia may be considered to be in the capillary. The term *inadequate* capillary blood flow is then more descriptive than the term *decreased* capillary blood flow. Capillary hypoxia is inevitably associated with either regional or general venous hypoxia.

Chronic alveolar hypoventilation

Hypoventilation is an important pathophysiologic aspect of certain clinical entities. The term *chronic alveolar hypoventilation* is used to describe this problem. As already implied, hypoventilation produces both hypoxemia and CO_2 retention. These blood-gas disturbances, if present for months to years, can result in a chain of serious consequences: respiratory acidosis, pulmonary arterial hypertension, and polycythemia. Hypercapnia produces somnolence. Polycythemia increases blood viscosity. Increased blood viscosity together with increased pulmonary arterial pressure increases the work of the right ventricle, leading to hypertrophy and eventual insufficiency.

Patients with extreme obesity may exhibit this chain of consequences. The symptoms of the fat boy were well described by Dickens and have been termed a "pickwickian syndrome." Another clinical example of chronic alveolar hypoventilation is

Table 8
Classification of hypoxia*

Type	Primary site of disturbance	Cause
Aerohypoxia	Inspired gas	1. Altitude 2. Decompression simulating altitude 3. Confined breathing space 4. Low O_2 breathing mixtures
Alveolar hypoxia	Alveolar gas	1. Alveolar hypoventilation not due to bronchopulmonary disease 2. Alveolar hypoventilation due to bronchopulmonary disease
Arterial hypoxia	Systemic arterial blood	1. Impaired alveolocapillary diffusion a. Loss of surface area b. Increased length of diffusion pathway 2. Venous-to-arterial shunts (intrapulmonary or cardiovascular) 3. Maldistribution of: a. Alveolar ventilation and/or pulmonary capillary blood flow b. Diffusion and/or pulmonary capillary blood flow
Capillary hypoxia	Systemic capillary blood	1. Decreased or inadequate capillary blood flow a. General b. Local 2. Reduced O_2 capacity a. Anemia b. Abnormal or bound hemoglobin (e.g., methemoglobin or carboxyhemoglobin) 3. Increased affinity of hemoglobin for O_2 a. Alkalosis b. Hypothermia
Histohypoxia	Tissues	1. Impaired diffusion due to tissue edema, fibrosis, or calcification 2. Increased tissue demand 3. Poisoning of intracellular enzymes

*Modified from Luft, U. C.: Aviation physiology—the effects of altitude, Handbook of physiology, Section 3, Respiration, vol. 2, Washington, D. C., 1965, The American Physiological Society, p. 1109.

kyphoscoliosis, in which thoracic deformity prevents adequate pulmonary ventilation.

Snorkel breathing

A snorkel (from German, "little snout") is a tube, or pair of tubes, housing air intake and exhaust pipes that can be extended above the surface of the water for operating submerged craft. The term also refers to a plastic breathing tube with a mouthpiece at one end and a valve at the other that admits air when projected above water, but closes when submerged. It is used for swimming near the surface with the head under water.

What is the maximum length of a snorkel tube through which a person can breathe? Several physiologic considerations are involved.* If the subject inspires through the tube but expires into the water around him, there is no problem of added dead space. However, if he expires through the snorkel tube, respiratory dead space is increased and he always reinspires some of his expired gas. The longer the tube the more the rebreathing. This phenomenon could be a depth-limiting factor, depending upon the volume of the tube.

If the tube is very narrow, the resistance to air flow is so great that an adequate ventilation rate cannot be achieved. Note that the ventilation rate necessary is increased by the increased work of breathing.

Another factor is the maximum inspiratory pressure a subject can exert in sucking in his breath. Beneath the surface the pressure of the water upon a subject's chest tends to deflate the lungs. If he dives while holding his breath, intrapulmonary pressure increases to the level of the hydrostatic pressure of the surrounding water as gas in the lungs is compressed. However, in breathing through a snorkel tube, intrapulmonary pressure is essentially the same as ambient pressure at the water surface. Reference to the pressure-volume diagram of chest wall and lungs in healthy man (Fig. 5-4) shows that he can exert, at maximum, an inspiratory pressure of about 100 mm Hg. This is about 1,350 mm of water and corresponds to a depth of about 1.33 M.

The heart is another very important consideration. Since the chest contents are essentially at atmospheric pressure whereas the body generally is subject to the pressure of the surrounding water, the heart must pump "uphill" into a vascular bed of very high resistance. Increased work of the heart could well be limiting in this circumstance. Lanari and Bromberger studied healthy submerged human subjects who were breathing through tubes; they found showers of ventricular premature systoles.

*This problem reminds us of our hero hiding in the water from his enemies. He is completely submerged and quietly breathing through a hollow reed that the motion picture film producer has conveniently provided for the purpose.

HYPERVENTILATION AND TETANY

Acapnia means a lack or absence of CO_2. *Hypocapnia* means lower than normal P_{CO_2}. Physiologically, acapnia is unknown. If an infinitely high ventilation rate were possible, it would bring alveolar gas to the concentration levels of tracheal gas and reduce the P_{CO_2} of arterial blood to zero. Hyperventilation moves alveolar and blood-gas tensions in the direction of inspired air (Fig. 14-2). Alveolar and arterial P_{O_2} values increase, but as already implied, no amount of hyperventilation could increase these P_{O_2} values beyond the P_{O_2} of inspired air.

The dizziness experienced on blowing up an air mattress is the result of reduced P_{CO_2}, not increased P_{O_2}. Hyperventilation lowers P_{CO_2}; if the alveolar ventilation rate is doubled, alveolar P_{CO_2} is halved. If alveolar P_{CO_2} decreases to the level of 20 or 25 mm Hg in a sea-level resident, he experiences dizziness and numbness and tingling of the extremities. Systemic arterial blood pressure falls and there is cerebral vasoconstriction. A decrease of alveolar P_{CO_2} to a level of 15 or 20 mm Hg may produce tetany. This condition is characterized by increased neuromuscular excitability, muscular tension, spontaneous twitching, and sustained involuntary muscular contractions. It is the result of acute respiratory alkalosis and the related decrease of Ca^{++} concentration. Hyperventilating subjects are prone to develop a particular spasm of the hands and feet, termed *carpopedal spasm.* At P_{CO_2} levels associated with dizziness, numbness, and tingling, there is usually loss of neuromuscular coordination and psychomotor performance. This performance decrement may be a serious matter if the hyperventilating subject is a jet aircraft pilot.

Hyperventilation can evoke abnormal

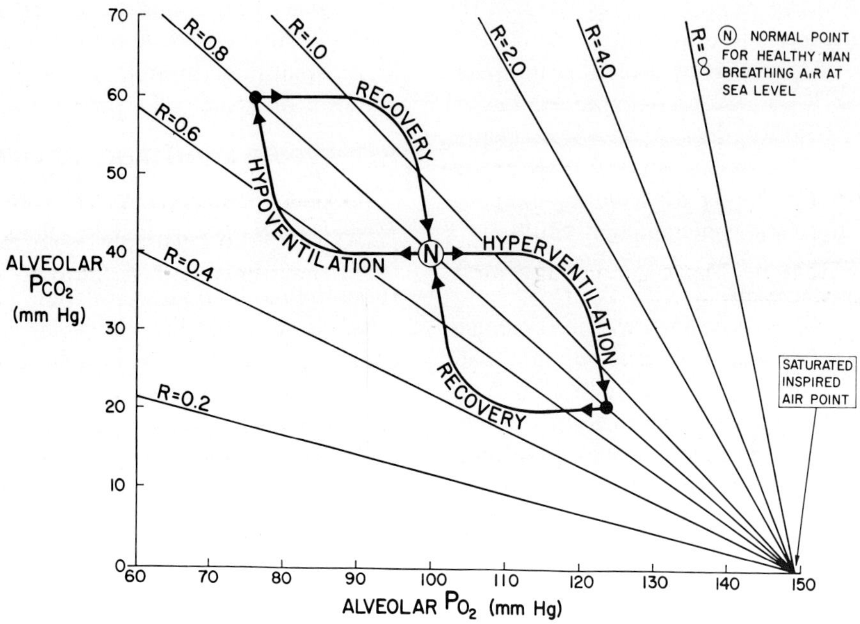

Fig. 14-2

O_2-CO_2 diagram, showing alveolar pathways during hyperventilation, hypoventilation, and recovery. (From Rahn, H., and Fenn, W. O.: A graphical analysis of the respiratory gas exchange, Washington, D. C., 1955, The American Physiological Society.)

electroencephalographic patterns. It is standard practice for EEG technicians to perform a hyperventilation test. The 3-per-second dome and spike pattern of petit mal epilepsy is sometimes discovered in this way.

Hyperventilation tends to be hypnotic. Some individuals cannot stop, even in tetany, unless commanded to do so. Amateur mountain climbers sometimes continue high ventilation rates into their rest periods. Such ventilation then constitutes hyperventilation because metabolic rate is lower at rest. P_{CO_2} falls and the climber feels dizzy. Experienced group leaders carry paper or plastic bags into which hyperventilators can rebreathe; this conserves CO_2, and the dizziness disappears.

Both the hypoxia of high altitude and the increased H^+ concentration of metabolic acidosis increase pulmonary ventilation. This hyperventilation reduces P_{CO_2}. If either hypoxia or acidosis persists, "acclimatization" to low P_{CO_2} occurs. Individuals so acclimatized develop increased resistance to the effects of low P_{CO_2}. After such acclimatization, tingling and dizziness may not occur until alveolar P_{CO_2} falls to a level of 15 or 20 mm Hg; tetany may not occur until alveolar P_{CO_2} drops to 10 mm Hg.

Hyperventilation is an important clinical problem. Aside from its occurrence in acidosis, massive hemorrhage, and salicylism, it commonly indicates emotional stress. Such stress may be of psychoneurotic origin or may occur in relation to the realistic problems of living. Hyperventilation is often observed in visitors to high altitude, where its symptoms complicate the usual responses. Hyperventilation of emotional origin may be sustained or episodic. The episodic type is sometimes of dramatically sudden onset, may involve extreme hyperventilation, and is rapidly productive of distressing symptoms. (See also the discussion of emotional stress pattern, p. 181.)

The symptoms of hyperventilation are often misdiagnosed as serious organic disease. Paradoxically, the patient often complains that he "can't get enough air." Dizziness, hypotension, and cerebral vasoconstriction can produce serious impairment of psychomotor performance, the implications of which should not be underestimated.

If hyperventilation is suspected, the diagnosis is usually simple: (1) measurable, if not perceptible, increase of minute volume of breathing; (2) reproducibility of symptoms by hyperventilation; (3) abolition of symptoms by rebreathing; and (4) arterial blood findings of increased P_{O_2} and pH in association with decreased P_{CO_2} (respiratory alkalosis).

ALTITUDE AND HYPOBARISM

The altitude-pressure table in the Appendix (p. 199) shows the relationship between altitude and barometric pressure. Note that 5,500 M, or 18,000 feet, corresponds to a barometric pressure of 380 mm Hg, or one half of the sea level value of 760 mm Hg, at which altitude atmospheric air is one half as dense as it is at sea level. Another value of particular interest is that at 19,200 M, or 63,000 feet, the barometric pressure is 47 mm Hg and equals the water vapor tension in the lungs at 37° C.

Responses and acclimatization

Unfortunately man is not endowed with any sensory mechanism to transduce falling P_{O_2} into a red alert. This lack is in striking contrast to the alarming dyspnea of rising CO_2 levels. Characteristic features of hypoxic accidents are the insidious onset of impairment and the victim's lack of awareness of danger.* Decompression chamber experiments have shown an interesting pattern of cerebral dysfunction as hypoxia becomes more severe. This pattern involves progressively more frequent and longer periods of cerebral uselessness interspersed between relatively lucid intervals.

If a newcomer to high altitude ascends above a critical level and remains there beyond a critical length of time, he may experience fatigue, headache, irritability, dizziness, palpitation, nausea, loss of appetite, coupled breathing, exertional dyspnea, abdominal cramps, impaired cerebration, insomnia, and, rarely, pulmonary edema (Fig. 14-3). Men are more likely to develop palpitation and dyspnea. A constellation of these symptoms is termed *acute mountain sickness.* The first day and night are usually the worst; after that the newcomer gradually feels better, but it may be many days before he is reasonably comfortable. Many newcomers feel dehydrated initially but have little desire to drink.

Hypoxia causes hyperventilation,† which reduces alveolar and arterial P_{CO_2}, producing respiratory alkalosis. Under the influence of reduced P_{CO_2} the kidney excretes HCO_3^-. However, this compensation is nullified by a further increase in ventilation on the second day. More HCO_3^- excretion is followed by still greater hyperventilation. After 7 to 10 days, ventilation no longer increases. The kidney continues to excrete HCO_3^-, and arterial blood pH falls toward normal.

---

*Women are more resistant (as usual) to the effects of hypoxia than men.

†E. B. Brown observed that about 3% of a male military population tended to faint during decompression simulating altitude and used the term "fainter" to describe these subjects. It appears that occasional individuals do not respond to hypoxia with the usual increase in pulmonary ventilation. The mechanism and implications of this observation for altitude acclimatization, anesthesia, and various cardiopulmonary diseases remain unexplored.

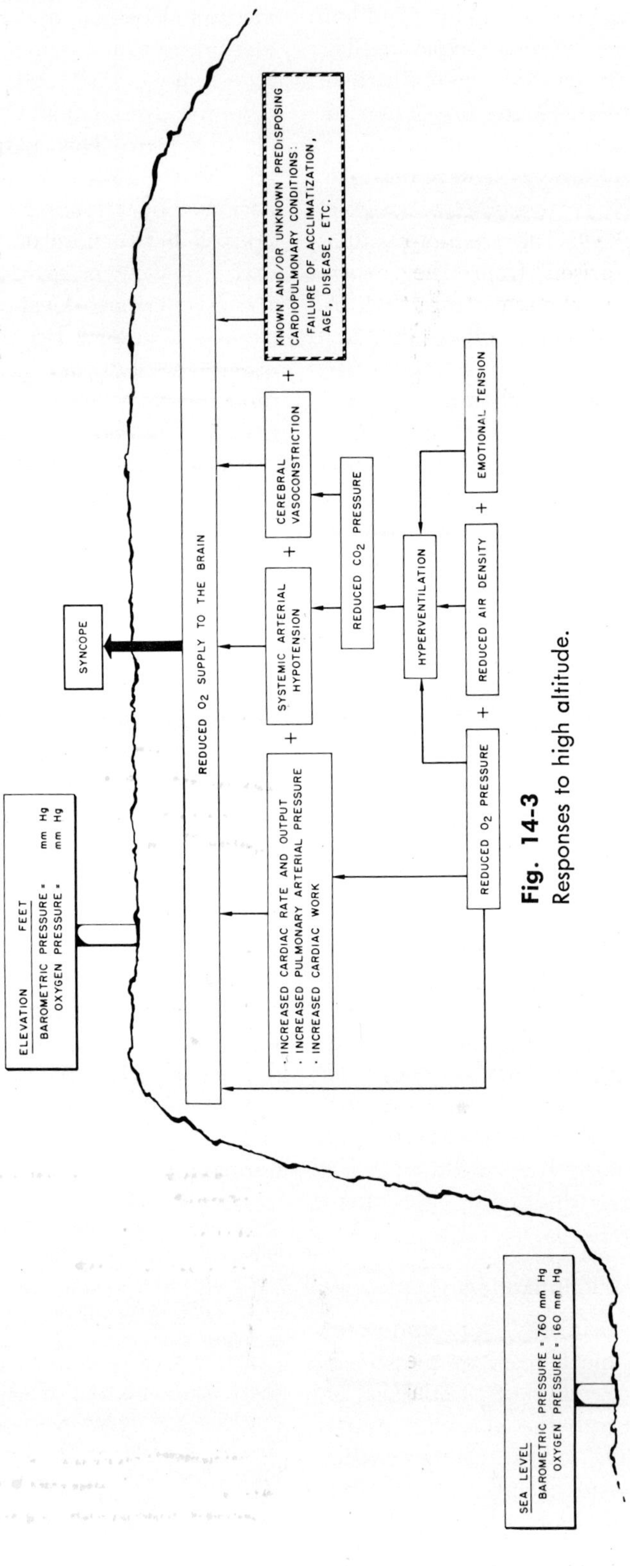

Fig. 14-3
Responses to high altitude.

The ventilatory events during altitude acclimatization result from an interplay between the central and peripheral chemoreceptors. Hypoxia initiates hyperventilation, and hyperventilation reduces P_{CO_2}, producing respiratory alkalosis both in blood and in the environment of the central chemoreceptors. The ventilatory drive that normally arises from the central chemoreceptors is depressed so that the chemical drive for breathing is then hypoxic. However, as the respiratory alkalosis of the central chemoreceptors is compensated for by gradual loss of HCO_3^-, ventilatory drive returns over a period of many days, gradually adding to the hypoxic drive to increase total ventilation.

Postulating a CO_2 dissociation curve for the fluid environment of the central chemoreceptors, we may speculate as follows. Carbon dioxide sensitivity increases because of the new low CO_2 dissociation curve. A small shift to the right (increasing P_{CO_2}) along this curve changes pH more than a similar shift along the higher, normal CO_2 dissociation curve. Recovery of the ability to respond to CO_2 despite continuous hyperventilation is an important aspect of altitude acclimatization. After acclimatization the pH of cerebrospinal fluid has been normal at all altitudes studied.

When the acclimatized subject descends from altitude, arterial P_{O_2} increases and the hypoxic drive is reduced or abolished. This decreases ventilation somewhat, as a result of which P_{CO_2} increases. However, the P_{CO_2} rise produces respiratory acidosis in the central chemoreceptors, increasing their ventilatory drive. Ventilation does not return to normal until this respiratory acidosis of the central chemoreceptors is compensated for by accumulation of HCO_3^-. After descent from acclimatized residence at high altitude, hyperventilation persists for several weeks.

A definite tolerance to low P_{O_2} develops as the newcomer remains at high altitude, and the minimum P_{O_2} that will sustain consciousness decreases. Altitude acclimatization involves acclimatization *both* to low O_2 and to low CO_2, the latter reflecting *sustained* hyperventilation in the successfully acclimatizing individual. Appetite and a sense of well-being gradually return.

Occasionally a high altitude dweller stops hyperventilating and may even hypoventilate. P_{CO_2} rises and P_{O_2} falls to levels inconsistent with useful performance. This has been suggested as an important mechanism in the development of *chronic mountain sickness.*

It is a mistake to assume that metabolic rate decreases on ascent to altitude merely because ambient P_{O_2} is low. Metabolic rate actually increases somewhat because of increased work of breathing, acclimatization to low temperature, and increased sympathetic nervous system activity. In a study of the acute effects of exposure to high altitude, Chidsey and Beckwitt found a 10% to 15% increase of basal metabolic rate. This increase returned to the normal control level at about the tenth day of the exposure. Increased O_2 uptake and BMR, norepinephrine, and free as well as total thyroxine were observed. Epinephrine remained essentially unchanged. These data suggest increased sympathetic nervous system activity rather than increased adrenal medullary activity.

Exposure to altitude increases thyroid function. This is presumably due to increased secretion of pituitary thyrotropic hormone (TSH). Under conditions of actual exposure at high altitude, therefore, the combined effects of hypoxia and cold probably both play a role in elevating the level of thyroid function. Experimental evidence suggests that hypothyroidism protects against the effects of altitude, presumably because it reduces the O_2 requirement of experimental animals. Hyperthyroid rats have been found to be more susceptible to altitude than normal rats. Glucocorticosteroids (GCS) also protect against the effects of altitude; smaller doses are necessary for protection of hypothyroid experimental animals.

Ascent to high altitude is associated with a prompt, slight rise of hematocrit, hemoglobin concentration, and erythrocyte count.* In man this increase is probably not a result of splenic contraction as it may be in the dog. A shift of fluid out of the vascular compartment, producing hemoconcentration, has been postulated.

Increased red blood cell production (erythropoiesis) in the bone marrow is stimulated by the hormone *erythropoietin*, which increases during hypoxia. The resulting polycythemia develops over a period of weeks to months. This polycythemia is marked in young people, is less pronounced among the middle-aged, and may be completely absent in the aged. The erythropoiesis-stimulating hormone, erythropoietin, is governed by P_{O_2}. The polycythemia of altitude acclimatization and the anemia of chronic hyperoxia are illustrative examples of this fact.

At one time some physiologists believed that hemoglobin produced at high altitude had a different oxyhemoglobin dissociation curve; however, it is now clear that hemoglobin produced at altitude is the same as hemoglobin produced at sea level (Hb A).

The myoglobin content and vascularity of muscle increase as a result of exposure to high altitude. Studies of chronically hypoxic rats indicate that this increased vascularity is due to increased number of capillaries, rather than simply increased patency of existing vessels. Although examples of anatomic and biochemical responses to altitude are known, much remains to be learned of the biochemistry of hypoxia- and pH-sensing organs, as well as the biochemistry of tissue responses.

During exercise at high altitude, healthy individuals show increased alveolar P_{O_2} but decreased arterial P_{O_2} and saturation. With this fact in mind, certain athletic teams competing at high altitude have breathed O_2 before performance. This has greater psychologic than physiologic value because the body is poorly equipped to store O_2. The solubility of O_2 at body temperature is low (Table 5). The lungs are the major site of O_2 storage but they lose their extra supply rapidly as soon as the athlete breathes air. At intermediate altitudes that boast competitive sports, arterial oxyhemoglobin saturation is relatively good—above 90%. Oxygen breathing can increase this saturation, but the volume of O_2 gained is small. Because of the shape of its dissociation curve, myoglobin remains saturated until P_{O_2} falls to extremely low values.

Oxygen breathing during exercise at high altitude has real value. It permits considerably higher metabolic rates than does breathing air at the same altitude. Oxygen breathing after exercise speeds recovery and improves the way an athlete feels.

The significance and extent of acclimatization can be seen from the fact that altitude-acclimatized mountain climbers can climb at ambient P_{O_2} levels which are too low to sustain the consciousness of sea-level residents. Altitude acclimatization, which includes the process of acclimatization to low CO_2 as well as to low O_2, decreases tolerance for high CO_2. After altitude acclimatization the capacity for breath-holding and underwater swimming is therefore greatly reduced.

The hazard of carbon monoxide intoxication is greater at altitude. It is estimated

*This increase of hemoglobin concentration is similar to the prompt increase observed with exercise, during which increases of 10% may occur within 5 minutes. Thus determination of hemoglobin concentration and O_2 capacity is relatively meaningless unless the conditions of physical activity and P_{O_2} are precisely stated.

that for every 1% carboxyhemoglobin present, altitude tolerance is reduced by about 335 feet. High altitude hypoxia also means that internal combustion engines produce larger amounts of CO because of less complete combustion. Smokers are more likely to feel the effects of CO poisoning than are nonsmokers because of both pulmonary dysfunction and the initial carboxyhemoglobin levels.

The following observations seem to indicate a relationship between hypoxemia or deficient systemic arterial blood flow and growth failure or weight loss, although the mechanisms are presently unknown:

1. Obesity is quite uncommon at high altitude. Mountaineers sojourning at very high altitude lose weight continuously. The mechanism of this weight loss is uncertain, although hypoxia, anorexia, dehydration, cold, and increased thyroid function probably all play a role. Weight loss may amount to as much as 30 to 40 pounds over a period of 6 weeks at extremely high altitude.
2. The birth weight of infants born at altitude is less, and the higher the altitude the less the weight. If we define prematurity as a birth weight of less than 2,500 grams, then the higher the altitude the higher also is the prevalence of prematurity.
3. Patients with severe pulmonary emphysema characteristically lose weight.
4. Congenital cardiovascular diseases with decreased cardiac output or with arterial hypoxemia are often associated with growth failure.

Summary of findings at 1-mile elevation

Many cities are situated at elevations considerably above sea level. In cities at 1 mile above sea level such as Denver, Colorado, Albuquerque, New Mexico, and Guadalajara, Mexico, the following physiologic effects may be observed in healthy acclimatized individuals:

1. Inspired P_{O_2} is about 130 mm Hg (dry) instead of 160 mm Hg (dry) as at sea level, resulting in a slightly hypoxemic arterial P_{O_2} of 75 mm Hg. Arterial blood O_2 saturation at rest is therefore 94% instead of 97% as at sea level.
2. There is slight hyperventilation at rest as well as for any higher metabolic level.
3. Slight respiratory alkalosis results from the chronic hyperventilation. Alveolar and arterial P_{CO_2} values are 36 mm Hg instead of 40 mm Hg as at sea level.
4. There is slight compensatory metabolic acidosis with whole blood total CO_2 content of 19 mM/L instead of 22 mM/L as at sea level.
5. Minute volume of breathing and alveolar ventilation decrease promptly when O_2-enriched gas mixtures are breathed, indicating abolition of tonic peripheral chemoreceptor activity.
6. Total circulating hemoglobin mass and concentration are slightly increased as a result of the hypoxemia.
7. Ventilatory capacity (expressed BTPS) is slightly increased (about 10%) as a result of decreased air density.
8. Visual dark adaptation is slightly impaired as a result of hypoxemia. Aircraft pilots should use supplemental O_2 during night flights above 1-mile altitude.
9. The mean electrical axis of the QRS complex of the electrocardiogram shows slight right deviation for subjects of comparable age as compared to data from sea level.
10. The birth weight of infants is slightly lower than at sea level.

Pulmonary arterial hypertension

High altitude dwellers are said to exhibit low systemic arterial blood pressure; however, strikingly high pulmonary arterial pressure is a confirmed fact, and during exercise, systolic pulmonary arterial pressure may rise to more than 100 mm Hg. Significant pulmonary arterial hypertension is found in otherwise healthy individuals living at or above an elevation of 10,000 feet.*

Significant species differences in response to the hypoxia of high altitude have been noted. Sheep have been found relatively unreactive in contrast to cattle, which resemble human subjects in their reaction.

The mean electrical axis of QRS in the frontal plane shows increasing right deviation in populations at progressively higher altitude. Age, somatotype, and functional residual capacity are also factors affecting the electrical axis of QRS. This right axis shift quite probably reflects the right ventricular hypertrophy resulting from pulmonary arterial hypertension. The following data show the relationship between altitude and mean QRS axis.

	Altitude (feet)	*Mean QRS axis (degrees)*
Lima, Peru	500	+55°
Denver, Colorado	5,300	+68°
Leadville, Colorado	10,200	+84°
Morococha, Peru	14,900	+125°

High altitude pulmonary edema. An acute pulmonary edema may occur in individuals at elevations above 9,000 feet. This condition has been noted to occur especially in those originally residing at high altitude who are returning after an interval at lower elevations. It has been observed in both sexes and in children as young as 5 years of age. It often follows exertion at altitude, but not necessarily. Patients with high altitude pulmonary edema should be given supplemental O_2 and removed to a lower altitude as rapidly as possible; the condition is reversible by prompt, vigorous therapy but is occasionally fatal. The clinical findings include pulmonary edema with bilateral patchy infiltrations in the chest roentgenogram, arterial hypoxemia, increased pulmonary arterial pressure, reduced cardiac output, but normal heart size. In fatal cases postmortem examination has shown thrombi in pulmonary capillary and precapillary vessels.

Interval studies have shown normal pulmonary artery wedge, as well as left atrial, pressure. However, Grover found tachycardia in patients subject to high altitude pulmonary edema. In studies of exercise at altitude such patients showed abnormally large changes in arterial P_{O_2}, alveoloarterial P_{O_2} gradient, and pulmonary arterial pressure in comparison with exercise studies of healthy subjects at altitude.

High altitude disease of cattle. Cattle living at elevations of 10,000 feet or more often develop a condition termed *brisket disease,* named for the edematous brisket of the affected animal. Pathophysiologically, it is a chronic pulmonary arterial hypertension, resulting in right ventricular failure. Brisket disease is an economically important problem and resembles chronic mountain sickness of human beings in almost all important respects. However, cattle residing at high altitude do not develop appreciable polycythemia and have been reported to show increased clotting time. It is also of interest that cattle fail to sustain hyperventilation at high altitude. Animals vary greatly in their individual response to the same hypoxemic stress, and different species vary even more so. For example, a comparable condition does not occur in sheep living at the same altitude.

Acclimatization as opposed to adaptation

There is no general agreement on terminology to describe the physiologic processes involved in a single individual's becoming accustomed to altitude over a period of days to years, as opposed to the tolerance observed in groups of people

*A relationship between residence at high altitude and the prevalence of the uncommon clinical entity, *essential pulmonary arterial hypertension,* has been suggested.

living at altitude for generations. We will refer to the first process as *acclimatization* and to the second process as *adaptation*. Adaptation includes, among other things, a restoration of fertility (adequately functioning germinal epithelium) that people merely acclimatized to altitude do not recover. There is evidence that the processes of altitude adaptation, occurring over many generations, result in pulmonary arterial hypertension of somewhat lesser degree.

By far the largest populations at high altitude live in the Andes mountains of South America. Some of these people live at what may be the upper limit for permanent human habitation—a village at 17,600 feet above sea level. Amerind natives of the high Andes are of short stature but are large chested and able to engage in vigorous ball games. When they act as porters, they run with their loads until tired or winded, at which time they sit down and rest before another cycle of activity.

The Sherpas of Nepal are known for their assistance as pack-bearers in numerous Himalayan climbing expeditions. Indeed, it is no exaggeration to say that without their assistance such expeditions would be impossible. It was Tenzing Norkey, a Sherpa, who together with Edmund Hillary first climbed Mount Everest (1953).

There is a popular belief that residents at high altitude are better equipped than sea-level residents to engage in high altitude athletics. Although this may be true for altitude-*adapted* individuals, it does not appear to be true for those who are merely *acclimatized* to high altitude. Grover and Reeves arranged for a track team from Leadville, Colorado (altitude 10,200 feet), to compete first at Leadville and then in Kentucky against a championship Kentucky track team. The Leadville team was defeated as badly at Leadville as it was in Kentucky.

To understand this a clear-cut distinction must be drawn between those athletic events that are extremely demanding but relatively brief (essentially anaerobic) and those events of longer duration that are essentially aerobic. Grover and Reeves showed that exhausting events of less than 1 minute's duration were done as well in Leadville as in Kentucky. However, as the time required for exhausting events increased, performance in Leadville fell progressively further short of performance in Kentucky.

Subatmospheric decompression and altitude chambers

It is convenient to distinguish two types of decompression—subatmospheric decompression to which aerospace travellers are exposed as opposed to the decompression from high pressure down to atmospheric level to which divers are exposed. Morbid consequences of the former are termed *altitude decompression sickness,** a term for all early sequelae of decompression from atmospheric level down to ambient pressures of 0.5 to 0.06 atm. These sequelae include the prompt effects of expanding gases trapped in body cavities as well as the delayed effects of gases, primarily nitrogen, that evolve from body fluids and tissue—but not the effects of hypoxia. Morbid consequences of the latter are termed *diver's decompression sickness,* or "caisson disease," from the submerged chambers used in underwater construction work.

In 1908 Boycott and Haldane suggested that exposure to ambient pressures of less than 300 mm Hg could cause decompression sickness. During World War I it was speculated that decompression sickness due

*Decompression of this type presents the same problems of aerobullosis, bends, chokes, and possible lung overinflation as does decompression during ascent from a dive. The term *hypobarogenous aerobulosis* has been suggested by Slonim as more descriptive of what occurs during decompression than the term *aeroembolism.* Actually, embolism is only a part of the pathology of decompression sickness.

to evolved gas could disable a flier. "Bends" precipitated by altitude chamber flights were first described in 1930. Neurocirculatory collapse complicating decompression sickness was first described in 1938, and during World War II aviator's decompression collapse became a well-known entity.

Altitude decompression sickness is usually self-limited, responding readily to a return to ground level or to recompression to 1 atm or more of pressure. Physical exertion promotes the appearance and growth of gas bubbles. A given subject tends to show the same pattern of recurrence of bubbles and symptoms if exposure is repeated. Although tissue deformation caused by the changing volume of trapped gases during ascent may cause intense pain and may even be followed by local inflammatory reaction, life itself is not threatened. The same is true for the effects commonly ascribed to evolved gases. Cerebral and coronary vessels usually show a great many bubbles in decompression sickness, so that symptoms of myocardial or cerebral ischemia can be expected. If circulatory or neurologic symptoms develop, the term *neurocirculatory collapse* is used to describe the symptom complex. Neurocirculatory collapse occurred 150 times during approximately 1,000,000 altitude chamber exposures, an incidence of 0.015%.

The complications of subatmospheric decompression can be minimized or avoided by preflight denitrogenation, by limiting the duration of exposure at altitudes over 20,000 feet, and by discontinuation of flights as soon as symptoms are identified. The recommended treatment for neurocirculatory collapse complicating altitude decompression sickness is prompt compression to 6 atm of pressure, absolute.

Decompression sickness is readily produced experimentally in dogs and other animals. Extensive decompression results in the appearance of gross bubbles in the venous circulation, pulmonary arterial hypertension and tachypnea. These objective signs of decompression sickness are reversed in anesthetized dogs by increasing the ambient pressure. Small increases in ambient pressure may be quite effective in reducing severe pulmonary arterial hypertension. The pulmonary arterial hypertension and tachypnea may be the result of simple mechanical blockage of the pulmonary vascular tree by bubbles,* since bubbles appear in the venous circulation before pulmonary arterial hypertension and tachypnea develop; however, pulmonary reflexes may be important.

Behnke cites rapid, shallow breathing, or tachypnea, as a sign pathognomonic of bubbles in pulmonary vessels after decompression. Exposed subjects with tachypnea should be suspected of aeroembolism before a diagnosis of hyperventilation is accepted, especially if other symptoms of decompression sickness are present.

Bubbles do not appear in the arterial system until circulatory collapse is imminent because intra-arterial pressure is relatively high and because bubbles tend to form in muscles, which they leave by way of the venous circulation. The high-pressure arterial system and the tissues it supplies are thus naturally protected against bubble emboli.

After decompression an experimental animal may appear perfectly stable for 5 to 30 minutes before showing signs of decompression sickness and then, within a minute, develop bubbles in the venous circulation, severe pulmonary arterial hypertension, and tachypnea.

During recompression, gas bubbles in the venous circulation diminish greatly in size but do not completely disappear. Bubbles do not disappear completely during recompression in vitro, either.

Altitude or decompression chambers, from which the air can be evacuated, have

*Injection of small bubbles into the venous circulation also causes pulmonary arterial hypertension and tachypnea.

been constructed in various sizes and shapes. These are used for simulating and testing the effects of altitude without actually going to altitude. In addition to the convenience that such chambers afford, a much more rapid "ascent" can be made than is possible on a mountain. Some chambers are constructed so that pressure can be reduced with extreme rapidity, so as to simulate the sudden decompression an aerospace traveller would encounter if his sealed, pressurized cabin suddenly disintegrated. The term *rapid decompression* is more descriptive than its synonym, explosive decompression.

DIVING AND HYPERBARISM

Diving expeditions are constantly extending our experience with the problems of hyperbarism. In one expedition off Cap Ferrat, France, under Jacques-Yves Cousteau, six men remained at a depth of 100 M for 3 weeks, breathing a 2% O_2–98% helium mixture. Decompressive ascent was accomplished over a period of 4 days. Dives without breathing equipment (free dives) to depths greater than 60 M have been recorded.

During a dive, gas volumes are compressed as predicted by the general gas law: $PV = nRT$—where P is pressure, V is volume, n is the number of moles of gas, R is the gas constant, and T is absolute temperature. At constant temperature if pressure is doubled, volume is halved. If total lung capacity (TLC) is 6 L, a diver who inspires fully at the surface and dives quickly to a depth of 20 M (3 atm total pressure) has only about 2 L of gas in his lungs. If residual volume occupies 1.5 L of his 6 L total lung capacity, this diver could exhale only 500 ml at the 20 M depth. Actually, he could blow out somewhat less, since gas leaves the lungs for the blood under these conditions of pressure.

A diver who fills his lungs with compressed air under a total pressure of 3 atm has three times as many molecules of gas in the lungs as he would have if he filled them at the surface. If he did not allow gas to leave the lungs during ascent, he would be in serious trouble. With open mouth and glottis and with no effort on his part, gas will escape continuously until he reaches the surface. If a diver cannot be certain his glottis is open during ascent, he should assure this by active, slow exhalation.

If a diver whose lungs contain 5% CO_2 holds his breath and plunges rapidly to a depth of 10 M (2 atm total pressure), the lungs still contain 5% CO_2, but since total lung volume is halved, the CO_2 molecules are packed closer together. Although the diver still has 5% CO_2 in the lungs, alveolar P_{CO_2} is doubled. However, the P_{CO_2} of arterial blood is not doubled. Carbon dioxide moves rapidly into the blood, as it would in CO_2 inhalation, and the CO_2 concentration in the lungs decreases.

If the metabolic rate of a diver does not change during a dive, the number of CO_2 molecules entering the venous circulation from the tissues remains constant. During a steady state, which is possible if a diver breathes from a self-contained underwater breathing apparatus (scuba), alveolar P_{CO_2} may be essentially the same as at the surface, but alveolar CO_2 *concentration* may be quite low. A diver at 5 atm pressure may have only 1% CO_2 in the lungs, but the alveolar P_{CO_2} is $0.01\ [(5 \times 760) - 47] = 37.5$ mm Hg.

Divers often show acclimatization to high CO_2 as a result of the increased density and P_{O_2} of breathing mixtures at depth. If they dive without a compressed gas supply, they may also show acclimatization to low O_2 as a result of breath-holding.

As ambient pressure increases, the partial pressure of the constituent gases in a mixture also increases. These increased partial pressures drive more gas into solution in body fluids and tissue than are normally dissolved. During brief exposures, equilibration is far from complete, but as exposure time increases, equilibrium is gradually achieved. The solubility of N_2 in fat is about five times as great as its solubility in body fluids, which explains the predilection of gas bubbles for fatty tissue.

The rapidity of safe ascent from depth depends not only upon depth but also upon the length of time spent at that depth. The greater the depth the greater are the pressures forcing gases into solution. The longer the time spent at depth the more nearly the dissolved gases will have achieved equilibrium. If ascent is too rapid, gases expand, wherever they may be, come out of solution,* cause pain and mechanical obstruction, and form emboli in the blood. If bubbles form in the joints, a diver experiences "bends." If they block the pulmonary circulation, he experiences "chokes." If gas bubble emboli coalesce in the left side of the heart or in the great arteries, they may interfere with cerebral or coronary circulation, a sometimes fatal condition.

When compressed air is breathed during a dive, decompression according to the Standard U. S. Navy Diving Tables is recommended. These tables give safe rates of ascent and should be consulted any time that decompression involves a pressure decrease to one half or less of the pressure experienced at depth, or for decompression following dives deeper than about 10 M. When the pressure decrease exceeds this 2:1 ratio, a diver must decompress gradually by spending time at intermediate depths in order to allow dissolved gas to come out of solution gradually.

Nitrogen is both relatively insoluble and the major atmospheric constituent. Because of its low solubility it leaves gas bubbles slowly. However, it is a mistake to assume that bubbles emerging during decompression consist of pure N_2. Carbon dioxide and O_2 diffuse into a bubble present anywhere in the body until the partial pressures of the gases in the bubble are in equilibrium with the surrounding fluid or tissue and water vapor saturates the bubble gas. Eliminating N_2 from the breathing mixture minimizes bubble formation. Experimental animals breathing pure O_2 are well protected against bubble formation during decompression from any pressure level, as compared to animals breathing N_2-containing mixtures; however, if O_2 is substituted for N_2, another serious problem is created.

Recompression is the treatment of choice for victims of decompression sickness. This may be accomplished either in a recompression chamber or by allowing the diver to descend again so that decompression can be accomplished more slowly.

Nitrogen narcosis

Most physiologists believe that "rapture of the deep," an intoxicated condition which a diver may experience, is *nitrogen narcosis*. Although chemically and physiologically inert at ordinary partial pressure, N_2 is narcotic at high pressure. Substitution of helium for N_2 in the diver's breathing mixture precludes this condition.

However, a few physiologists believe that the symptoms attributed to N_2 are actually due to CO_2 accumulation. The greatly increased density of a breathing mixture at depth increases the work of breathing; for a given effort a smaller volume is ventilated than would be the case if air were being breathed at the surface. According to the CO_2 accumulation theory, it is the increased P_{CO_2} resulting from this hypoventilation that produces the symptoms in question.

***Hypobarogenous aerobullosis* is a neologism proposed by Slonim to mean the generalized emergence and growth of gas bubbles from solution in fluids and tissues throughout the body as a result of decompression. This term should be distinguished from aeroembolism, which has been used in this sense, but as the term suggests, aeroembolism should mean the *intravascular* emergence, growth, and *transport* of gas bubbles as a result of decompression.

The theory continues that substitution of helium for N_2 protects against these symptoms because the less dense helium mixture is easier to breathe. Proponents of the nitrogen narcosis theory suggest that if CO_2 produces light-headed intoxication at depth, then CO_2 inhalation should produce the same effect in the laboratory—and it does not!

HYPEROXIA

Oxygen therapy is often a lifesaving modality in clinical medicine. In general, O_2 should be used in sufficient concentration to restore arterial blood and tissue tensions to normal or, at most, somewhat higher values.

A gram of hemoglobin can combine chemically with a maximum of 1.36 ml (STPD) of O_2. At a normal P_{O_2} of 100 mm Hg, arterial hemoglobin is 97% saturated, so that little additional O_2 can be added to hemoglobin by increasing P_{O_2}. On the other hand, each 100 ml of plasma contains only 0.3 ml of dissolved O_2 at normal alveolar pressures. If exposed to 100% O_2 at 1 atm of pressure, each 100 ml of plasma would dissolve approximately 2.4 ml of O_2, whereas at 3 atm the dissolved O_2 content is more than 6 vol %, exceeding the normal arteriovenous blood O_2 difference of man at rest. Reducing the temperature of plasma would increase dissolved O_2 further for any given P_{O_2}.

Within minutes after a subject starts to breathe an O_2-enriched mixture (e.g., 60% O_2), there is a decrease of as much as 1 gm % in hemoglobin concentration of the circulating blood. Breathing O_2-enriched mixtures decreases cardiac rate, cardiac output, and cardiac work. By direct action increased P_{O_2} produces systemic arterial vasoconstriction, thus increasing diastolic blood pressure. Cerebral vasoconstriction also occurs. As expected, high P_{O_2} also constricts the placental artery, which does not have an autonomic nerve supply. Increased P_{O_2} dilates the pulmonary vasculature, thus exerting an action *opposite* to that which it has on the systemic vasculature. This action may be a part of the mechanism that regulates $\dot{V}_A/\dot{Q}_c$ ratios in the lung, since it tends to increase perfusion where ventilation is good.

Normobaric and hypobaric hyperoxia

The effect of hyperoxia upon the living cell is biochemical and must be understood in biochemical terms. Hyperoxia inhibits a number of intracellular enzymes, including succinic dehydrogenase, catalases, hydrogenases, urease, arginase, and succinic oxidases. It also inhibits a pyridine nucleotide system, decreasing ATP; sodium succinate appears to protect the ATP supply.

When a sea-level resident breathes pure O_2, ventilation decreases initially but then rises gradually to level off at about 15% above resting, control ventilation. This may occur because the increased amounts of *dissolved* O_2 available to and used in metabolism mean that less oxyhemoglobin is reduced to hemoglobin and more unbuffered H^+ stimulate the peripheral chemoreceptors, increasing breathing.

Carbon dioxide narcosis. In patients whose ventilatory drive depends upon hypoxia as a result of CO_2 retention and decreased responsiveness to CO_2, pulmonary ventilation may decrease seriously, or they may even become apneic, when an O_2-enriched breathing mixture is administered. This clinical situation is termed *carbon dioxide narcosis.* The cerebral complications of stupor, coma, and increased cerebrospinal fluid pressure (*pseudotumor cerebri*) are manifestations of increased P_{CO_2}, rather than O_2, and can be relieved by increasing alveolar ventilation to remove CO_2. The term "oxygen poisoning" has been used, but is not descriptive and should be abandoned. Carbon dioxide narcosis is never a contraindication for O_2 but, rather, an indication for providing *both* O_2 and the required ventilatory assistance.

Oxygen toxicity. Although pure O_2 at

normobaric or hypobaric pressures can be breathed for minutes to hours without *apparent* adverse effects, O_2 is clearly toxic to living cells when they are exposed to more than twice the normal P_{O_2} (more than 40% O_2 at sea level) for considerable periods of time. Indeed, one is tempted to call a discussion of O_2 toxicity "too much of a good thing." Excessive concentrations or, more relevantly, excessive partial pressures of O_2 are already known to have a variety of toxic effects. Toxic manifestations range from mucous membrane irritation, pulmonary congestion, loss of pulmonary surfactant, atelectasis, hyaline membrane formation, ocular damage, and impaired fertility to convulsions and death. Susceptibility to these toxic effects varies with species, the tissue exposed, and age. However, the lung, the central nervous system, and one of its ontogenetic derivatives, the eye, are particularly susceptible to hyperoxic damage.

Rahn and Farhi kept mice in a 100% O_2 atmosphere at about 200 mm Hg for 60 days, during which time they conceived and delivered apparently normal young. However, there is evidence that the fertility of both male and female mice is impaired by P_{O_2} in excess of 500 mm Hg for 2 weeks. Ulvedal kept roosters at a P_{O_2} of 380 mm Hg for 22 days. Sperm motility, total sperm count, and ejaculate volume decreased during the first week. Spermatogenesis was impaired and testicular atrophy was noted. The mechanism of these changes may be either a direct cytotoxic effect of O_2 or an indirect endocrine effect.

Dogs and other mammals die after normobaric exposure to pure O_2 for periods ranging from 1½ to 3 days. At autopsy the lungs show vascular congestion and consolidation, and the alveoli are filled with fluid and lined with a hyaline membrane. Animals sacrificed prior to spontaneous death show atelectatic areas in the lungs. These pulmonary findings can be produced unilaterally if one lung breathes pure O_2 while the other lung breaths air. They are prevented or delayed by hypophysectomy or adrenalectomy. These *pulmonary* effects are not observed in animals living in pure O_2 at 0.5 atm.

Guinea pigs and rats show progressive loss of pulmonary surfactant after 5 to 7 days of 100% O_2 breathing at 1 atm. As a result of this loss, surface tension in the alveoli increases, promoting alveolar collapse and progressive atelectasis together with vascular engorgement, pulmonary edema, hyaline membrane formation, and alveolocapillary diffusion block.

The eye is another organ that shows great sensitivity to the toxic effects of hyperoxia. Exposure to 100% O_2 at 1 atm pressure for more than 24 hours depresses the electroretinogram (ERG). Normobaric hyperoxia exerts a selective action upon the endothelium of developing retinal vessels but does not affect immature cerebral or meningeal vessels or directly injure other retinal structures. The mature eye is also sensitive, but the visual cells, rather than the vascular bed, are the target tissue.

Retrolental fibroplasia is a clinical example of the toxic action of O_2 on the immature eye. High P_{O_2} causes an arteriolar spasm in the retina of premature infants, which is followed by a retinal fibrosis, termed *retrolental fibroplasia.* This complication of O_2 therapy can be avoided by keeping the inspired O_2 concentration less than 40% (assuming a normal alveoloarterial gradient) and limiting the use of O_2 in premature infants to a maximum of 7 days. However, in the presence of cardiopulmonary disease, such as pulmonary hypoperfusion syndrome, the concentration of inspired O_2 must be high enough to achieve normal arterial P_{O_2}.

Some think that high O_2 is less dangerous to man than it is to the more commonly used experimental animals. This idea may be the result of clinical experience with O_2 therapy in which high concentrations are seldom actually achieved, and where continuous exposure does not occur. However, human subjects exposed to high O_2 atmospheres show signs and symptoms of toxicity. Pratt observed pulmonary vascular congestion and hyaline membranes at autopsy in patients given 100% O_2 at atmospheric pressure preterminally. Such membranes impair gas diffusion and, paradoxically, produce or aggravate hypoxemia. Further study of the effects of long-term exposure to high O_2 atmospheres in man is needed.

Hyperbaric hyperoxia

Hemoglobin becomes almost fully saturated when exposed to a normal P_{O_2} of 100 mm Hg during passage through the pulmonary capillaries. If additional O_2 is forced into the blood at higher tensions, it enters solution in the aqueous or plasma compartment. Because of its relative insolubility at body temperature, O_2 in physical solution increases only 3 vol % in the aqueous compartment of blood for each 1,000 mm Hg rise in P_{O_2}. Nevertheless, more O_2 can be forced into physical solution during practical hyperbaric exposure than the normal volume of O_2 extracted from arterial blood by the tissues. The arterial blood P_{O_2} of normal animals and man breathing pure O_2 at 3 atm of pressure is about 2,000 mm Hg. It should be noted, however, that pulmonary gas exchange is inefficient in the presence of a right-to-left shunt; as a result, the arterial blood P_{O_2} increase is comparatively modest, even at 3 atm.

During hyperbaric hyperoxia, cardiac rate, cardiac output, and regional blood flow to certain organs decrease in normal man; vasoconstriction causes increased peripheral vascular resistance. The content and tension of O_2 rise in venous blood, suggesting that more O_2 is available for utilization despite concomitant vasoconstriction. After total interruption of blood flow to an organ, normal function persists longer if an animal has been hyperoxygenated prior to the induction of ischemia. However, neuropathologic studies suggest that when total circulatory standstill is induced in an animal, hyperoxygenation confers less than 5 minutes of additional protection to the central nervous system. Furthermore, pathologic evidence shows that despite hyperbaric hyperoxia, an intact circulation peripheral to a nonperfused zone does not prevent necrosis of the adjacent ischemic tissue.

Hyperbaroxic toxicity. When rising O_2 tension reaches a critical level, convulsions occur. In man this level usually results from breathing pure O_2 at a pressure of about 3 atm. However, symptoms may appear in less than 15 minutes at 4 atm pressure. The clinical sequence includes restlessness, pallor, convulsions, coma, and finally death if exposure continues. Fortunately, prompt and complete recovery follows removal of a victim from the high O_2 tension environment. The seizures occur at irregular intervals and are of abrupt onset and spontaneous cessation. The frequency of these convulsions increases as the duration of exposure increases. Adding low concentrations of CO_2 to the breathing mixture accelerates the onset of convulsions and potentiates other neurotoxic effects because CO_2 increases cerebral circulation and exposes the brain to higher P_{O_2} levels. However, high concentrations of CO_2 inhibit O_2 convulsions.

Experimental animals breathing 100% O_2 at 3 atm show a loss of pulmonary surfactant after 4 to 5 hours of exposure. Depression of the electroretinogram (ERG) is maximal after 3 to 5 hours of exposure to 100% O_2 at 3 atm, and irreversible retinal injury occurs regularly after 5 to 6 hours. After exposure to 100% O_2 at 3 atm for more than 4 hours, human subjects show progressive contraction of visual fields and impairment of central vision. In the rabbit, an animal with an avascular retina, death of visual cells has been described.

Dogs exposed to 100% O_2 at 3 atm pressure for more than 4 hours develop a selective retinal lesion termed a *cytoid body*. This lesion consists of segmental degeneration of axons in the nerve fiber layer of the retina around the optic nerve head. They appear similar to the cytoid bodies of the "cotton wool" spot, which are characteristic of human retinal vascular disease. This lesion is not observed in dogs subjected to shorter periods of hyperbaric hyperoxia ranging from ¾ to 2 hours. These ocular lesions can be prevented by the use of a 98% O_2–2% CO_2 breathing mixture. However, when this is used, the resulting cerebral vasodilatation exposes the central nervous system to the toxic effects of O_2, as shown by neurologic deficits and neuronal necrosis.

Such high O_2 tensions produce retinal vasocontriction and decrease retinal blood flow. It is not known whether a hyperoxia-induced ischemia is the paradoxical cause of the damage or whether direct cytotoxic action of high P_{O_2} together with high tissue susceptibility is the explanation. Although the strong vasoconstrictive reaction of the retina to hyperbaric O_2 suggests the possibility of ischemic damage, it is difficult to accept ischemia as a likely causative mechanism.

Hyperbaric oxygenation. Many medical and research centers in Europe and America now have chambers in which the pressure can be increased to several atmospheres. Small chambers are used for hyperbaric studies of experimental animals, and large chambers accommodate patients who can be given pure O_2 to breathe. Surgery can thus be performed under hyperbaric conditions while a patient breathes O_2 at a tension somewhat below that which would produce convulsions, and while the surgical team breathes the compressed air that fills the chamber. Locks are installed between chamber and outside in which all personnel may decompress.

Hyperbaric oxygenation involves appreciable hazards, not only to the patient but also to the personnel; all are subject to the dangers of toxicity, explosion, decompression, aeroembolism, and nitrogen narcosis. For reasons of safety, hyperbaric pressures in large chambers are usually generated by compressed air. Special respiratory assemblies are then used to deliver pure O_2 to the patient. As already discussed, exposure to O_2 at 3 atm pressure for as brief a time as 30 minutes can produce convulsions, although this effect appears completely reversible with prompt decompression. However, with prolonged exposure the direct toxic chemical effect of O_2 on the cerebral tissues can lead to permanent central nervous system damage, paralysis, and death.

There are also difficulties associated with compression and decompression. Rapid pressurization is well tolerated if pressures in the paranasal sinuses and middle ear equalize well. The absorption of gases from any cavity is more rapid when it is filled with O_2 than when it is filled with air. This fact favors pulmonary atelectasis, retraction of the tympanic membrane, or pain from the gas space beneath a dental filling. If the negative pressure in a closed body space exceeds plasma osmotic pressure, fluid and plasma protein will transude into the space.

To avoid obvious toxicity, hyperbaricists limit uninterrupted therapeutic exposures to 5 hours or less at a P_{O_2} not exceeding 3 atm. Because of the possibility of nitrogen narcosis, physicians should probably not attempt to perform complicated tasks, such as cardiovascular surgery while breathing air at more than 4 atm. However, this limit can be greatly extended by replacing nitrogen in the inspired gas mixture with helium. The most serious hazard of hyperbaric oxygenation is decompression sickness as a result of rapid decompression. This may occur in a mild form, including arthralgia and transient skin rash, or in a severe form with neurologic deficit, paralysis, coma, and fatal termination. It also carries the risk of arterial aeroembolism due to rapid expansion of lung gas if a subject does not exhale during decompression. The risk of serious decompression sickness can be virtually eliminated by application of tested decompression schedules and by prompt recompression should symptoms appear.

Since O_2 is the most flow-limited substance required in cellular metabolism, improving O_2 transport to an ischemic organ confers real benefit. The rationale of hyperbaric oxygenation rests upon the assumption that exposure to high tensions of O_2 can prevent or reverse tissue hypoxia without inflicting serious damage upon a patient. However, the clinical effectiveness of hyperbaric oxygenation is limited by failure to deliver O_2 through defective blood vessels and by the brevity of tolerated exposures.

Clinically, hyperbaric oxygenation appears promising for treatment of circulatory shock, carbon monoxide poisoning, cyanide intoxication, serious anaerobic infections—such as infection with *Clostridium welchii*—and as a potentiator of ionizing radiation in the therapy of certain malignancies. It may also prove useful in cardiovascular surgery, cerebral ischemic episodes, and circulatory arrest. Organs that have been harvested for later transplantation lose viability rather quickly because of ischemia. Hyperbaric oxygenation, together with hypothermia, can be used to maintain tissue integrity for longer periods of time. Hyperbaric oxygenation is being evaluated for prevention of ischemic damage to vulnerable tissues during surgical transplantation.

RESPONSES TO CO_2-CONTAINING ATMOSPHERES

The excitatory and depressant effects of CO_2 upon ventilation were considered in Chapter 12. In concentrations up to about 12% (sea level), CO_2 behaves as a powerful stimulant. Carbon dioxide tensions above 120 mm Hg inhibit hyperbaric O_2 convulsions. Human subjects breathing 25% CO_2 are conscious but unable to perform simple tasks, such as removing the respiratory valve and mouthpiece from their own mouth. They may think great thoughts but cannot recall these at the end of the experiment. Tunnel vision is common. Recovery from such exposure is accompanied by a variety of psychologic reactions that depend upon the personality of the subject. However, most subjects report that the experience is not unpleasant and state that they would be willing to repeat it. It has been reported that brief exposure to high CO_2 may improve reading speed and retention, as well as mathematical computation speed and accuracy, for a period of hours following exposure. However, Porteus' maze test shows decreased ability to plan ahead following CO_2 exposure.

In concentrations of 30% and above, CO_2 is anesthetic. High CO_2 has been used as a somatic therapy in psychiatry for a variety of disorders; however, the extreme subjectivity and the problem of establishing satisfactory controls make the results of such treatment difficult to evaluate.

Because high CO_2 depresses the central nervous system its concentration should not be allowed to rise unmonitored in closed spaces where people may be exposed. Carbon dioxide accumulation in coal mines is a well-known hazard. Crashes have been attributed to the use of CO_2 fire extinguishers in pressurized aircraft.

Carbon dioxide produces local vasodilatation in denervated areas, but its central action is opposite and dominant. High CO_2 breathing mixtures produce blanched skin through a wide concentration range; conservation of circulation by this mechanism may explain, in part, how CO_2 increases cerebral and coronary blood flow.

Administration of high CO_2 produces a rapid fall of body temperature. Not only is metabolic rate reduced but also shivering is inhibited and heat loss by evaporation from the upper respiratory tract is increased, because of increased pulmonary ventilation. High CO_2 reduces the rectal temperature of rats even when ambient temperature is high. Peripheral vasoconstriction retards heat gain from the hot environment while evaporation of water removes heat from blood perfusing the respiratory tract and slowly metabolizing body core.

High CO_2 is lethal if breathed for long periods of time; the higher the concentration of CO_2 the shorter is the survival time. Carbon dioxide also synergizes with both hypoxia and hyperoxia in shortening survival time. Barley, grown in O_2 in a closed, dark container, dies when the CO_2 concentration reaches 30% (sea level). High CO_2 atmospheres prevent the decay of meat at room temperature.

Acclimatization

Chronic exposure to an atmosphere containing a low concentration of CO_2 results in certain responses that increase tolerance to the effects of this gas. The ventilatory response to CO_2 decreases with such exposure; breath-holding time and alveolar P_{CO_2} at the breath-holding breaking point are both increased. The initial respiratory acidosis is more rapidly compensated if inspired CO_2 concentration is high than if it is low! Initial euphoria is followed by lassitude and impaired performance, which tend to persist despite acclimatization. Upon emerging from a CO_2 atmosphere, subjects report a smell of ammonia.

As in altitude acclimatization, an interplay between central and peripheral chemoreceptors during CO_2 acclimatization gradually decreases ventilation and CO_2 sensitivity. Initially, increased P_{CO_2} produces respiratory acidosis in blood and in the central chemoreceptors. Hydrogen ions and, perhaps, CO_2 produce a sustained increase in ventilation by stimulation of peripheral chemoreceptors. This is augmented by the respiratory acidosis in the central chemoreceptors. However, as HCO_3^- accumulates in the cerebrospinal fluid, the ventilatory drive of the central chemoreceptors decreases. Carbon dioxide sensitivity is reduced, and the breath-holding, breaking-point curve is elevated because P_{CO_2} increments along the new high CO_2 dissociation curve now produce less pH change than similar increments produced along the normal CO_2 dissociation curve.

Return to air breathing produces respiratory alkalosis in the central chemoreceptors and reduces peripheral chemoreceptor drive. Total ventilation is thus depressed until HCO_3^- loss restores normal central chemoreceptor pH.

SPECIAL ATMOSPHERES

Aerospace cabin and submarine chamber atmospheres

Prolonged exposure to high P_{O_2} atmospheres suppresses erythropoiesis, producing anemia. This fact is of obvious practical importance in selecting atmospheres for aerospace cabins and submarine chambers and in planning routine periodic examinations of exposed personnel. The atmospheres within manned aerospace capsules launched by the United States thus far have consisted of 100% O_2 at 0.34 atm. This means an inspired P_{O_2} of about 250 mm Hg. However, atmospheres consisting of gas mixtures would have certain advantages for prolonged space missions. Among other inert gases, helium has been considered as a replacement for nitrogen. The advantages of helium include its low density, higher thermal conductivity, and reduced hazards of aerobullosis and nitrogen narcosis.

Despite their relative chemical unreactivity, the noble gases can exert certain effects upon biologic systems. The viability of chick embryos incubated in 21% O_2–79% helium is reduced by 50%. Further tests of appropriate mammalian systems are needed to assess the advisability of using helium as a component of cabin or chamber atmospheres. Latterell reported studies of the effects of acute anoxia on the hydrated seeds of Prolific rye. The postexposure growth of survivors of prolonged anoxia is much less than that of controls grown in air. He found that prolonged exposure to acute anoxia causes a progressive reduction in viability of the seeds and that for equal exposures of 9 days or longer, mortality was significantly higher in helium than in nitrogen. The main difference between the two experimental series was in the time lapse before the apparent threshold of lethality was reached: 5 to 7 days in helium and 7 to 9 days in nitrogen.

Artificial gills

The coming exploration and habitation of undersea regions will require devices that permit man to breathe under water. Perhaps the most attractive answer to this problem involves the efficient and rapid extraction of dissolved O_2 from sea water, although electrolysis also deserves consideration. To accomplish extraction, energy will be required to circulate both water and air. The average O_2 content of ocean water from surface to a depth of 1,000 M is about 4 ml/L, whereas below that depth 7 to 8 ml/L are usually present. The partial pressures of O_2 and other dissolved gases increase slightly with depth.

Bodell showed that silicone rubber membranes (Silastic), which allow diffusion of O_2 and CO_2, can be used to make artificial gills capable of extracting dissolved O_2 from water. Two thousand feet of thin-wall, fine-caliber tubing were capable of extracting 136 ml/hr of O_2. An adult rat was sealed in a flask and the atmosphere circulated at a rate of 400 ml/min through the gill tubing, while tap water was circulated over the gill coils at a rate of 4,000 ml/min. Although a control rat that was simply sealed in a flask died in 1 hour, the experimental rat was still living after 25 hours. The flask atmosphere reached equilibrium at a P_{O_2} of 75 mm Hg and P_{CO_2} of 15 mm Hg.

Liquid respiration and submerged survival

Kylstra studied mice and dogs respiring hyperbarically oxygenated electrolyte solutions and demonstrated survival. Chambers containing pools of saline or Ringer's solution were filled with O_2 at several atmospheres of pressure. When the experimental animals sank into the saline, their breathing movements continued and they respired the hyperbarically oxygenated solution. The P_{O_2} of the saline solutions was sufficient to drive adequate volumes of O_2 across the alveolocapillary membrane and into the pulmonary capillaries. Such animals survived the ordeal of breathing hyperbarically oxygenated saline and sometimes the ordeal of emerging to return to air breathing. However, pulmonary complications usually occur within a few days because the aqueous electrolyte solution washes out pulmonary surfactant, or because the inhaled saline is contaminated with excreta or bacteria from the body surface. Kylstra suggested that pulmonary gas exchange in liquid-ventilated lungs is diffusion limited. Viscosity and temperature are important variables, as well as the diffusion rates of O_2 and CO_2 through the respired liquid.

Oxygen and CO_2 are very soluble in certain organic liquids of viscosity near that of water and of relative biologic inertness. Clark and Gollan showed that both silicone oils (polymethylsiloxanes) and fluorocarbon liquids (perfluorobutyltetrahydrofurans), equilibrated with O_2 at atmospheric pressure, can support respiration in mice and cats. Arterial P_{O_2} was well maintained, but CO_2 elimination was impaired, with consequent respiratory acidosis. Animals that had breathed silicone oil died shortly after return to air-breathing, whereas those that had breathed fluorocarbon liquid survived for weeks. The addition of an anesthetic, Fluothane, arrested the swimming motions of submerged mice, but the animals survived. Pulmonary damage was observed in all animals. They also showed that goldfish can survive under silicone oil for several weeks. The fluorocarbon liquid FC-80 is superior to the silicone oils and has the advantage over aqueous liquids of higher solubility for O_2 and CO_2, higher diffusion coefficient for these gases, and somewhat lower viscosity.

Atmospheric pollution

Of all living things, we alone are in the process of polluting our natural environment and even have the power to destroy it. Atmospheric pollution is actually only an aspect of the larger problem of environmental pollution, truly one of the pressing health problems of our times. What this exposure lacks in intensity is more than made up for by its chronicity. Where pollution is present, every breath is affected. Atmospheric pollution is largely the result of modern industrial technology and transportation. Motor vehicle fumes and exhausts are a large contributor in many instances.

The chemistry of air pollution is often complex and varies from region to region. Pollutants may be gaseous, liquid, or particulate. The chief noxious ingredients are commonly SO_2, NO_2, O_3, CO, and assorted hydrocarbons, several of which are known to be carcinogenic.

Nitrogen oxides are not only themselves toxic but, with other pollutants, breed ozone. In the presence of ultraviolet radiation, certain hydrocarbons catalyze the oxidation of nitric oxide (NO) to nitrogen dioxide (NO_2), which in turn with ultraviolet dissociates to yield oxygen atoms, or free radicals.* These free atoms combine with molecular oxygen to form ozone as follows:

$$\ddot{O} + O_2 \rightleftharpoons O_3$$

These free atoms also react with hydrocarbons and nitrogen oxides to form peroxyacetylnitrate (PAN), according to the following crude composite equation:

$$\ddot{O} + \text{Hydrocarbons} + NO_x \rightarrow \text{PAN}$$

Two simple ways of decreasing the nitrogen oxide effluent from the internal combustion engine are available—either recirculation of exhaust through the intake manifold, thus decreasing O_2 concentration, P_{O_2}, and peak combustion temperature, or the use of water to decrease combustion temperature.

Although obnoxious and irritating, urban air pollution is not known to cause a specific disease entity. It does, however, aggravate the symptoms of patients with respiratory tract disease. Under certain conditions, breathing polluted air can impair pulmonary function temporarily or even permanently. Air pollution is probably a significant causative factor in lung cancer and in certain chronic bronchopulmonary diseases. Is prolonged exposure to oxidant air pollutants a cause of the increasingly prevalent bronchitis-emphysema syndrome? Is it a cause of accelerated aging of the exposed respiratory tract?

An important meteorologic phenomenon that can produce sudden increases in the concentration of atmospheric pollutants is the *atmospheric temperature inversion.* When the normal relationship of *warmer,*

*A free radical is an uncharged reactive fragment consisting of one or more atoms.

lower air to *colder, higher* air is reversed, there is little or no tendency for dilution and dissipation of atmospheric pollutants by convection currents. This inverted relationship is known as an atmospheric temperature inversion. Death has occasionally resulted in individuals with chronic cardiopulmonary diseases when atmospheric temperature inversion produced sudden increases in the concentration of air pollutants.

Studies of the effects of air pollution on human populations are necessarily epidemiologic in nature and suffer from the problems and limitations of this approach. The subject is as important as it is complex, and doubtless various synergistic mechanisms will be discovered as research proceeds.

Tobacco smoking. The prevalence of tobacco smoking and its serious implications for human health require a definitive statement. Tobacco smoking is a large topic with economic, psychosocial, and medical aspects. It is easily oversimplified. However, certain *medical* aspects of cigarette smoking are abundantly clear; cigarette smoke is a complex chemical mixture that produces inflammation of the respiratory tract. In certain individuals it produces allergic disease as well. Continued inhalation of cigarette smoke almost always results in gradual loss of pulmonary function in all its aspects. The precise nature and extent of pulmonary functional loss vary considerably from individual to individual. At present the resulting clinical picture is indistinguishable from bronchitis-emphysema syndrome, of which cigarette smoking must therefore be considered an important causative factor.

Because cigarette smoke contains numerous potent carcinogenic chemical substances, as well as radioactive polonium-210, long-term inhalation greatly increases the probability of bronchopulmonary malignancy in any given individual. Because these carcinogenic chemical substances find their way from the respiratory tract into the stomach and urinary bladder, cigarette smokers are also exposed to appreciably increased risk of malignancy of these organs.

Cigarette smoking produces tachycardia and increased systemic vascular resistance, both of which increase cardiac work. Smokers are also exposed to increased risk of certain vascular diseases, including coronary artery disease. While smoking and inhaling cigarettes, from 2% to 10% of the smoker's hemoglobin combines with carbon monoxide of the smoke to form the relatively stable, but physiologically useless, carboxyhemoglobin.

Cigarette smoking has been properly termed a tranquilizer or "psychologic crutch," although the term "neurosis-sparing device" is more descriptive. It is especially important to note that the habit of smoking cigarettes often becomes deeply entrenched, so that individuals either are unable to stop smoking or find it a difficult, continuing struggle.

Noxious gases

Ozone. Ozone, or O_3, is a highly reactive oxidant gas of characteristic odor. It is produced in O_2-containing atmospheres by electric discharge or by ionizing radiation and is thus a natural constituent of the atmosphere. The interaction of solar ultraviolet radiation with O_2 in the upper atmosphere produces an appreciable quantity of ozone, which shields the surface of the earth by absorption of certain ultraviolet frequencies. Exposure to ozone is increasing as a result of modern technology. New sources include electric appliances and equipment and artificial ultraviolet light and other ionizing radiation. Commerically available "air purifiers" and "deodorizers" generate sufficient ozone to be hazardous under certain conditions of use, e.g., inadequate room ventilation.

Ozone, known to be poisonous since its

discovery in 1840, is toxic at levels of less that 1 ppm. In man low concentrations—from 0.6 to 0.8 ppm for 2 hours—reduce both pulmonary ventilatory and diffusing capacity. Industrial exposure to concentrations of 9 ppm has produced severe pneumonia. Thickening of alveolar walls by edema fluid is the most likely cause of this decreased diffusing capacity. In laboratory animals, concentrations of approximately 4 to 30 ppm for 3 to 4 hours produce fatal pulmonary edema. Experimental animals exposed to concentrations of ozone of from 1 to 50 ppm over many months show atrophy of alveolar walls, especially in alveoli evaginating from respiratory bronchioles and alveolar ducts.

Measurable tolerance to otherwise lethal doses of ozone develops after sublethal exposures. Cross-tolerance between ozone, nitrogen dioxide, and other oxidant irritants also occurs. Tobacco plants show an ozone-type injury when exposed to mixtures of O_3 and SO_2 at subthreshold concentrations, suggesting a synergism between the toxic effects of these two noxious gases.

Cyanide. The main toxic effect of cyanide involves inhibition of the intracellular enzyme cytochrome oxidase. Oxygen transport and O_2 tension are usually adequate during cyanide poisoning, but the cellular utilization of O_2 is diminished (hypoxidosis). The usual treatment consists of amyl nitrite, sodium nitrite ($NaNO_2$), or sodium thiosulfate ($Na_2S_2O_3$). Sodium nitrite converts hemoglobin to methemoglobin, which then effectively binds cyanide to form the relatively stable cyanmethemoglobin. Sodium thiosulfate is used as a substrate by the enzyme rhodanese, which detoxifies cyanide by converting it to thiocyanate. In mice, sodium thiosulfate, when administered alone, appears more effective than sodium nitrite. In combination the protective effect is additive in mice but synergistic in dogs. Normobaric O_2 and hyperbaric O_2 have been reported to be of some value in cyanide poisoning; ECG changes are reversed by O_2. Although hyperoxia alone has slight effect, striking enhancement of prophylactic protection has been reported when mice given potassium cyanide were treated with hyperoxia plus sodium nitrite and sodium thiosulfate. The optimum O_2 tension and the biochemical mechanism of action are presently unknown.

CHAPTER 15 Clinical evaluation of pulmonary function

What is pulmonary function? In a clinical sense the term *pulmonary function* refers only to the role of the bronchopulmonary system in respiratory gas exchange; it does not refer to the other functions of the lung—metabolic, endocrine, hematologic, immunologic, self-cleansing, and heat and water eliminative. Clinical studies of the lungs are of three general types, and pulmonary function refers to the first two: (1) physiologic measurements, which are quantitative and the results are averaged (e.g., expiratory minute volume under stated conditions); (2) capacity, load, or stress tests, which are quantitative and the best values are reported (e.g., vital capacity); and (3) diagnostic tests and procedures, which are essentially nonquantitative and the results are interpreted (e.g., chest roentgenogram).

Chronic bronchopulmonary diseases are increasing rapidly in prevalence and will continue to do so for the foreseeable future because of age trends in the population and because of the inescapability of noxious respiratory exposures. The importance of pulmonary function evaluation for both clinical diagnostic and research purposes will increase accordingly. Various methods are used to evaluate the pulmonary function of patients with respiratory symptoms. These include the clinical history, physical examination, and, in certain cases, function fluoroscopy. In function fluoroscopy the patient is instructed to perform various respiratory maneuvers that permit evaluation of thoracic and diaphragmatic structure, mobility, and excursion. Thus an estimate can be made of ventilatory capacity, and such abnormalities as weakness or paradoxical motion of a hemidiaphragm or trapping of air during forced expiration can be detected. Chest roentgenographic examination with posteroanterior and lateral views in both inspiration and expiration often yields important diagnostic information but lacks any appreciable correlation with pulmonary function. Perhaps the most informative examination is the direct observation of a patient during and immediately following exercise. For this purpose nothing more complicated than a well-trained physician, a stethoscope, and a flight of stairs is required.* However, pulmonary function tests are indicated when the symptoms or degree of incapacity is greater than expected on the basis of clinical findings, where the diagnosis seems unsatisfactory or uncertain, and for preoperative evaluation of surgical and anesthesia risk in patients suspected of bronchopulmonary disease.

SIGNIFICANCE OF PULMONARY FUNCTION TESTS

A large number of pulmonary function tests are now available with which to

*Of these, the well-trained physician is easily the most complicated.

determine the nature and extent of pulmonary dysfunction. These tests are important both to physiology and to clinical medicine, just as cardiovascular, renal, and hepatic function tests are necessary for understanding and treatment in their respective areas. Pulmonary function tests have made, and continue to make, a valuable contribution in the following five areas: (1) basic physiologic knowledge of pulmonary function in healthy man as affected by sex, size, age, and physical training status; (2) information regarding pathophysiology, the natural history of cardiopulmonary diseases, and clinicopathologic correlations; (3) diverse research, which has important implications for the rational therapy of disease, including the evaluation of various therapies and analysis of the results of surgery; (4) early detection, diagnosis, and differential diagnosis of disease; and (5) guidance for management and therapy of various cardiopulmonary diseases.

All pulmonary function tests are *diagnostic* in nature. They are quantitative measures of the various aspects of bronchopulmonary function by means of which we define the normal and determine the nature and extent of bronchopulmonary dysfunction. However, pulmonary function tests cannot indicate that a lesion exists, unless it impairs bronchopulmonary function sufficiently to produce clear-cut deviation from normal values; they cannot tell *where* a lesion is, much less *what* a lesion is; they make neither *clinical* nor *pathoanatomic* diagnoses.

For example, pulmonary function tests can reveal the existence of a right-to-left circulatory shunt but cannot indicate whether such a shunt is intracardiac or intrapulmonary. They can reveal impaired diffusion across the alveolocapillary membrane but cannot distinguish either interstitial edema from intra-alveolar fluid, or reduced surface area from lengthened diffusion pathway. Pulmonary function tests cannot detect slight loss of functioning pulmonary tissue or the presence of small regions in the lungs that have neither ventilation nor perfusion. They may, therefore, be within normal limits in patients with minimal or even cavitary pulmonary tuberculosis or pulmonary neoplasm, unless these lesions happen to be strategically located so that they disturb bronchopulmonary function to a measurable extent. To cause detectably diminished *total lung capacity*, disease processes must be either diffuse or advanced. It is thus clear that pulmonary function tests do not reveal dysfunction in all types of bronchopulmonary disease.

Pulmonary function is measured for a variety of clinical purposes (Fig. 15-1). These include medical diagnosis, preoperative surgical and anesthesia risk evaluation, symptom or disability evaluation for legal or insurance compensation purposes, public health survey, and clinical research. Pulmonary function tests are often necessary for clinical evaluation of *symptoms* such as dyspnea, cough, and wheezing, or *signs* such as digital clubbing and cyanosis, or abnormal laboratory and chest roentgenographic findings. The definitive diagnosis of polycythemia always requires information about blood O_2 tension and saturation and, if arterial hypoxemia is present, evaluation of pulmonary function. It is therefore clear that pulmonary function tests supplement but do not replace other clinical diagnostic procedures.

Quantitative assessment of all aspects of pulmonary function requires a variety of tests. As with physiologic tests of other organ systems, no single pulmonary function test yields all the information desired in every patient, nor are all tests necessary for the management of every patient.

The results of pulmonary function tests may or may not reflect the status of the respiratory apparatus. They do so only

Indications for pulmonary function tests

I. Medical diagnostic
  A. To measure effect of any disease on pulmonary function
  B. To follow the course of any disease affecting pulmonary function
  C. Evaluation of symptoms, signs, or laboratory findings
    1. Dyspnea, orthopnea, wheeze, cough, palpitation, chest pain, cyanosis, digital clubbing, polycythemia, chest x-ray, ECG
  D. Physical fitness selection or evaluation
  E. To reassure physician and/or patient
II. Surgical diagnostic
  A. Preoperative risk evaluation re anesthesia and surgery
  B. Postoperative evaluation of thoracic surgical results
III. Disability evaluation
  A. Rehabilitation
    1. Industrial medical
    2. Vocational rehabilitation
  B. Insurance
    1. Private
    2. Government compensation laws
  C. Legal
    1. Social security oasi
    2. Personal injury lawsuit
    3. Other legal purposes (e.g., criminal charge of "driving under the influence"*)
IV. Public health
  A. Epidemiologic survey
V. Research unlimited

Fig. 15-1

Classification of indications for referral of patients to a pulmonary function laboratory. *After imbibition, ethanol is either metabolized or excreted by the kidneys and lungs. Exhalatory breath tests for alcohol intoxication, based on a correlation of breath alcohol with blood alcohol concentration, are widely used. Unfortunately, there is not yet sufficient information regarding the validity of such tests in individuals who have chronic, diffuse bronchopulmonary disease. It is hard to believe that severe disturbances of pulmonary function do not affect the results of exhalatory breath tests for alcohol intoxication.

if the subject is cooperative and the performance-limiting factors are respiratory. Subjects may fail to cooperate fully because of nonrespiratory factors such as communication barriers (language, sensory deficit, altered state of consciousness resulting from hypoxia, drugs, psychosis, or metabolic disturbances, etc.), pain, anxiety, or actual malingering. The desire for financial compensation is an increasingly prevalent factor affecting cooperation. Nonbronchopulmonary, performance-limiting factors include neurologic, muscular, and skeletal disorders and obesity.

Failure of a patient to cooperate results in data that may suggest respiratory dysfunction. The following points are useful in assessing the *validity* of pulmonary function test data that appear to indicate a deficit:

1. The cardiopulmonary technologist's impression and report of the subject's cooperation
2. The reproducibility, regularity, and maintenance of effort as determined from simple visual inspection of the spirographic record
3. Internal consistency of the various test results
4. Spirographic signs, when present
   a. Elevation of the respiratory level of the spirographically recorded maximal voluntary ventilation
   b. Airway collapse pattern
   c. Air-trapping sign

Pulmonary function tests at altitude require special consideration. Altitude differs from sea level mainly with respect to ambient barometric pressure, oxygen partial pressure, and air density. However, differences with respect to temperature, humidity, concentration, and chemical nature of gaseous and particulate air pollutants, intensity and pattern of solar radiation, and background intensity of ionizing radiation may also be of physiologic importance.

With regard to all tests of ventilatory capacity the following considerations apply. The volume flow rate of a gas increases with driving pressure and decreases with resistance. During laminar or streamlined flow the rate varies inversely as the gas viscosity. Tracheobronchial gas flow during normal quiet breathing is laminar in the small airways and turbulent in the large ones. During tests of ventilatory capacity, turbulence increases so that the flow rate is almost directly proportional to the square root of the driving pressure and inversely proportional to the square root of the gas density. Air density decreases with altitude, resulting in both decreased turbulence and increased flow rates for any given driving pressure or effort. Proper use and, even more especially, development of prediction tables for tests of ventilatory capacity at altitude require a good grasp of these considerations.

Pulmonary function tests performed by a well-trained cardiopulmonary technologist upon a cooperative subject compare favorably, both with respect to *reproducibility* and *accuracy*, to other routine clinical tests available in a general hospital.

Pulmonary function tests of various racial groups reveal significant differences. Prediction equations must thus take account of race, as well as sex, age, body size, and environmental factors such as altitude. When pulmonary function studies are repeated in the same patient within a relatively short period of time (e.g., 1 month), it is usually proper to use the predicted values that were calculated in relation to the first study for the second study as well. What is usually sought in such instances is a change in *found* values. The use of the same *predicted* values causes the values for *percent predicted* to reflect this information directly.

SPIROMETRY

Spirometry provides information about ventilatory capacity and vital capacity. Although O_2 uptake can also be measured spirometrically, this method is less accurate than the open-circuit expired gas method. Spirographic records of quiet breathing, forced expired and inspired vital capacity, maximal voluntary ventilation, and vital capacity provide a permanent basis for comparison with later studies.

In the sedentary individual, spirometry can detect obstruction to expiration before dyspnea and wheezing are clinically apparent. In this connection the tendency of cigarette smokers to deny symptoms of cough, expectoration, dyspnea, and wheezing is of interest.

Measures of ventilatory capacity

The effect of gas density on all measures of ventilatory capacity requires consideration. Gas density decreases with altitude and may also vary under experimental conditions or in artificial cabin atmospheres. Subjects performing maximal voluntary ventilation efforts where argon or helium has been substituted for atmospheric nitrogen can readily detect the changed respiratory resistance. Increased ventilatory capacity is measurable at elevations of 1 mile or less above sea level.

Maximal voluntary ventilation (MVV). Maximal voluntary ventilation is the maximal volume of gas that can be ventilated by voluntary effort during a given number of seconds, expressed as L/min. The subject is instructed to breathe as deeply and rapidly as he can through a low resistance system for an arbitrarily chosen period of time, ranging from as little as 12 seconds to as much as 30 seconds. This test, also termed *maximal breathing capacity* (MBC), differs from other measures of ventilatory capacity in that (1) it involves both inspiratory and expiratory phases of ventilation; (2) it requires voluntary, sustained, maximal effort; and (3) it requires neuromuscular coordination. The graphic record provided by spirometry permits analysis of breathing frequency, tidal volume, and midposition, or end-expiratory level. The Collins 13.5 L spirometer (Respirometer) is not inferior to low resistance, low inertia, open-circuit methods with Douglas-type gas bag or the 120 L Collins Gasometer when used for patients with appreciable ventilatory deficit.

MVV is a valuable test when conscientiously performed and properly interpreted. It is both more complex and less sensitive than the maximal midexpiratory flow. It is more liable to both practice effects and fatigue effects. Thus the MVV is generally less suitable for evaluating the effects of drugs or other medical therapy as well as for public health screening or survey work. With some asthmatic patients the exertion of the MVV itself produces bronchospasm.

However, the spirographically recorded MVV may reveal breathing patterns of diagnostic value such as elevation of midposition, or end-expiratory level, and airway collapse pattern. Although the expiratory phase of the MVV is always *some* portion of the forced expired vital capacity, and often an early portion, calculation of the MVV from data such as the forced expired volume at 1 second ($FEV_{1.0}$) obscures more than it illuminates.

Usually, maximal ventilation is only achieved by voluntary effort. However, during exhausting exercise the ventilation rates of healthy, trained subjects may exceed the MVV, probably because of airway dilatation associated with the stress.

Forced expired vital capacity (FEVC). The FEVC is a simple, rapidly performed, reproducible, quantitative maneuver involving only the expiratory phase of ventilation (Fig. 15-2). From it are derived a number of useful measurements characterizing the process of forced expiration, a process that is commonly affected by diffuse bronchopulmonary disease. The subject is instructed to inspire maximally and then to blow out as hard and fast as he can until maximum expiration is achieved.

Even when diffuse bronchopulmonary obstruction affects the expiratory phase of ventilation greatly, it affects the inspiratory phase only slightly. Sustained elevation of end-expiratory level during the spirographically recorded MVV is a sensitive semiquantitative indicator that a loss of ventilatory capacity is due to obstruction rather than restriction. Calculation of the MVV from data obtained from the forced expired vital capacity curve demonstrates a degree of relationship that does indeed exist, but it should be noted that the spirographically recorded MVV provides considerable information of practical value which the FEVC cannot.

Of the entire FEVC curve, the terminal portion is predictably the most sensitive indicator of diffuse obstructive bronchopulmonary disease. Unfortunately, the terminal portion is also relatively variable due to nonbronchopulmonary factors present during this phase of the expiratory effort. The terminal phase involves neuromuscular factors, such as maintenance and coordination of effort. Similarly, nonbronchopulmonary factors are present during the initial phase of the FEVC curve. The initial phase involves not only neuromuscular factors but also mechanical

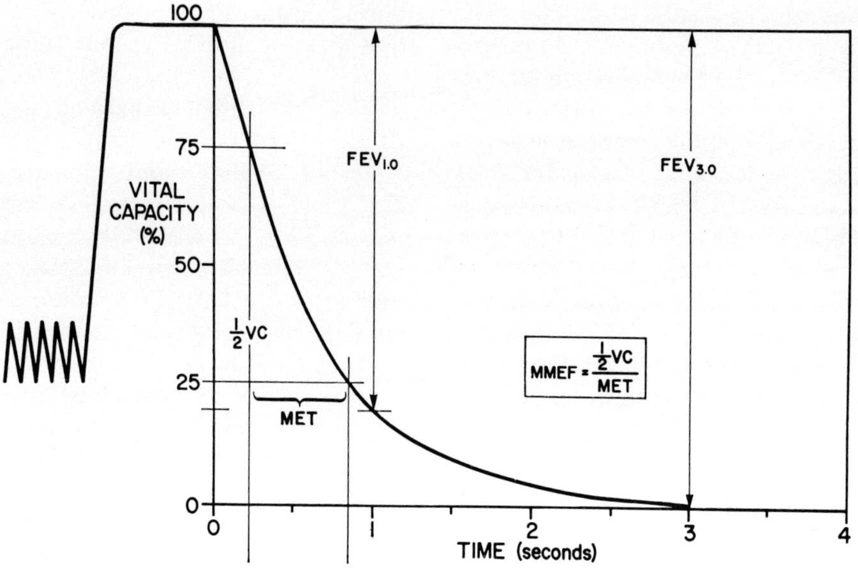

Fig. 15-2
Forced expired vital capacity.

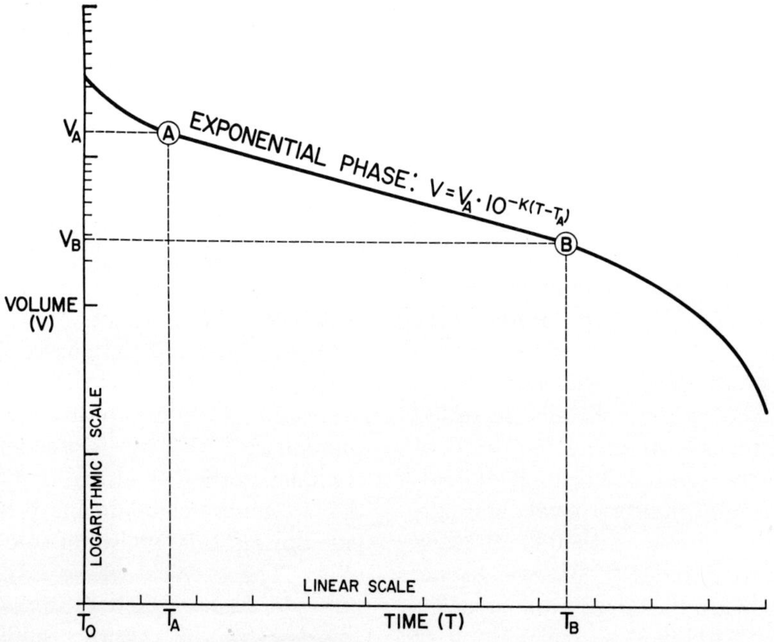

Fig. 15-3
Forced expired vital capacity spirographic curve replotted on a log-linear graph: bronchitis-emphysema syndrome. (An illustrative drawing, not an actual replot of data from a patient's spirographic record.)

equipment factors as well, such as inertial distortion. Measurements that avoid both initial and terminal phases of the expiratory effort, such as the maximal midexpiratory flow, are therefore the most reliable indicators of diffuse, obstructive bronchopulmonary disease.

When patients with chronic, diffuse, obstructive bronchopulmonary disease have appreciable obstruction to expiration, the FEVC curves are essentially exponential in nature; at any given point in the process of forced expiration the flow rate is directly proportional to the volume. This mathematical characteristic is readily seen when the spirographically recorded FEVC is replotted on a log-linear graph (Fig. 15-3).

Maximal midexpiratory flow (MMEF). The most sensitive quantitative spirometric tests for expiratory obstruction are the MMEF and midexpiratory time. Although MMEF is slightly less reproducible than other commonly used measurements of ventilatory capacity, its sensitivity more than makes up for this disadvantage. Indeed, one sees occasional patients in whom MMEF and MET are clearly abnormal, whereas MVV, $FEV_{1.0}$, and $FEV_{3.0}$ are all within normal limits.

Midexpiratory time (MET). MET is defined as the time required to expel the middle half of the vital capacity during a maximally deep and rapid expiration. MET is both simple and valuable as a test of slowed expiration and is largely independent of body size. However, the MET cannot be fully interpreted without reference to the magnitude of the vital capacity.

A healthy subject can expel the entire vital capacity from the lungs in about 3 seconds, and the middle half of the vital capacity in about 0.5 second (MET). In patients with severe obstructive disease the MET may be as long as 8 to 10 seconds.

Vital capacity (VC)

Vital capacity and its subdivisions can also be measured with volume recorders such as the spirometer. Expiratory vital capacity is measured by asking the subject to inspire maximally and then to expire completely into the spirometer. In this test no time limit is imposed upon the subject. Unless otherwise stated, the term *vital capacity* is generally understood to mean expiratory vital capacity. In cardiac insufficiency an accentuation of the physiologic reduction of vital capacity upon changing from erect to supine position is sometimes observed. Oxygen breathing reduces vital capacity, probably by dilatation of pulmonary blood vessels. In patients with obstructive bronchopulmonary disease who trap air during forceful expiration, inspiratory vital capacity may greatly exceed expiratory vital capacity.

Spirometric signs

Analysis of the spirographic record. Analysis of the spirographic record should begin with simple visual inspection, from which certain inferences may be drawn regarding subject cooperation and data interpretability, and from which an estimate can be made regarding normality or abnormality of ventilatory capacity and vital capacity. In addition to the usual constructions and measurements that are applied to the spirographic record, five spirographic signs containing valuable information can be readily appreciated by simple visual inspection: emotional stress pattern, elevation of end-expiratory level during the spirographically recorded MVV, airway collapse pattern, air-trapping sign, and penmanship sign.

Emotional stress pattern (ESP). Emotional stress, whether realistic or psychoneurotic, produces a hyperventilation characterized by increased rate and depth of breathing, irregularity, and frequent, deep, sighing inspirations, often of in-

SPIROGRAM - SUPINE

SH: CPL - 1600M

PSYCHONEUROSIS, SYMPTOMATIC

BRONCHITIS - EMPHYSEMA SYNDROME, SLIGHT

POSSIBLE ANGINA PECTORIS

61 WMM CARPENTER, Height-62. WEIGHT-123.

PAROXYSMAL DYSPNEA, 4½ years, episodes lasting seconds to minutes

PAST HISTORY: NASAL SURGERY

MVV_{20} = 90
MMEF = 1.627
MET = 1.08
VC_{I-SU} = 3.464
RV = 2.108
TLC = 5.572
RV/TLC = 37.8

[A] SUPINE, REST, NO MEDICATION

[B] SUPINE, AWAKE, 15 min after PROMAZINE 25 mgm IV

[C] SUPINE, ASLEEP, 45 min after PROMAZINE 25 mgm IV

COLLINS 13.5 LITER SPIROMETER, without CO_2-ABSORBING CANISTER or FLUTTER VALVES

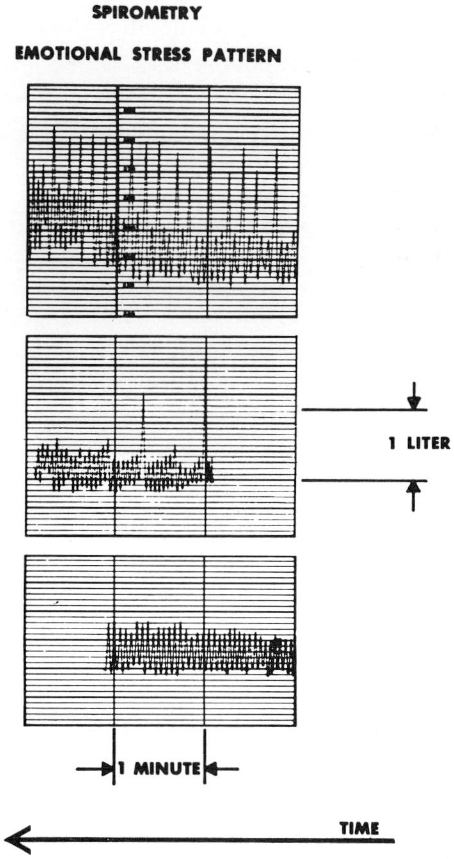

Fig. 15-4
Emotional stress pattern.

spiratory capacity magnitude. The resulting spirographic representation is termed *emotional stress pattern* (Fig. 15-4). This pattern is accentuated by anything that heightens emotional stress, such as provocative interrogation during a polygraph ("lie detector") test, and is diminished by anything that reduces emotional stress, such as human warmth, or tranquilizers like meprobamate or promazine. Emotional stress pattern is an objective spirographic sign containing valuable information, which is readily appreciated by simple visual inspection of the spirographic record.

Elevation of respiratory level (ERL) during the spirographically recorded MVV. Elevation of respiratory level during the spirographically recorded MVV is a valuable spirographic sign of obstruction to expiration and increased airway resistance, which can be readily appreciated by simple visual inspection. This elevation occurs during the first few breaths of the patient's MVV effort, and if this effort is vigorous and well sustained, the elevation may be remarkably constant throughout the entire MVV effort (Fig. 15-5). In patients with severe obstruction to expiration, elevation is quite definite and of considerable extent.

Where vital capacity and inspiratory capacity are reduced, there is less room for such elevation to occur and smaller elevations are noted. In such cases each unit of elevation, whether measured in millimeters of spirometer chart paper or in milliliters of lung volume, is more significant of increased airway resistance than the same unit in patients with nor-

SPIROGRAM - ERECT

RJE: CPL - 2186 M

BRONCHITIS-EMPHYSEMA SYNDROME

40 WMM PHARMACIST, Ht.-70, Wt.-142

EXERTIONAL DYSPNEA
PRODUCTIVE COUGH
OCCASIONAL WHEEZING

PAST HISTORY: MULTIPLE ALLERGIES
CHRONIC BRONCHITIS

MVV_{20}	=	82
MMEF	=	1.491
MET	=	1.25

VC_{I-SU}	=	3.727
RV	=	2.736
TLC	=	6.463
RV/TLC	=	42.3

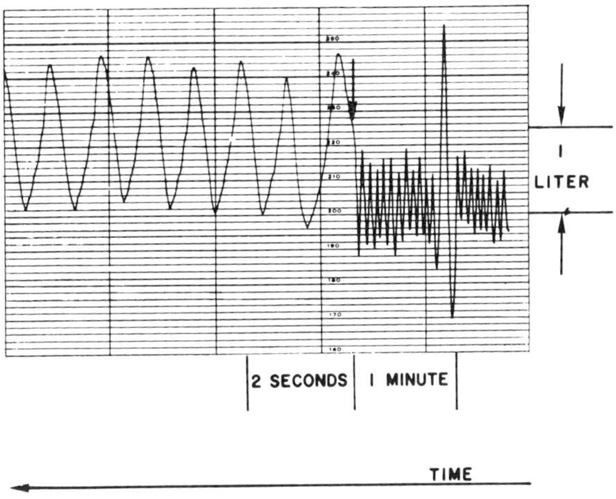

Fig. 15-5
Elevation of respiratory level during spirographically recorded MVV.

mal vital capacity. Indeed, it seems likely that if appropriate correction is made for reduced vital capacity or inspiratory capacity, an appreciable, positive correlation would be found between airway resistance and the extent of ERL.

During the MVV, ERL results in use of a higher and more favorable portion of the FEVC curve. This gives a better MVV than if ERL did not occur and, at the same time, provides the basis in these patients for comparison of MVV with $FEV_{0.75}$ or $FEV_{1.0}$. The invariably more favorable shape of the early portion of the FEVC curve, together with ERL during MVV, explains the fact that the MMEF is a more sensitive measure of ventilatory capacity than the MVV. As a further consequence of ERL, the MVV in terms of percent predicted is always greater than the MMEF expressed in similar terms, if MVV effort is vigorous and well sustained and if inspiration is not selectively impaired. Conversely, when significant obstruction to expiration is present and MVV in terms of percent predicted is less than MMEF expressed in similar terms, this indicates failure to produce or sustain the MVV effort for any of various reasons, except in those unusual cases where something selectively interferes with the inspiratory phase of ventilation and diminishes MVV without affecting FEVC and MMEF. Sustained ERL is a sensitive semiquantitative indicator of expiratory obstruction and increased airway resistance that can be seen when MVV expressed in numerical terms, $FEV_{1.0}$, and $FEV_{3.0}$, are still within normal limits. Patients with restrictive, as opposed to obstructive, ventilatory impairment have abnormal tests of ventilatory capacity but do not show ERL during the spirographically recorded MVV.

SPIROGRAM - ERECT

GRD: CPL - 1802 M

BRONCHITIS - EMPHYSEMA SYNDROME

COR PULMONALE

KYPHOSCOLIOSIS

FUSION OF RIBS (5), RIGHT

33 WMM GUARD, Ht. - 65, Wt. - 123

DYSPNEA, WHEEZING, COUGH,

EXPECTORATION

MVV_{20}	=	53
MMEF	=	0.271
MET	=	5.31
VC_{I-SU}	=	2.651
RV	=	2.067
TLC	=	4.717
RV/TLC	=	43.8

SPIROMETRY

AIRWAY COLLAPSE PATTERN

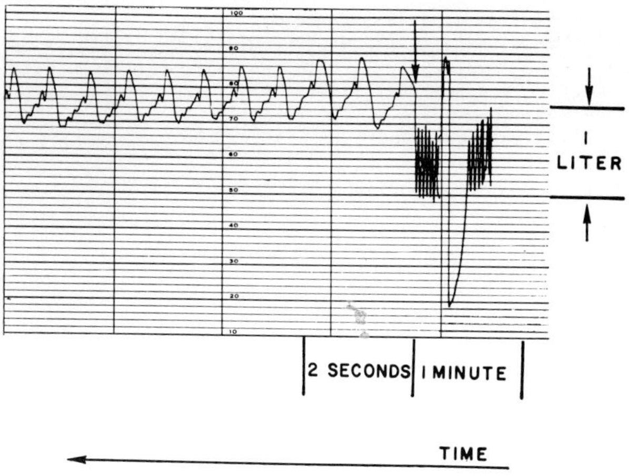

COLLINS 13.5 LITER SPIROMETER, without
CO_2-ABSORBING CANISTER or FLUTTER VALVES

Fig. 15-6
Airway collapse pattern.

Elevation of respiratory level during the spirographically recorded MVV is a simple, objective, reproducible, valuable spirographic sign of obstruction to expiration and increased airway resistance that is not easily simulated and that, when present, validates the measures of ventilatory capacity which may appear abnormal due solely to deficient cooperation or actual malingering.

Airway collapse pattern (ACP). Airway collapse pattern consists of both notching and inflection of the initial expiratory portion of the spirographically recorded MVV and FEVC curve (Fig. 15-6). Occasionally, two or even three notches occur. The notches represent momentary near cessation of air flow, and the inflection indicates resumption of air flow following collapse at a definitely slower rate. This spirographic pattern results during forceful expiration when the intrathoracic pressure, and therefore transairway pressure difference, becomes supraoptimal and collapses the airway.

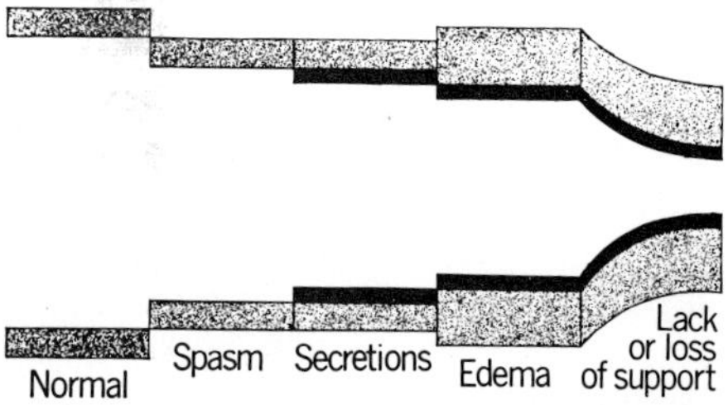

Fig. 15-7
Diagrammatic representation of conditions affecting airway.

Any lack or loss of normal airway support and/or diminution of normal airway stiffness predisposes to airway collapse

SPIROGRAM - SUPINE, Rest

AWS: CPL - 1367 F

RADIATION FIBROSIS, LUNGS
SARCOMA, EPICARDIUM

65 WMF HOUSEWIFE, Ht. - 58, Wt. - 87
DYSPNEA, COUGH
DEPENDENT EDEMA
PAST HISTORY: THORACOTOMY - Oct. 1964
MEDICATION: PREDNISONE

MVV_{20} = 56
MMEF = 1.845
MET = 0.33

VC_{I-SU} = 1.120
RV = 1.408
TLC = 2.528
RV/TLC = 55.7

REST: $S_{a_{O_2}}$ = 78
CO_2 = 22.8 mM/L
pH = 7.50

OXYGEN: $S_{a_{O_2}}$ = 85

SPIROMETRY

PENMANSHIP SIGN

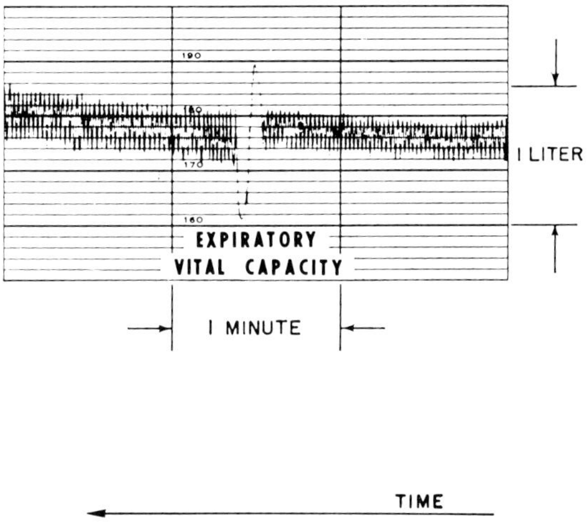

COLLINS 13.5 LITER SPIROMETER, without CO_2-ABSORBING CANISTER or FLUTTER VALVES

Fig. 15-8
Penmanship sign.

(Fig. 15-7). Bronchitis-emphysema syndrome of moderate to severe degree is the clinical entity most commonly associated with ACP. ACP is almost always seen together with ERL during the spirographically recorded MVV because obstruction to expiration is a factor common to both and is reflected earlier by ERL. Although notching may occur during forceful expiration as a result of supraoptimal force and intrathoracic pressure in healthy subjects, inflection does not.

Airway collapse pattern is a reproducible, valuable sign of chronic, diffuse, obstructive bronchopulmonary disease with abnormal airway collapsibility that is readily appreciated by simple visual inspection of the spirographic record. Because it is not easily simulated, ACP yields objective evidence of obstruction to expiration and reduced ventilatory capacity, validating other findings that may be abnormal solely as a result of deficient cooperation or actual malingering.

Air-trapping sign (ATS). The normal mechanics of inspiration and expiration are such that localized or diffuse obstructive bronchopulmonary processes tend to manifest themselves during expiration before inspiration and, first of all, during forceful expiration. When the magnitude of several forced expired vital capacities is clearly less than the magnitude of several expiratory vital capacities performed without regard to time, this disparity is termed *air-trapping sign.* Because ATS is the result of obstructive airway disease, it is almost always seen with elevation of the respiratory level during the spirographically recorded MVV and is often associated with airway collapse pattern.

Air-trapping sign is reproducible, valuable evidence of air-trapping in the lungs during forceful expiration that is readily appreciated by simple visual inspection of the spirographic record. Because it is not easily simulated, ATS yields objective evidence of obstruction to expiration and reduced ventilatory capacity, validating other findings that may be abnormal solely as a result of deficient cooperation or actual malingering.

Penmanship sign. A spirographic pattern of rapid, extremely regular respirations of low tidal volume is termed *penmanship sign* for its resemblance to a penmanship exercise. It is seen in patients who have greatly diminished vital capacity and diffuse bronchopulmonary fibrosis (Fig. 15-8).

Tests of airway reactivity

It is sometimes desirable to test the sensitivity or reactivity of the airway, often in relation to the clinical diagnosis of asthmatic bronchitis. For this purpose, spirometry is repeated after the administration of bronchodilators such as isoproterenol (Isuprel) or after the administration of bronchoconstrictors such as histamine or acetylcholine. Inasmuch as these are potent drugs with powerful cardiopulmonary effects, they are always used under the supervision of a physician, and only after a specific order by the patient's physician.

Isoproterenol may be given sublingually, by nebulizer, or by intermittent positive pressure breathing (IPPB) using compressed air instead of oxygen. When isoproterenol is given by IPPB, it should be noted that two things are actually being done to the patient—intrabronchial instillation of a bronchodilator, and forced inflation of the lungs. Isoproterenol, as prescribed, together with a suitable volume of sterile water, is given by IPPB at the required mask pressure, using compressed air, until the entire dose has been given. As in giving medication by any other route of administration, a certain dose is prescribed, and administration should be complete before the postbronchodilator tests are done. Isoproterenol should be administered as quickly as is compatible with the patient's comfort and spirometry repeated soon thereafter because its effects are transient.

DETERMINATION OF FUNCTIONAL RESIDUAL CAPACITY (FRC) BY THE OPEN-CIRCUIT NITROGEN WASH-OUT METHOD

The *concentration-dilution* principle of elementary chemistry is applied: $C_1V_1 = C_2V_2$ or $V_1 = C_2V_2/C_1$. Lung nitrogen* is washed out (diluted) with almost pure oxygen in such a manner that nitrogen is neither added to nor lost from the system. Initial lung nitrogen *concentration* is assumed, and final lung nitrogen *concentration* (alveolar gas sample) is actually measured. Initial *volume* is FRC, and final *volume* is FRC plus bag volume. Correction is made both for the small nitrogen content of the almost pure oxygen and for the body nitrogen that is brought to the lungs from the tissues by the circulation during the period of oxygen breathing. The result of this process is represented by a simple concentration-dilution equation containing one unknown—FRC, which is accordingly determined.

*Actually, *nonabsorbable* gas, mostly nitrogen.

Functional residual capacity (FRC) is calculated according to the following equation:

$$FRC = \frac{(V_B)(N_B - N_C) - C}{81 - (N_A - N_C)} \bullet \frac{P_B}{P_B - 47}$$

where FRC is the functional residual capacity in milliliters (BTPS); V_B is the measured volume of gas in the Douglas-type gas bag in milliliters (BTPD); N_B is the measured nitrogen concentration of gas in the Douglas-type gas bag in percent; N_C is the analyzed correction for nitrogen content of the almost pure oxygen in percent; C is the estimated correction for body nitrogen in milliliters (BTPD) that is brought to the lungs from the tissues by the circulation during 7 minutes of pure oxygen breathing, varying with body size and calculated for the fasting, resting subject from the linear equation $C = (BSA)(96.5) + 35$; 81 is the assumed initial alveolar nitrogen concentration of the fasting, resting subject in percent; N_A is the measured nitrogen concentration of alveolar gas after 7 minutes of oxygen breathing in percent; and P_B is barometric pressure in millimeters of Hg.

Methods involving wash-out or wash-in of inert gas measure *communicating* lung volume, as distinguished from the body plethysmograph, which measures total thoracic gas volume. The difference between the two—*noncommunicating* thoracic gas volume—is made up of the volume of any regions in the lung that are not ventilated during the test, plus the volume of any gas that is extrapulmonary but intrathoracic.

After intensive therapy of diffuse, obstructive bronchopulmonary conditions that involve a reversible inflammatory component, inert gas wash-out or wash-in often reveals slightly increased residual volume, total lung capacity, and RV/TLC ratio. This seeming paradox is explained by the fact that previously obstructed regions of lung are less so following treatment, and so contribute to the volume that is measured by the inert gas methods. Simultaneous measurement of thoracic gas volume with the body plethysmograph shows the difference between communicating and noncommunicating lung volume prior to treatment in such cases.

Patients with chronic, diffuse, obstructive bronchopulmonary disease may trap air to a variable extent during forceful expiration. Spirographic evidence of such air trapping is a useful laboratory sign. However, for calculation of TLC it is best to avoid air trapping by using *inspiratory* vital capacity, rather than the usual *expiratory* vital capacity. FRC is actually greater in the erect than in the supine position because of a shift of the midposition, or end-expiratory level (Fig. 4-2). However, subtraction of the appropriate expiratory reserve volume gives an accurate residual volume that is almost the same for the two different body positions. The comparative reproducibility of TLC is greater than that for RV because vital capacity with its high reproducibility comprises a large fraction of the TLC.

INTERPRETATION OF CARDIOPULMONARY LABORATORY DATA

Before cardiopulmonary laboratory data are interpreted, they should be examined for *internal consistency* and *credibility*. Data are internally consistent if there are no internal contradictions and credible if they are within bounds of the possible. Such examination sometimes leads to a question about a particular value in a set of data, so that certain tests can be repeated or calculations checked.

1. The respiratory exchange ratio (R_E) as calculated from measurement and analysis of expired gas provides interesting and valuable information in fasting subjects. Because it is appreciably affected by both composition and quantity of food taken prior to study, interpretation is a

complex matter in nonfasting subjects. The respiratory exchange ratio, which equals the respiratory quotient (R) during steady state conditions, varies from about 0.70 to 0.86 in fasting subjects at rest. Factors that increase R_E are as follows:

a. Hyperventilation, before attainment of a steady state of respiratory alkalosis or during recovery from hypoventilation
b. Exercise, where increase is the result of increased CO_2 exhalation, as metabolic acidosis develops, and, later, of preferential carbohydrate utilization by working muscles after achievement of a nearly steady state
c. Postabsorptive metabolic conversion of nutrient substances, a process that is accelerated by exercise

Factors that decrease R_E are as follows:

d. Hypoventilation, before attainment of a steady state of respiratory acidosis or during recovery from hyperventilation
e. Exercise, before attainment of a steady state
f. Loss of CO_2 when expired gas is permitted to stand in Douglas-type gas bags

If an expired gas sample is simply mixed with atmospheric air, then calculated CO_2 output, O_2 uptake, and R_E all remain unchanged because F_{ECO_2} and F_{EO_2} are affected proportionately.

2. MVV in terms of percent predicted exceeds the MMEF expressed in similar terms, except in cases where the process of inspiration is selectively affected or where the subject cannot or will not sustain the MVV effort.
3. Arterial blood O_2 saturation cannot exceed 100% under any conditions including rest, hyperventilation and breathing high O_2 mixtures. In cases where the calculated value does exceed 100%, this may be the result of incorrect values for (1) total whole blood O_2 content, (2) total whole blood O_2 capacity, (3) either of their respective corrections for dissolved O_2, or (4) any combination of these.
4. Hemoglobin concentration as calculated from O_2 capacity almost always decreases promptly when high O_2 mixtures are breathed and increases promptly during exercise.
5. If analyses are correct, the CO_2 content of simultaneously drawn mixed venous blood must exceed that of systemic arterial blood, which must in turn exceed that of a capacity blood sample prepared by the multiple air-equilibration method.
6. During exercise a metabolic acidosis characterized by decreased arterial blood pH and CO_2 content is almost always seen. This pattern may be complicated in certain cases by hyperventilation during exercise, producing concomitant respiratory alkalosis, or by superimposed respiratory acidosis in patients with severe ventilatory deficit.

To facilitate the interpretation of data obtained by study of its patients, each laboratory should make an effort to develop a concept of its own normal values for healthy subjects. Normal values vary from laboratory to laboratory because of differences with respect to location, equipment, and personnel. The concept of normal values should include measures of central tendency (arithmetic means), reproducibility of the various test procedures (standard deviations), and comparative reproducibility of one test procedure with another (coefficients of variation, or dispersion relative to the mean).

ARTERIAL BLOOD STUDY

Analysis of arterial blood for CO_2, O_2, and pH provides basic information about cardiopulmonary function. Although somewhat more difficult to obtain than capillary or venous samples, arterial blood is essential for this purpose and there is no satisfactory substitute. Arterial blood, with rare exceptions, is a stream of uniform composition. It has the further advantage of reflecting cardiopulmonary function more directly than capillary or venous blood possibly can because these latter sources are subject to the complicating effects of changing regional and tissue conditions.

Arterial puncture and placement of an indwelling cannula is a procedure requiring aseptic technic and involving the potential hazards of hematoma, nerve trauma, and infection. Obviously, this is a procedure for the physician. With proper technic, complications are extremely rare and almost never constitute a contraindication to this vital source of information.

Principles of blood-gas and pH analysis

It must be stressed that collection, storage, and analysis of blood for CO_2, O_2, and pH present unique problems that are not encountered when blood is used for other clinical chemical determinations. Competency in clinical blood chemistry does not necessarily imply competency in blood analysis for CO_2, O_2, and pH. Indeed, it often happens that familiarity with clinical blood chemistry breeds contempt for the necessary precautions that are termed *anaerobic technic.* Anaerobic technic is based on knowledge of the physical chemistry and physiology of blood as a tissue. This technic comprises all those methods and devices which ensure that blood composition with respect to the interdependent parameters of CO_2, O_2, and pH does not suffer violence from the time of withdrawal from the circulation to the time of analysis. Time and again, individuals without adequate instruction or understanding of the relevant principles collect, prepare, or store blood samples in such a manner that they are totally worthless.

Blood samples should be drawn with the least possible traction, suction, or pulling force. Evacuated containers that draw blood samples into a vacuum are worthless for this purpose. In drawing systemic arterial samples, it is often possible to avoid traction completely. Blood samples with air bubbles should be discarded. Blood samples should be analyzed immediately. If this is impossible, maximum immersion of the syringe up to, but not above, the flange or shoulder in ice water with immediate and continuous refrigeration is imperative. When blood is allowed to stand after removal from the circulation, the erythrocytes sediment at a rate that is characteristic for each subject. Before withdrawal of any aliquot for analysis, the whole blood sample must be thoroughly mixed by shaking or rotation to assure identical composition of each. Transfer of the blood sample should also be done quickly to avoid such separation. In general, blood should be handled with care because erythrocytes are fragile and hemolysis produces complex changes that may be undesirable. If blood samples contain anesthetic gases, such as nitrous oxide, or volatile liquids, appreciable analytic errors can result because of their solubility in, or reaction with, absorbent solutions. Account of their presence should be taken.

Blood pH is a function of temperature. The pH of human whole blood rises with falling temperature 0.0147 pH unit/° C. The relationship of hemoglobin oxygenation to blood pH should not be ignored. If the pH of a highly saturated arterial blood sample is measured and its hemoglobin then completely reduced, holding P_{CO_2} constant, pH increases 0.06 to 0.07 unit. The P_{O_2} decreases as whole blood stands. This decrease is largely due to the metabolism of the white blood cells. As whole blood stands, metabolic acidosis develops—fixed acids increase and pH falls. Initially, the pH decrease is about 0.001

pH unit/min. Subsequent changes are less predictable and also depend upon whether fluoride has been added. Sodium fluoride should not be added to blood samples for pH determination because pH should be determined within minutes anyway and because the addition of sodium salts aggravates the glass electrode sodium error. Large P_{CO_2} gradients from blood sample to room air are always present and favor loss of CO_2, or respiratory alkalosis. *Dried* heparin minimizes dilution of the blood sample.

Several systems are commercially available, incorporating pH, P_{CO_2}, and P_{O_2} electrodes, for clinical service and research use. The *Astrup micromethod* for blood-gas and pH analysis is a widely used system in which P_{CO_2} is estimated from a nomogram, rather than measured directly. This method involves the use of the *Siggaard-Andersen curve nomogram,* which is discussed on p. 116. A correction must be made when the oxyhemoglobin saturation of the blood sample is less than 100%: for each gram percent of unsaturated hemoglobin the pH-log P_{CO_2} line is moved 0.005 pH unit to the left. The Astrup micromethod gives values for CO_2 content that are about 2 mM/L lower than the results of standard methods. This problem is still unsolved and may be due to metabolic acidosis, respiratory alkalosis, hemoglobin oxygenation, or the use of an assumed pK (6.11) that is too high. If *cutaneous* blood* must be used in place of the preferred *arterial* sample, the hand should be immersed in hot water for 3 to 5 minutes before puncture. Squeezing and consequent *dilution* of the cutaneous blood sample with tissue juice results in characteristic errors.

Blood O_2 capacity

Blood samples for determination of O_2 capacity must be obtained in relation to blood samples drawn for O_2 content not only at rest but also for each different physiologic state. For example, hemoglobin concentration and O_2 capacity may undergo considerable change during exercise or O_2 breathing. Arterial blood samples should be used for determination of blood O_2 capacity whenever possible. Samples of venous blood are less satisfactory for this purpose due to their lower and more variable initial O_2 content.

By exposure in a closed container to a volume of O_2, or by exposure to successive volumes of fresh air, the blood sample is brought toward equilibrium with the water vapor–saturated gas. The multiple air-equilibration method is preferable (1) because air has a sufficiently high P_{O_2} when ambient pressure is approximately that at sea level for almost complete saturation of the hemoglobin, (2) because air is readily available, and (3) because the composition of air is precisely known.

Note that this method of measuring blood O_2 capacity involves the near equilibration of whole blood with saturated air at *ambient* pressure and *room* temperature. Such blood samples are therefore different from blood samples drawn anaerobically from a subject. Dissolved O_2 content is larger at any given P_{O_2} than that in blood samples with the same P_{O_2} at body temperature.

Blood O_2 saturation

In calculation of oxyhemoglobin saturation, both total O_2 content and total O_2 capacity are corrected by subtraction of their respective values for dissolved O_2. The following three methods for obtaining dissolved O_2 are in general use:

1. Dissolved O_2 can be obtained by the estimation and assumption of standard values.

2. Calculation of approximate saturation can be made by dividing the uncorrected content by the uncorrected capacity. The resulting quotient is then used to-

*Try to get the cutaneous blood sample from the *arterial* end of the capillaries.

gether with arterial pH to find P_{O_2} from the oxyhemoglobin dissociation curve (Fig. 7-2). This method can only be used when P_{O_2} is below 100 mm Hg, where the slope of the oxyhemoglobin dissociation curve is appreciable.

3. After actual measurement of P_{O_2} with an O_2 electrode, dissolved O_2 can be calculated by multiplication with the factor for the appropriate temperature (Table 5).

O_2 method for detection of venous-to-arterial circulatory shunts

The brachial or radial arteries of either upper extremity may be used, giving a choice of four possible sites. Although the femoral arteries are larger, they are less desirable if exercise is anticipated because exercise is awkward with the indwelling cannula in this location.

Venous-to-arterial circulatory shunts, also termed right-to-left shunts, can be detected by failure to achieve full arterial blood O_2 tension and saturation after 15 minutes of O_2 breathing. Thebesian vein blood from the coronary circulation empties into the left ventricle, constituting a tiny physiologic right-to-left shunt. Pathoanatomic right-to-left shunts include intrapulmonary (arteriovenous fistula), intracardiac, and bronchial artery-to-pulmonary vein types. Pathoanatomic shunts may be quite large, diverting a sizable fraction of the cardiac output away from contact with alveolar gas. In chronic hepatic disease, shunts may occur that result in arterial O_2 saturation values of less than 90%. Anatomic localization of large venous-to-arterial shunts is possible in many cases with angiography; however, their existence and functional significance can be determined by the oxygen method.

The subject is given a high-O_2 breathing mixture for a period of 15 minutes, with a deep breath each minute. The temptation to cut this period short must be resisted, or equivocal data will result in certain cases, and the question of venous-to-arterial shunt will remain unanswered. Concentrations of O_2 from 60% to 100% may be used for the test. Lower O_2 concentrations, such as 60%, are advantageous where only O_2 content, capacity, and saturation are measured and where a standard correction for dissolved O_2 is used. In this case the error introduced by assuming a value for dissolved O_2 is minimized because dissolved O_2 is a smaller value than that obtained if higher O_2 concentrations were breathed. Furthermore, if O_2 saturation is used, it is important to note that hemoglobin concentration and O_2 capacity decrease during O_2 breathing.

Actual measurement of P_{O_2} with an O_2 electrode is considerably more sensitive than measurement of O_2 content, capacity, and saturation. The correction for dissolved O_2 can then be calculated for each individual subject. Breathing 100% O_2 at sea level can be calculated to produce a maximum alveolar P_{O_2} of 673 mm Hg. Water vapor tension and CO_2 tension are subtracted from the barometric pressure: $760 - 47 - 40 = 673$ mm Hg. However, actual found values for arterial P_{O_2} in healthy subjects breathing 100% O_2 at sea level range from 610 to 660 mm Hg. When pulmonary function is tested for clinical purposes, the highest arterial P_{O_2} achieved is used, and a value less than 550 mm Hg is considered to indicate a venous-to-arterial shunt.

Formulas have been proposed for estimation of the magnitude of right-to-left shunts. These require arterial, mixed venous, and pulmonary end-capillary O_2 data. Such calculations ignore the effects of any $\dot{V}_A/\dot{Q}_c$ or diffusion abnormality that may be present, relying upon the fact that their interference is minimized during high O_2 breathing. Determination of mixed venous blood O_2 involves right heart catheterization, and calculation of absolute values for shunt flow requires simultaneous measurement of cardiac output.

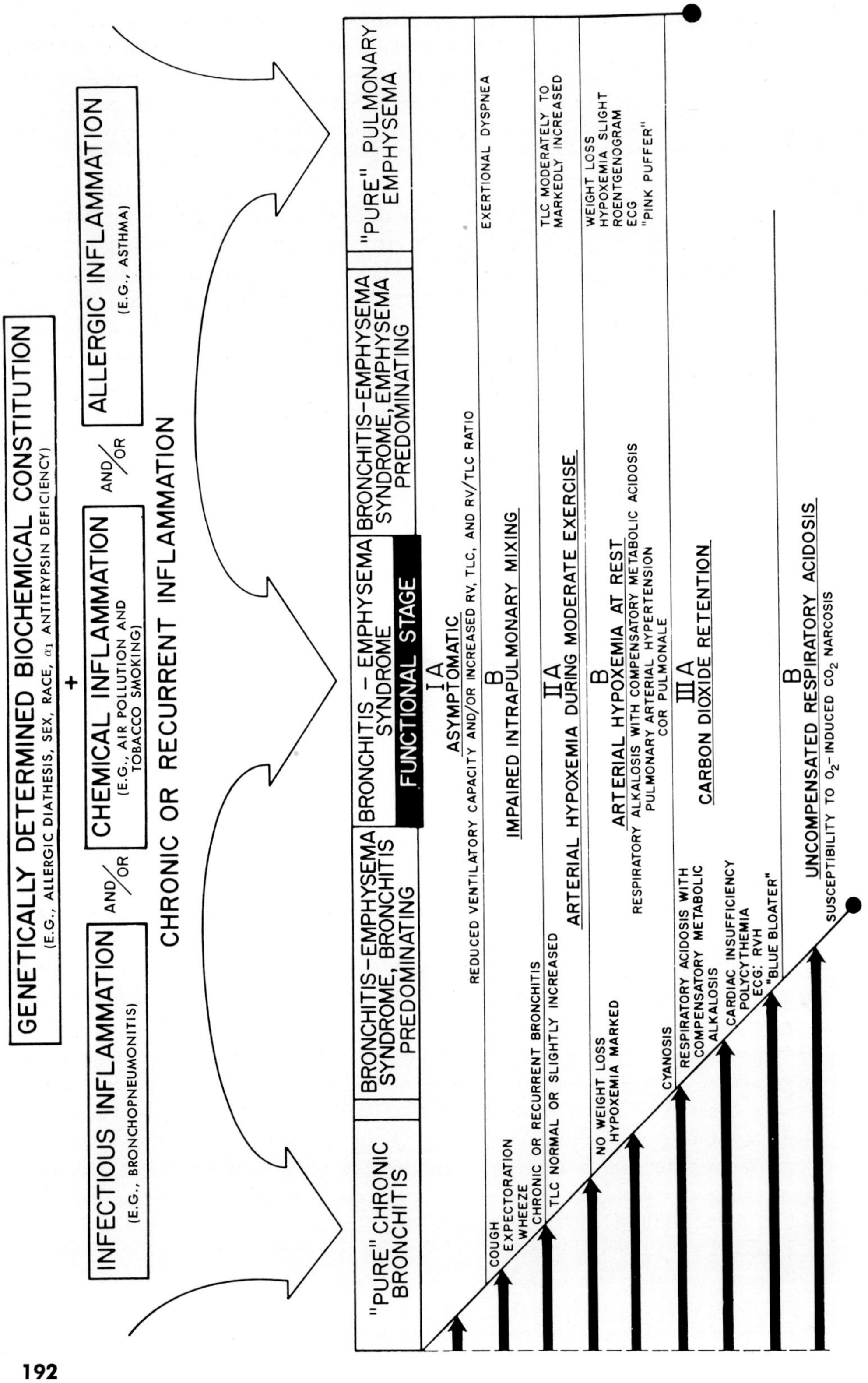

Fig. 15-9
Spectrum of the bronchitis-emphysema syndrome, a chronic, obstructive bronchopulmonary syndrome of multifactorial causation.

Table 9

Functional classification of cardiopulmonary insufficiency in bronchitis-emphysema syndrome (a chronic, obstructive bronchopulmonary syndrome of multifactorial causation)

Functional stage		Pathologic physiology: Pulmonary function evaluation	Pathologic physiology: Comment	Clinical manifestations: Bronchitis	Clinical manifestations: Emphysema
I	A	Reduced ventilatory capacity and/or Increased residual volume, total lung capacity, and RV/TLC ratio	Low MMEF may be the only spirometric evidence of reduced ventilatory capacity Elevation of respiratory level seen in spirographically recorded MVV	May be asymptomatic	May be asymptomatic
	B	Impaired intrapulmonary mixing		Cough Expectoration Wheeze Chronic or recurrent bronchitis	Exertional dyspnea
II	A	Arterial P_{O_2} falls during moderate exercise	Arterial hypoxemia during moderate exercise, but not at rest	TLC normal or slightly increased	TLC moderately or greatly increased
	B	V_A/Q_c abnormality Arterial P_{O_2} and S_{O_2} low at rest Arterial P_{CO_2} low or WNL	Arterial hypoxemia at rest Airway collapse may occur during forced expiration Air trapping may occur during forced expiration	Respiratory alkalosis with compensatory metabolic acidosis Pulmonary arterial hypertension Hypoxemia marked Cyanosis	Respiratory alkalosis with compensatory metabolic acidosis Weight loss Pulmonary arterial hypertension Hypoxemia slight "Pink puffer"
III	A	Arterial P_{CO_2} high Arterial CO_2 content high Arterial pH WNL	CO_2 retention, slight to moderate	Respiratory acidosis with compensatory metabolic alkalosis Cor pulmonale Cardiac insufficiency Polycythemia "Blue bloater"	
	B	Arterial pH low	CO_2 retention, severe Uncompensated respiratory acidosis	Susceptibility to O_2-induced CO_2 narcosis	

If the subject's condition permits, he is next exercised by means of a bicycle ergometer or treadmill, erect or supine, at a steady work rate judged to be safe by the physician. The exercise period should be of at least 5 minutes' duration and, if possible, should be standardized with respect both to work rate and duration. In follow-up studies it is highly desirable for purposes of comparison that any given subject repeat the same work stint done in the prior study. Treadmill work rate is determined by grade and speed. Bicycle ergometer work rate is determined by load setting and RPM. When venous-to-arterial shunts are present, exercise produces a further decrease of arterial P_{O_2} and saturation because the shunted mixed venous blood then contains even less O_2.

DIFFERENTIAL DIAGNOSIS OF ARTERIAL HYPOXEMIA

Arterial hypoxemia is a clinically important manifestation, the differential diagnosis of which involves basic physiologic principles. The four causes of arterial hypoxemia are usually present in one or another combination, but in certain instances may occur in almost pure form. They follow in order of their clinical frequency: (1) abnormality of $\dot{V}_A/\dot{Q}_c$ ratios, (2) alveolar hypoventilation, (3) loss of pulmonary diffusing capacity, and (4) pathoanatomic venous-to-arterial shunts.

It is possible to test for item 4 quite readily. Arerial blood samples are drawn for O_2 analysis both before and after the patient breathes 60% to 100% O_2 for 15 minutes with a deep breath every minute. The resulting increased alveolar P_{O_2} is sufficient to overcome any bronchopulmonary factor, so that full arterial blood O_2 tension and saturation result, unless pathoanatomic venous-to-arterial shunts are present.

Two important clinical observations are as follows: First, arterial hypoxemia *always* precedes CO_2 retention in the course of chronic, diffuse bronchopulmonary disease. Second, patients with sufficiently impaired pulmonary diffusing capacity demonstrate arterial hypoxemia, yet have arterial P_{CO_2} values that are either low, due to hyperventilation, or within normal limits. The explanation of these two observations involves the physiologic significance of $\dot{V}_A/\dot{Q}_c$ ratios, the slope of the two dissociation curves for O_2 and CO_2, and the fact that CO_2 is about twenty times as diffusible as O_2 across the alveolocapillary membrane.

In hypoxemia, rational clinical treatment includes efforts to increase alveolar ventilation, as with a mechanical respirator, and the use of increased concentrations of O_2 sufficient to restore arterial P_{O_2} to normal or near normal levels (70 to 100 mm Hg). This can often be accomplished with O_2 administered at low flow rates, such as 1 to 3 L/min.

As already mentioned, the prevalence of chronic bronchopulmonary disease is increasing rapidly. The largest single clinical entity contributing to this increase is the *bronchitis-emphysema syndrome*,* a spectrum of chronic conditions of multifactorial causation. Because of its prevalence and the wide range of pathophysiologic problems it produces, we present Fig. 15-9 and Table 9, which give the basis for etiologic analysis and functional classification of patients.

**Chronic bronchitis* is characterized pathologically by hyperplasia and hypertrophy of the bronchial mucous glands, chronic inflammatory cell infiltration and edema of the bronchial mucosa, and squamous metaplasia of the respiratory epithelium. *Pulmonary emphysema* is characterized pathologically by widespread focal degeneration of elastic tissue, reticulum and collagen formation at the sites of elastic fiber damage, attenuation and disappearance of alveolar capillaries, and the fenestration and dissolution of alveolar septa.

Appendix

SYMBOLS AND ABBREVIATIONS FOR RESPIRATORY PHYSIOLOGY
(Based on standardization of definitions and symbols in respiratory physiology, Fed. Proc. 9:602, 1950)

1. Primary variables

Symbol	Definition
C	Concentration of gas in blood phase
D	Diffusing capacity in general; volume per unit time per unit pressure difference
F	Fractional concentration in dry gas phase
f	Breathing frequency; breaths per unit time
P	Gas pressure in general
$\bar{P}$	Mean gas pressure
Q	Volume of blood
$\dot{Q}$	Rate of blood flow
R	Respiratory exchange ratio in general—$\dot{V}_{CO_2}/\dot{V}_{O_2}$ (Use small upper case subscript E when R is based upon analysis of mixed expired gas.)
S	Saturation of hemoglobin with oxygen or carbon monoxide in percent
V	Gas volume in general (Pressure, temperature, and water vapor tension must also be given.)
$\dot{V}$	Gas volume per unit time; rate of gas flow

2. Secondary symbols for the gas phase

Symbol*	Definition
A	Alveolar gas
B	Barometric
D	Dead space gas
E	Expired gas
I	Inspired gas
L	Lung
T	Tidal gas

*All symbols under item 2 are small upper case letters.

3. Secondary symbols for the blood phase

Symbol	Definition
a	Arterial blood (specify exact location)
b	Blood in general
c	Capillary blood (specify exact location)
v	Venous blood (specify exact location)
$\bar{v}$	Mixed venous blood

4. Other secondary symbols and abbreviations

Symbol or abbreviation	Definition
ATPD*	Ambient temperature, ambient pressure, dry
ATPS*	Ambient temperature, ambient pressure, saturated with water vapor
BTPD*	Body temperature, ambient pressure, dry
BTPS*	Body temperature, ambient pressure, saturated with water vapor
STPD*	Standard temperature, standard pressure, dry
s	Subscript to denote the steady state
$\bar{X}$	Dash above any symbol used to indicate a mean value
$\dot{X}$	Dot above any symbol used to indicate a rate

*Small upper case letters.

5. Abbreviations for pulmonary function tests and measurements

A. For lung volume and its subdivisions

Abbreviation	Definition
ERV	Expiratory reserve volume; maximal volume that can be expired from resting expiratory level
FRC	Functional residual capacity; volume of gas in lungs at resting expiratory level
IC	Inspiratory capacity; maximal volume that can be inspired from resting expiratory level
IRV	Inspiratory reserve volume; maximal volume that can be inspired from end-tidal inspiratory level
RV	Residual volume; volume of gas in lungs at end of maximal expiration
TLC	Total lung capacity; volume of gas in lungs at end of maximal inspiration
VC	Vital capacity; maximal volume that can be expired after maximal inspiration

B. For ventilatory capacity

Abbreviation	Definition
	Single breath tests*
FEVC	Forced expiratory vital capacity; following maximal inspiration, entire vital capacity volume is expelled as rapidly as possible
FEV_T†	Forced expiratory volume, timed; volume which has been expired at any time T during forced expiratory vital capacity
FEV_T%†	Percent of vital capacity volume which has been expired at any time T during forced expiratory vital capacity
MEFR	Maximal expiratory flow rate; average rate of flow during expulsion of liter from 200 to 1,200 ml during forced expiratory vital capacity
MET	Midexpiratory time; time required for expulsion of middle half of vital capacity during forced expiratory vital capacity
MMEF	Maximal midexpiratory flow; average rate of flow during expulsion of middle half of vital capacity during forced expiratory vital capacity
PEFR	Peak expiratory flow rate
	Multiple breath tests
MBC_T† or MVV_T†	Maximal breathing capacity or maximal voluntary ventilation calculated from an effort of T seconds' duration
MVV_f	Maximal voluntary ventilation at designated breathing frequency

*To abbreviate corresponding *inspiratory* measurements, substitute I for E.

†Subscript T is a small upper case letter.

USEFUL DATA AND CONSTANTS

Absolute zero, 0° K = − 273.16° C

Water vapor tension, P_{H_2O} = 47.067 mm Hg at 37.0° C

Avogadro's number = 6.023 × 10^{23} molecules/mole

Gas constant, R = 8.31432 × 10^7 ergs/°K/mole

Gram-molecular volume of an "ideal" gas = 22,414 ml (STPD)

Gram-molecular volume of CO_2 = 22,260 ml (STPD); hence,

$$CO_2 \text{ content (mM/L)} = \frac{CO_2 \text{ content (vol \%)}}{2.226}$$

Air density (STPD) = 1.2929 gm/L

Mercury density at 0° C = 13.5955 gm/ml

Mercury density at 25° C = 13.5340 gm/ml

Water density, maximum at 3.98° C = 1.0000 gm/ml

Velocity of sound in air (STPD) = 1087.1 feet/sec or 33,136 cm/sec

Acceleration due to gravity, g, at sea level and 45° latitude = 32.172 feet × sec^{-2} or 980.62 cm × sec^{-2}

1 atmosphere = 760 mm Hg; 29.9 inches Hg; 1.03 kg/cm^2; 14.7 pounds/square inch

1 gallon of water weighs approximately 8.3 pounds

1 cubic foot of water weighs approximately 62.4 pounds

Hydrostatic pressure increases with water depth by approximately 0.1 atm/M, the exact value depending upon salinity, temperature, and latitude

Heat of fusion of water at 0° C = 79.71 cal/gm

Heat of vaporization of water at 100° C = 539.55 cal/gm

Whole blood: specific gravity = 1.055

Hemoglobin: 1 gram capable of combining with 1.36 ml of O_2 (STPD)

CONVERSION TABLE FOR UNITS OF MEASURE

1 inch	2.54001 centimeters
1 centimeter	0.39370 inch
1 foot	0.30480 meter
1 meter	3.28083 feet; 39.3700 inches
1 pound	0.45359 kilogram
1 kilogram	2.20462 pounds
1 ounce	28.34953 grams
1 gram	0.03527 ounce
1 quart	0.94633 liter
1 liter	1.0561 quarts

1 micron (μ) = 10^{-4} centimeter
1 angstrom unit (Å) = 10^{-8} centimeter
1 watt (absolute) = 10^{7} ergs/sec
1 watt (absolute) = 0.10197 kg-m/sec

MATHEMATICAL CONSTANTS

π	3.14159
e	2.71828
$\log_{10}$ e	0.43429
$\ln_e$ 10	2.30259
1 radian	57.29578° or 57° 17′ 45″
1 degree	0.01745 radian

Number	Square root
2	1.41421
3	1.73205
5	2.23607
6	2.44949
7	2.64575
8	2.82843
10	3.16228

VALUES PECULIAR TO EACH DIFFERENT LABORATORY

The value generally used to convert pressure from units of mm Hg to CGS units of dynes/cm² is 1,330 (mercury density × acceleration due to gravity). This value varies slightly with temperature (mercury density varies with temperature), altitude, and latitude (acceleration due to gravity, g, varies with *both* altitude and latitude).

Predicted values for certain pulmonary function tests vary somewhat from laboratory to laboratory, depending upon technic and equipment. Altitude, in particular, affects certain tests.

ALTITUDE-PRESSURE TABLE*

Altitude (M)	Altitude (feet)	P_B† (mm Hg)	$(P_B - 47)$‡ (mm Hg)	$0.209\ (P_B - 47)$¶ (mm Hg)
0	0	760	713	149
610	2,000	707	660	138
1,220	4,000	656	609	127
1,830	6,000	609	562	118
2,440	8,000	564	517	108
3,050	10,000	523	476	100
3,660	12,000	483	436	91
4,270	14,000	446	399	83
4,880	16,000	412	365	76
5,490	18,000	379	332	69
6,100	20,000	349	302	63
6,710	22,000	321	274	57
7,320	24,000	294	247	52
7,930	26,000	270	223	47
8,540	28,000	247	200	42
9,150	30,000	226	179	37
9,760	32,000	206	159	33
10,370	34,000	187	140	29
10,980	36,000	170	123	26
11,590	38,000	155	108	23
12,200	40,000	141	94	20
12,810	42,000	128	81	17
13,420	44,000	116	69	14
14,030	46,000	106	59	12
14,640	48,000	96	49	10
15,250	50,000	87	40	8
19,215	63,000	47	0	0

*From Rahn, H., and Fenn, W. O.: A graphical analysis of the respiratory gas exchange, Washington, D. C., 1955, The American Physiological Society, p. 41. (Source of data: W. G. Brombacher, Nat. Adv. Com. Aer. Report 538, 1935.)

†P_B = barometric pressure.

‡$(P_B - 47)$ = (a) total pressure of the dry gases after the inspired gas has been saturated with water vapor at 37° C and (b) inspired O_2 tension, $P_{I_{O_2}}$, when pure oxygen is inspired.

¶$0.209\ (P_B - 47)$ = inspired O_2 tension, $P_{I_{O_2}}$, when air is breathed.

RESPIRATORY CALCULATIONS

The ability to represent a relationship or problem in mathematical terms and the power to manipulate and solve it are invaluable. Mathematical manipulation of biologic data is a valuable exercise and sometimes leads to discovery of important facts and relationships. However, the results of such manipulation must always be finally interpreted in terms of what is biologically meaningful, what is biologically possible, and what is cause (independent variable) and what is effect (dependent variable).

1. General gas law describing "ideal gas":

   A. PV = nRT

For calculating change of state, mass remaining constant:

$$B.\quad \frac{P_1V_1}{T_1} = \frac{P_2V_2}{T_2}$$

The following formulas for conversion of gas volume are merely special cases of B:

$$C.\quad V_{STPD} = V_{ATPS} \cdot \frac{(P_B - P_{H_2O}) \times 0.35942}{(T^\circ\ C + 273.16)}$$

$$D.\quad V_{BTPS} = V_{ATPS} \cdot \frac{310.16}{273.16 + T^\circ\ C} \cdot \frac{P_B - P_{H_2O}}{P_B - 47.067}$$

$$E.\quad V_{BTPD} = V_{ATPS} \cdot \frac{310.16}{273.16 + T^\circ\ C} \cdot \frac{P_B - 47.067}{P_B}$$

2. For calculation of O_2 *uptake* (A) or CO_2 *output* (B) from measurement of volume and analysis of composition of mixed expired gas while breathing any mixture of O_2 and CO_2 in nitrogen or other inert gas (all gas volumes are STPD):

$$A.\quad \dot{V}_{O_2} = \dot{V}_E \cdot \frac{[F_{I_{O_2}}(1 - F_{E_{CO_2}}) - F_{E_{O_2}}(1 - F_{I_{CO_2}})]}{(1 - F_{I_{O_2}} - F_{I_{CO_2}})}$$

$$B.\quad \dot{V}_{CO_2} = \dot{V}_E \cdot \frac{[F_{E_{CO_2}}(1 - F_{I_{O_2}}) - F_{I_{CO_2}}(1 - F_{E_{O_2}})]}{(1 - F_{I_{O_2}} - F_{I_{CO_2}})}$$

Equation B divided by equation A gives the *respiratory exchange ratio* for expired gas:

$$C.\quad R_E = \frac{\dot{V}_{CO_2}}{\dot{V}_{O_2}} = \frac{[F_{E_{CO_2}}(1 - F_{I_{O_2}}) - F_{I_{CO_2}}(1 - F_{E_{O_2}})]}{[F_{I_{O_2}}(1 - F_{E_{CO_2}}) - F_{E_{O_2}}(1 - F_{I_{CO_2}})]}$$

For the special case where CO_2 may be considered negligible in the inspired gas, equations A, B, and C reduce to simpler forms. If measurements are made in the steady state, then $R_E = R_s =$ metabolic respiratory quotient.

3. For calculation of *respiratory dead space* (all gas volumes are BTPS):

$$A.\quad V_D = \left(V_T - \frac{\dot{V}_A}{f}\right) \text{ or } \dot{V}_A = (V_T - V_D)\,f$$

Bohr equation for *respiratory dead space to any gas, G:*

$$B.\quad V_{D_G} = \frac{(F_{E_G} - F_{A_G})\,V_T}{(F_{I_G} - F_{A_G})}$$

4. For calculation of *alveolar O_2 pressure* while breathing any mixture of O_2 with inert gas at any ambient pressure:

$$P_{A_{O_2}} = F_{I_{O_2}}(P_B - P_{A_{H_2O}}) - P_{A_{CO_2}}\left[F_{I_{O_2}} + \frac{(1 - F_{I_{O_2}})}{R_A}\right]$$

This equation is sometimes called the "alveolar equation," although it applies equally well to any portion of expired gas that has undergone respiratory exchange. It is useful for determining equivalent altitudes and O_2 requirements for cabin or chamber atmospheres.

5. For calculation of *alveolar ventilation* from respiratory gas exchange:

$$\dot{V}_A = \frac{\dot{V}_{CO_2}}{F_{A_{CO_2}}} = \frac{R_A}{F_{A_{CO_2}}} \cdot \dot{V}_{O_2} = (P_B - P_{A_{H_2O}}) \cdot \frac{R_A}{P_{A_{CO_2}}} \cdot \dot{V}_{O_2}$$

6. For calculation of *pulmonary diffusing capacity* to O_2 by the Bohr method:

$$D_{L_{O_2}} = \frac{\dot{V}_{O_2}}{P_{A_{O_2}} - \bar{P}_{c_{O_2}}}$$

where $\bar{P}_{c_{O_2}}$ is the mean O_2 pressure in pulmonary capillary blood obtained by graphic integration of the oxyhemoglobin dissociation curve.

7. For calculation of *pulmonary blood flow* by the Fick principle:

$$\dot{Q}_b = \frac{\dot{V}_{O_2}}{(C_{a_{O_2}} - C_{\bar{v}_{O_2}})}$$

This equation assumes a steady state of the circulation and respiration and assumes that the two blood samples are simultaneously drawn midway during the mixed expired gas collection.

8. For calculation of the ratio of *alveolar ventilation* to *pulmonary blood flow:*

$$\frac{\dot{V}_A}{\dot{Q}_b} = R_s\,(P_B - P_{A_{H_2O}}) \cdot \frac{(C_{a_{O_2}} - C_{\bar{v}_{O_2}})}{P_{A_{CO_2}}}$$

This equation assumes a steady state of the circulation and respiration and assumes that no circulatory shunt exists so that right ventricular output is equal to left ventricular output.

9. *van der Waals' equation:*

$$(P + \frac{a}{V^2})\ (V - b) = RT$$

where P and V are the pressure and volume at any constant temperature, and a and b are constants; R is the gas constant and T is the absolute temperature. For values of R, a, and b, consult appropriate tables.

10. *Laplace's law* for bubbles:

$$A.\ P = \frac{4T}{r}$$

where P is pressure in dynes/cm^2 due to surface tension in a bubble of mean radius r cm for a liquid whose surface tension is T dynes/cm.

Laplace's law for drops:

$$B.\ P = \frac{2T}{r}$$

11. *Hydrostatic pressure:*

$$P = hdg$$

where d is the density of the liquid and h is the depth below the surface.

Total force on an area A due to hydrostatic pressure:

$$F = PA = Ahdg$$

If h is in cm, d in gm/cc, and g in cm × sec^{-2}, then force will be in dynes and pressure in dynes/cm^2.

12. *Poiseuille's law* for laminar flow rate of fluids through a tube:

$$\dot{V} = \frac{\pi \times \Delta P \times r^4}{8 \times L \times N}$$

where L is the length of the tube, r is its radius, ΔP is the driving pressure, N is the coefficient of viscosity, and $\dot{V}$ is the volume flow rate per second. If L and r are in cm, ΔP in dynes/cm^2, and n in poises or dyne × sec × cm^{-2}, then volumetric flow rate is in cc/sec. Note that density does not appear in this equation.

13. *Reynold's number calculation:*

$$N_R = \frac{v \times d \times 2r}{n}$$

where N_R is Reynolds' number indicating the tendency to turbulence, v is *average linear velocity* of gas in the airway, r is the radius of the airway, d is gas density, and n is absolute gas viscosity. If consistent units are used, the results are dimensionless.

14. *Bernoulli's law:* at any point in a tube through which a liquid is flowing, the sum of the pressure energy, potential energy, and kinetic energy is constant:

$$P + hdg + \tfrac{1}{2}dv^2 = a\ constant$$

where P is pressure, h is height above a reference plane, d is density of the liquid, and v is velocity of flow.

Diminution of pressure at the side of a moving stream:

$$P = \tfrac{1}{2}dv^2$$

for a fluid of density d, moving with a velocity v, the diminution of pressure P, neglecting viscosity, due to motion.

15. To prepare a gas mixture containing any intermediate concentration (F_3) of a gas (G) from two gas mixtures containing G in higher (F_1) and lower (F_2) concentrations, respectively.*†

Case 1: $F_2 > 0$

a. $F_1V_1 + F_2V_2 = F_3V_3$

b. $V_1 + V_2 = V_3$

c. $\frac{V_1}{V_2} = \frac{F_3 - F_2}{F_1 - F_3}$

Case 2: $F_2 = 0$

a. $\frac{V_1}{V_2} = \frac{F_3}{F_1 - F_3}$

*Resulting intermediate concentration will be only approximate, so that chemical analysis is required for accurate determination of concentration.

†Gasometer dead space must be considered.

GREEK ALPHABET

Greek character		Greek name	Greek character		Greek name
Α	α	alpha	Ν	ν	nu
Β	β	beta	Ξ	ξ	xi
Γ	γ	gamma	Ο	ο	omicron
Δ	δ	delta	Π	π	pi
Ε	ε	epsilon	Ρ	ρ	rho
Ζ	ζ	zeta	Σ	σ	sigma
Η	η	eta	Τ	τ	tau
Θ	θ	theta	Υ	υ	upsilon
Ι	ι	iota	Φ	φ	phi
Κ	κ	kappa	Χ	χ	chi
Λ	λ	lambda	Ψ	ψ	psi
Μ	μ	mu	Ω	ω	omega

ALPHABETICAL TABLE OF THE ELEMENTS

International atomic weights

The atomic weights listed are those adopted in 1963 by the International Commission on Atomic Weights.

Element	Symbol	Atomic number	Atomic weight	Element	Symbol	Atomic number	Atomic weight
Actinium	Ac	89	227*	Californium	Cf	98	249*
Aluminum	Al	13	26.98	Carbon	C	6	12.01115
Americium	Am	95	243*	Cerium	Ce	58	140.12
Antimony	Sb	51	121.75	Cesium	Cs	55	132.905
Argon	Ar	18	39.948	Chlorine	Cl	17	35.453
Arsenic	As	33	74.9216	Chromium	Cr	24	51.996
Astatine	At	85	210*	Cobalt	Co	27	58.9332
Barium	Ba	56	137.36	Copper	Cu	29	63.54
Berkelium	Bk	97	247*	Curium	Cm	96	247*
Beryllium	Be	4	9.0122	Dysprosium	Dy	66	162.50
Bismuth	Bi	83	208.980	Einsteinium	Es	99	254*
Boron	B	5	10.811	Erbium	Er	68	167.26
Bromine	Br	35	79.909	Europium	Eu	63	151.96
Cadmium	Cd	48	112.40	Fermium	Fm	100	253*
Calcium	Ca	20	40.08	Fluorine	F	9	18.9984

*Mass number of the isotope of longest known half-life or a better known one.

ALPHABETICAL TABLE OF THE ELEMENTS—cont'd
International atomic weights—cont'd

Element	Symbol	Atomic number	Atomic weight	Element	Symbol	Atomic number	Atomic weight
Francium	Fr	87	223	Polonium	Po	84	210*
Gadolinium	Gd	64	157.25	Potassium	K	19	39.102
Gallium	Ga	31	69.72	Praseodymium	Pr	59	140.907
Germanium	Ge	32	72.59	Promethium	Pm	61	147*
Gold	Au	79	196.967	Protactinium	Pa	91	231*
Hafnium	Hf	72	178.49	Radium	Ra	88	226*
Helium	He	2	4.0026	Radon	Rn	86	222*
Holmium	Ho	67	164.930	Rhenium	Re	75	186.2
Hydrogen	H	1	1.00797	Rhodium	Rh	45	102.905
Indium	In	49	114.82	Rubidium	Rb	37	85.47
Iodine	I	53	126.9044	Ruthenium	Ru	44	101.07
Iridium	Ir	77	192.2	Samarium	Sm	62	150.35
Iron	Fe	26	55.847	Scandium	Sc	21	44.956
Krypton	Kr	36	83.80	Selenium	Se	34	78.96
Lanthanum	La	57	138.91	Silicon	Si	14	28.086
Lawrencium	Lr	103	257*	Silver	Ag	47	107.870
Lead	Pb	82	207.19	Sodium	Na	11	22.9898
Lithium	Li	3	6.939	Strontium	Sr	38	87.62
Lutetium	Lu	71	174.97	Sulfur	S	16	32.064†
Magnesium	Mg	12	24.312	Tantalum	Ta	73	180.948
Manganese	Mn	25	54.9380	Technetium	Tc	43	99*
Mendelevium	Md	101	256*	Tellurium	Te	52	127.60
Mercury	Hg	80	200.59	Terbium	Tb	65	158.924
Molybdenum	Mo	42	95.94	Thallium	Tl	81	204.37
Neodymium	Nd	60	144.24	Thorium	Th	90	232.038
Neon	Ne	10	20.183	Thulium	Tm	69	168.934
Neptunium	Np	93	237*	Tin	Sn	50	118.69
Nickel	Ni	28	58.71	Titanium	Ti	22	47.90
Niobium	Nb	41	92.906	Tungsten	W	74	183.85
Nitrogen	N	7	14.0067	Uranium	U	92	238.03
Nobelium	No	102	256*	Vanadium	V	23	50.942
Osmium	Os	76	190.2	Xenon	Xe	54	131.30
Oxygen	O	8	15.9994	Ytterbium	Yb	70	173.04
Palladium	Pd	46	106.4	Yttrium	Y	39	88.905
Phosphorus	P	15	30.9738	Zinc	Zn	30	65.37
Platinum	Pt	78	195.09	Zirconium	Zr	40	91.22
Plutonium	Pu	94	242*				

*Mass number of the isotope of longest known half-life or a better known one.

†Because of natural variations in the relative abundance of the isotopes of sulfur, the atomic weight of this element has a range of ±0.003.

Questions and problems

QUESTIONS

1. What information do pulmonary function tests provide?
2. How may pulmonary function tests be classified?
3. How can the validity of pulmonary function test results be evaluated?
4. Define ATPS, STPD, BTPS, and BTPD.
5. What are the subdivisions or compartments of the total lung capacity? Which ones do not overlap?
6. Define hyperventilation. What other definitions are possible?
7. What is the difference between an inspiratory vital capacity and the usual expiratory vital capacity? Why may it differ? How is this fact of use in measuring total lung capacity?
8. What usually happens to the midposition, or end-expiratory level, when a subject changes from the supine to an erect position? What does this imply for functional residual capacity as determined in sitting as opposed to supine position?
9. What is the difference between a closed-circuit and an open-circuit breathing system as used in cardiopulmonary function testing?
10. Name all possible sources of alveolar N_2 during prolonged breathing of pure O_2.
11. What factors affect the distribution of inspired gas at altitude?
12. Why must blood samples for CO_2, O_2, and pH analysis be immersed in ice water if they cannot be analyzed immediately?
13. Using the oxyhemoglobin dissociation curve, explain why the saturation readings obtained with certain oximeters may be higher than those determined by a definitive method, such as the Van Slyke manometric method.
14. Using the oxyhemoglobin dissociation curve, explain the Bohr shift.
15. Why is an arterial blood study necessary for complete evaluation of pulmonary function?
16. What are the four primary causes of arterial hypoxemia? What physiologic tests can be used to distinguish among them?
17. Explain why blood drawn from a venous source cannot be prepared as a capacity sample in exactly the same way as arterial blood.
18. During the arterial blood study, under what conditions would 60% O_2 be preferable to pure O_2 as a test for venous-to-arterial shunt?
19. What are the physiologic effects of breathing O_2-enriched gas mixtures?
20. What are the respiratory responses to mild or moderate muscular exercise?
21. Discuss the direct Fick method for determination of pulmonary blood flow. Include the Fick equation. Why are blood samples drawn *simultaneously* from a systemic artery and from a mixed venous source midway during the mixed expired gas collection?
22. Define metabolic acidosis, metabolic alkalosis, respiratory acidosis, and respiratory alkalosis. What are some common clinical causes of each?
23. What is the carbonic acid–bicarbonate buffer system? What is its importance to respiratory physiology?
24. What are the effects of hyperventilation on alveolar and arterial P_{CO_2} and body stores of CO_2? What is the physiologic compensatory response?
25. Distinguish between in vitro buffer capacity and in vivo effective buffer capacity. What is the problem in comparing buffer capacity at different pH levels?
26. What is the biochemistry of physiologic O_2 sensors? pH sensors?
27. Discuss the regulation of pulmonary ventilation during muscular exercise.

28. What is the physiologic importance of the central chemoreceptors?
29. **Q.** When are ventilatory assistance and control clinically indicated in the management of respiratory failure?
    A. When patients are extremely dyspneic and fatigued, or when arterial blood values are pH less than 7.25, P_{CO_2} greater than 60 mm Hg, and P_{O_2} less than 50 mm Hg.
30. **Q.** What are the indications for *pressure-* as opposed to *volume*-cycled mechanical respirators?
    A. Both *pressure-* (IPPB) and *volume*-cycled respirators can achieve adequate alveolar ventilation under certain conditions. In patients who require high inflation pressure (e.g., greater than 30 mm Hg), volume-cycled respirators are needed. Note, however, that mechanical respirators are not a substitute for other measures, such as treatment of airway obstruction.
31. **Q.** If it is necessary to control a patient's pulmonary ventilation with a respirator, are venous blood pH and P_{CO_2} with ear oximeter saturations adequate for monitoring?
    A. These methods are far less satisfactory than *arterial* pH, P_{CO_2}, and P_{O_2}. Arterial puncture is a simple, rapid, and safe procedure that should be mastered by every physician.
32. **Q.** What are critical acute changes in arterial blood pH, P_{O_2}, and P_{CO_2} of human subjects, for example, patients with respiratory failure?
    A. Although no rigid criteria can be defined, an arterial blood pH less than 7.25, P_{O_2} less than 50 mm Hg, and P_{CO_2} greater than 60 mm Hg are considered to be urgent indications for treatment.

PROBLEMS

1. A sample of gas is withdrawn from a spirometer and analyzed in a Scholander Micrometer Gas Analyzer. The CO_2 concentration is found to be 4.00%. The spirometer temperature is 26.0° C, and the barometric pressure is 620.0 mm Hg. What is the CO_2 tension of the gas within the spirometer?

   Step A. The gas within a water-filled spirometer or gasometer is saturated with water vapor. Obtain the total dry gas pressure by subtracting the water vapor tension at the applicable temperature from the barometric pressure: 620.0 mm Hg − 25.2 mm Hg = 594.8 mm Hg.

   Step B. The CO_2 tension is next found by multiplying the fractional concentration of CO_2 (dry gas basis) by the total dry gas pressure: CO_2 tension = 0.0400 × 594.8 mm Hg = 23.8 mm Hg.

2. You accept a position in a cardiopulmonary laboratory that is located at ground level on the planet Mars. Ambient pressure at ground level on Mars is approximately one-tenth that of the average barometric pressure at sea level on Earth. Inside the ground-level plastic chamber the pressure is maintained at a level 24 mm Hg higher than the ambient pressure outside, and the temperature inside the chamber is exactly 16° C. An automatic humidifier holds the water vapor tension within the chamber at 5 mm Hg. The artificial chamber atmosphere has the following composition, all on a dry gas basis: (a) it is enriched to 80% O_2 from the liquid O_2 supply; (b) CO_2 concentration is maintained at exactly 5.00% by a special lightweight $Li(OH)_2$-absorbing system; and (c) N_2 to argon ratio is 2:1. Calculate the percent concentration on a dry gas basis and the partial pressure of each gas in the chamber atmosphere.

   Step A. The ambient pressure at ground level on Mars is $\frac{1}{10}$ × 760 mm Hg = 76 mm Hg.

   Step B. The total gas pressure inside the plastic chamber is 76 mm Hg + 24 mm Hg = 100 mm Hg.

   Step C. The total *dry* gas pressure inside the plastic chamber is the total gas pressure minus the water vapor tension: 100 mm Hg − 5 mm Hg = 95 mm Hg.

   Step D. The partial pressure of O_2 is its fractional concentration on a dry gas basis multiplied by the total dry gas pressure: 0.80 × 95 mm Hg = 76 mm Hg.

   Step E. The partial pressure of CO_2 is its fractional concentration on a dry gas basis multiplied by the total dry gas pressure: 0.050 × 95 mm Hg = 47.5 mm Hg.

   Step F. N_2 and argon together must account for the remaining 15% of the dry gas. Their ratio is 2:1 or 10:5, so that N_2 = 10%, and Ar = 5%.

   Step G. The partial pressure of each of these two gases is its fractional concentration on a dry gas basis multiplied by the total dry gas pressure:

Composition of the artificial chamber atmosphere

Gas	Concentration (%)	Pressure (mm Hg)
H_2O		5
DRY GAS BASIS		
O_2	80	76*
CO_2	5.00	4.75*
N_2	10*	9.5*
Ar	5*	4.75*
Total	100%	100 mm Hg

*Calculated value.

N_2 pressure = 0.10 × 95 mm Hg = 9.5 mm Hg. Argon pressure = 0.05 × 95 mm Hg = 4.75 mm Hg.

3. Find the theoretic maximum value for dissolved O_2 in a capacity blood sample prepared by exposure in a sealed syringe to successive volumes of air, so that the blood sample approaches the P_{O_2} of the gas phase, which is saturated with water vapor. The ambient pressure is 760.0 mm Hg, and the temperature of the syringe is 24° C.

Step A. In a sealed syringe the gas phase is saturated with water vapor at the given temperature. Note that unless the plunger of the syringe is stuck, its contents will be at ambient pressure. Subtract the water vapor tension at 24° C from the ambient pressure: 760.0 mm Hg − 22.4 mm Hg = 737.6 mm Hg.

Step B. Multiply this dry gas pressure by the fractional concentration of O_2 in dry air to obtain the P_{O_2} of the gas phase: 737.6 mm Hg × 0.2093 = 154.4 mm Hg.

Step C. Multiply this P_{O_2} by the solubility factor for dissolved O_2 in whole blood at 24° C (Table 5, p. 80) to obtain the theoretic maximum value for dissolved O_2 in the capacity blood sample: 154.4 mm Hg × 0.00411 vol %/mm Hg = 0.63 vol % of dissolved O_2. Such a value for dissolved O_2 is subtracted from the total O_2 content of the capacity blood sample for calculation of both hemoglobin and oxyhemoglobin saturation.

4. A fasting 30-year-old Nepalese skin diver, clad in a wet suit, hovers quietly at a depth of 17 feet below the surface of a cold Himalayan mountain lake at 18,000 feet elevation. He holds his breath for 60 seconds at this level. At the end of this time, what is the:
   a. Approximate intrapulmonic pressure?
   b. Intrapulmonic water vapor tension?
   c. Nitrogen tension, if alveolar N_2 concentration is 83%?
   d. Chest volume relative to same at 30 seconds?

Glossary

acidosis A disturbance of acid-base balance resulting from an increase of acidic chemical substances (proton donors) or loss of alkaline chemical substances (proton acceptors). If the accumulating substance is CO_2 (which reacts with water to form carbonic acid), the condition is termed *respiratory acidosis*. If the accumulating acidic substance is other than CO_2 or if alkaline substances are lost, the condition is termed *metabolic acidosis*. Homeostatic body mechanisms that attempt to correct an acidosis result in *pH compensation*. Such compensation may be complete (pH within normal limits) or only partial (pH remaining low). Acidosis is sometimes termed *acidemia*.

alkalosis A disturbance of acid-base balance resulting from an increase of alkaline chemical substances (proton acceptors) or loss of acidic chemical substances (proton donors). If the lost substance is CO_2 (which reacts with water to form carbonic acid), the condition is termed *respiratory alkalosis*. If the lost acidic substance is other than CO_2 or if alkaline substances increase, the condition is termed *metabolic alkalosis*. Homeostatic body mechanisms that attempt to correct an alkalosis result in *pH compensation*. Such compensation may be complete (pH within normal limits) or only partial (pH remaining high). Alkalosis is sometimes termed *alkalemia*.

alveolar gas The gas mixture present within the lungs reflecting the effects of respiratory gas exchange, as distinguished from *dead space gas*. The definition of alveolar gas composition is complicated by the discontinuous nature of lung ventilation, by lung perfusion, and by the nonuniform matching of these aspects of lung function. Alveolar gas is assumed to be saturated with water vapor at 37° C.

anaerobic Of or pertaining to the exclusion or absence of atmospheric air.

anemia Generally, a quantitative or qualitative lack or loss of blood. A qualitative lack is usually expressed as a deficiency of hemoglobin or red blood cells.

angiocardiography Visualization of the cardiovascular system by roentgenography following intravascular injection of a radiopaque contrast medium.

apnea Cessation of breathing movements, as in anesthetized animals following hyperventilation.

atelectasis Failure of the lungs to expand normally at birth, or collapse of an expanded lung as gas is absorbed following obstruction of an airway.

blood buffer curve A curve or line on any graph of the Henderson-Hasselbalch equation describing the pH and CO_2 content changes in blood resulting from addition or removal of CO_2. In essence, a line describing the titration of blood with carbonic acid. The slope of a blood buffer line is a measure of blood buffer capacity. It is also called CO_2 dissociation curve.

bronchiole Any of several generations of the smallest ramifications of the branching tracheobronchial tree.

carbonic anhydrase An enzyme present in various tissues, especially red blood cells, which catalyzes the reaction: $CO_2 + H_2O \rightleftharpoons H_2CO_3$. Important in CO_2 transfer from tissues to systemic capillary blood and from pulmonary capillary blood to alveolar gas.

closed-circuit A type of breathing system used in cardiopulmonary technology in which the contained gas mixture is rebreathed, either directly or after recirculation. **Example:** spirometer.

CO_2 output The rate at which CO_2 is exhaled from the lungs as determined by measurement and analysis of expired gas, with correction for any inspired CO_2. Expressed as a rate in volume units per unit time. **Distinguish:** *CO_2 production*, which is the rate at which CO_2 is produced by the metabolizing tissues. When a steady state of respiration and circulation exists, *CO_2 ouput* equals *CO_2 production*.

CO_2 retention The result of impaired pulmonary CO_2 elimination as in disease or hypoventilation. *Hypercapnia* refers to increased CO_2 tension in lung gas and blood and may be associated with either *CO_2 retention* or inhalation of CO_2-containing gas mixtures. *Respiratory acidosis* refers to the pattern of pH and electrolyte changes resulting from *hypercapnia*.

cyanosis A bluish discoloration of the skin, mucous membranes, and nail beds resulting from oxygen deficiency in the blood. It has been empirically determined that cyanosis first becomes apparent when arterial blood oxygen saturation decreases to about 83%. In other terms, cyanosis first becomes apparent when the concentration of reduced hemoglobin in the capillary blood of the skin, mucous membranes, or nail beds exceeds about 5 gm %.

dead space *Anatomic dead space* is the total volume of all nongas-exchanging airway passages. It consists of the upper airway and bronchial tree as far as the respiratory bronchioles. *Physiologic dead space* is a calculated, not a topographic, volume. By comparison with the anatomic dead space it expresses the nonuniformity of $\dot{V}_A/\dot{Q}_c$ ratios in the lung.

diffusing capacity The rate of gas transfer through a unit area of a permeable membrane in relation to the gas pressure difference across it. *Pulmonary diffusing capacity* is usually measured with O_2 or carbon monoxide and is expressed as milliliters of gas transferred per mm Hg pressure difference per minute.

dissolved gas That gas which is in simple physical solution, as distinguished from that which is chemically combined or which has reacted chemically with solutes or solvent.

distribution The concept or mathematical description of the manner in which the volume of inspired gas is distributed to the large number of ventilatory lung units. The theoretically perfect distribution of a nonexchanging gas, in which each alveolus receives the same volume of inspired gas from the tidal volume in relation to its original volume as does every other alveolus. Also, the distribution of the volume of pulmonary blood flow. The *matching* of these two distributions is a subject of great physiologic importance.

dysbarism Any morbid condition or disease resulting from exposure to a change of ambient pressure and, therefore, usually sudden exposure or great change.

dyspnea The uncomfortable awareness or consciousness of the need for increased breathing. Dyspnea is subjective by definition; it is a symptom, not a sign, usually related to decreased ventilatory capacity and increased work of breathing. This sensation probably is not experienced by healthy, trained individuals.

erythrocyte A red blood cell. Human erythrocytes are biconcave, hemoglobin-containing disks about 1 μ thick and about 7.7 μ in diameter. There are normally about 5 million in each cubic millimeter of blood. The average life-span is about 120 days. Erythrocytes are important in both O_2 and CO_2 transport. Circulating erythrocytes of mammals have no nuclei.

febrile Of or pertaining to fever; feverish.

fibrosis The formation of fibrous tissue within an organ such as the lungs or heart; usually, a reaction to some identifiable condition, such as inflammation or hypoxia, which injures or destroys cells. Because of its stiffness, relative impermeability, and tendency to shrink, fibrous tissue not only is an important aspect of the healing process but also has importance for cardiopulmonary function. Although the term *fibrosis* is often loosely used to describe certain chest roentgenographic patterns or diminished lung volume, it is properly a histopathologic diagnosis requiring tissue examination by a pathologist.

gradient The rate of increase or decrease of any variable, or the curve that represents it; usually with reference to pressure. Often, the term *gradient* is mistakenly used to refer to a simple pressure difference between two points.

hyberbaric Of or pertaining to pressure in excess of ambient or atmospheric pressure. **Example:** hyperbaric oxygenation.

hyperbarism Any condition, especially morbid, or disease resulting from exposure to increased ambient pressure. Usually it is the result of sudden exposure or significant increase in pressure.

hyperpnea Increased rate and/or depth of breathing. **Example:** hyperpnea of exercise.

hyperventilation Generally, an increased pulmonary ventilation rate beyond the actual requirement for respiratory gas exchange. It may result from increased rate or depth of breathing, or any combination of these. Usually, hyperventilation is best expressed in terms of *alveolar* ventilation rate. It results in *increased* alveolar and arterial blood O_2 tension, and *decreased* alveolar and arterial blood CO_2 tension. Hyperventilation may produce dizziness, numbness, tingling, and significant psychomotor impairment if continued and is a cause of *respiratory alkalosis.*

hypobarism Any condition, especially morbid, or disease resulting from exposure to decreased ambient pressure. Hypobarism usually results from sudden exposure or significant decrease in pressure.

hypobarogenous aerobullosis A neologism; generalized emergence and growth of gas bubbles from solution in fluids and tissues throughout the body as a result of decompression. **Distinguish:** Aeroembolism has been used in this sense, but as the term suggests, it should mean the *intravascular* emergence, growth, and *transport* of gas bubbles as a result of decompression.

hypokalemia Deficiency of blood potassium; blood serum potassium ion concentration below the normal range of 3.5 to 5.5 mEq/L.

hyponatremia Deficiency of blood sodium; blood serum sodium ion concentration below the normal range of 135 to 147 mEq/L.

hypoventilation Generally, a reduced pulmonary ventilation rate below that actually required for respiratory gas exchange. It may result from decreased rate or depth of breathing, or any combination of these. Usually, hypoventilation is best expressed in terms of *alveolar* ventilation rate. It results in *decreased* alveolar and arterial blood O_2 tension, and *increased* alveolar and arterial blood CO_2 tension. If continued, hypoventilation produces hypoxemia, hypercapnia, CO_2 retention, and *respiratory acidosis. Chronic alveolar hypoventilation* is an important clinical syndrome. The combination of hypoxemia with respiratory acidosis constricts the pulmonary vascular bed to produce pulmonary arterial hypertension.

hypoxemia Low blood O_2 tension or oxyhemoglobin saturation.

hypoxia Low or reduced O_2 concentration or tension at any specified point in the transfer system from inspired gas to the metabolizing tissues. Also, insufficient O_2 tension or insufficient concentration of free O_2 molecules to meet the requirements of aerobic metabolism. **Histohypoxia:** Refers to reduced or insufficient P_{O_2} at the tissue or cellular level. **Hypoxidation:** A state or condition of reduced aerobic metabolism in association with the reduced energy requirements of hypothemia hibernation, hypothyroidism, or the effect of certain drugs. **Hypoxidosis:** A state or condition of impaired aerobic metabolism in hypoxia, enzyme deficiency or dysfunction, substrate lack, or excessive accumulation of metabolites. Paradoxically, hypoxidosis may result from hyperbaric oxygenation.

isobar A line connecting points of equal pressure or tension on a graph. **Example:** the lines connecting points of equal CO_2 tension on the pH-bicarbonate diagram.

midposition The end-expiratory or end-tidal level or position of the lung-chest system under any given conditions, defining the functional residual capacity. Sometimes called *respiratory level.* Do not confuse with midcapacity.

minute volume of breathing The volume of gas inspired or expired per minute under any given conditions. Usually, *expiratory minute volume* expressed as expired gas volume/min at BTPS. Note that *expired* gas usually differs from *inspired* gas with regard to temperature, and water vapor, CO_2, and O_2 contents.

open-circuit A type of breathing system used in cardiopulmonary technology in which gas is inspired through a limb or breathing branch connected to the gas source and is expired through a directional valve into a collecting reservoir or vented so that rebreathing does not occur. **Compare:** closed-circuit.

orthopnea Dyspnea decubitus; difficult breathing in a supine position relieved by sitting upright.

O_2 uptake The rate at which O_2 is *removed* by the blood from alveolar gas. Also termed *O_2 intake.* **Distinguish:** the rate at which O_2 is *used* by the metabolizing tissues, termed *O_2 consumption.* When a steady state of the respiration and circulation exists, *O_2 uptake* equals *O_2 consumption.* **Compare:** *CO_2 output* as opposed to *CO_2 production.*

partial pressure The *pressure* or *tension* exerted by any constituent gas in a mixture; the most significant measurement with respect to the physicochemical and physiologic behavior of a gas. As described by Dalton's law, the *total* pressure of a gas mixture is the arithmetic sum of all the *individual* partial pressures of the constituent gases.

plethysmograph An instrument for measuring volume or volume changes, especially those due to circulation; the *body plethysmograph* ("body box") for measuring thoracic gas volume.

pneumoperitoneum The presence of air or gas within the peritoneal cavity of the abdomen. It may be *spontaneous,* as from rupture of a hollow gas-containing organ, or *induced* for diagnostic or therapeutic purposes.

pneumothorax The presence of air or gas within either or both pleural cavities, resulting in corresponding lung collapse. *Spontaneous* pneumothorax results from unexpected rupture of a lung. Chest injury, such as that producing lung puncture, may result in *traumatic* pneumothorax. If the lung is torn in such a way that a tissue flap forms a directional valve favoring passage of air from bronchus to pleural space, an emergency termed *tension* pneumothorax results. When gas or air is deliberately injected into the pleural space for diagnostic or therapeutic purposes, the condition is termed *induced* or *artificial* pneumothorax.

polycythemia An excess of blood, especially its formed elements, usually expressed in terms of hemoglobin concentration or erythrocyte count. *Polycythemia vera* or *erythremia* is a disease characterized by excessive blood formation with increased blood volume and increases of all formed elements in the blood. *Erythrocytosis* refers to increased red blood cell count. Other polycythemias include those secondary to hypoxemia in the following conditions: (1) normal fetal condition, (2) altitude exposure, (3) chronic, diffuse bronchopulmonary disease, or (4) chronic alveolar hypoventilation. Hypoxemia has been found to increase production of the bone marrow–stimulating hormone, erythropoietin. **Compare:** anemia.

pressure breathing The use of various mechanical devices to *assist* spontaneous respiration for O_2 therapy or delivery of aerosol medication or to *control* and *regulate* pulmonary ventilation. Such breathing devices may be *pressure-cycled* or *volume-cycled,* and may employ *continuous* or *intermittent, positive* or *negative* (subatmospheric) pressure. These devices vary with respect to their dynamic flow-pressure characteristics, and their proper selection and application in a given clinical problem are a challenge to the knowledge and skill of the inhalation therapist.

pulmonary artery wedge pressure The pressure recorded through the tip of a catheter wedged in a small branch of the pulmonary artery; believed to reflect changes in left atrial pressure.

pulmonary edema A clinical term referring to a transudate of body fluids within the alveolar spaces of the lung. Usually it is the result of increased intravascular pressure. Such fluid may interfere greatly with respiratory gas exchange. **Compare:** *pulmonary interstitial edema,* which usually occurs earlier and is an accumulation of transudate fluid within the pulmonary tissues.

shunt A circulatory communication that bypasses alternate channels. Shunts may be (1) physiologic and intermittently open, (2) the result of trauma, (3) the result of abnormal fetal development, or (4) the result of failure of normal fetal communications to undergo postnatal closure.

stethomeiotic A neologism; any condition causing or associated with a reduction of chest volume below its normal value. Such condition may be congenital, acquired, temporary, or permanent.

surface tension A property of liquids that is due to intermolecular attractive forces, or cohesion, and to the specific orientation of molecules at the boundary of a liquid. A force exerted in the plane of the interface that acts to preserve the integrity of the surface of separation and to resist rupture of the surface film. The tension upon the surface of a liquid in contact with another fluid with which it does not mix. An exposed liquid surface tends to contract to the smallest possible area, forming spheroidal drops (one surface) or bubbles (two surfaces). Laplace's law relates surface tension and radius to pressure. Surface tension is expressed as dynes/cm or as ergs/cm^2.

surfactant A generic term for compounds that orient themselves at the phase boundary between two fluids, for example, the boundary between alveolar gas and the liquid alveolar lining layer. Pulmonary surfactants in the alveolar lining layer concentrate at the gas-hypophase boundary, altering the surface tension of the liquid in which they reside.

tension See ***partial pressure.***

"***true oxygen***" The calculated concentration as either percent or fraction, which, when multiplied by the expiratory minute volume at STPD, gives the O_2 uptake.

Valsalva maneuver A forceful expiratory effort against a closed glottis, producing various cardiopulmonary physiologic changes. **Example:** straining at stool or straining during childbirth. **Compare:** *Müller maneuver,* which is a forceful inspiratory effort against a closed glottis.

ventilation-perfusion ratio *Matching* of pulmonary *blood* distribution (perfusion) with pulmonary *gas* distribution (ventilation) in the lung. When the measured quantities, *ventilation* and *perfusion,* are expressed in the same units, an average ratio, $\dot{V}_A/\dot{Q}_c$, can be calculated. The *variability* of ventilation-perfusion ratios from one lung unit to another is termed unevenness, inequality, or nonuniformity. Ventilation-perfusion ratio is a subject of great physiologic importance. See ***distribution.***

Selected bibliography

GENERAL

Bates, D. V., MacKlem, P. T., and Christie, R. V.: Respiratory function in disease, ed. 2, Philadelphia, 1971, W. B. Saunders Co.

Caro, C. G., editor: Advances in respiratory physiology, Baltimore, 1966, The Williams & Wilkins Co.

Cherniack, R. M., and Cherniack, L.: Respiration in health and disease, Philadelphia, 1961, W. B. Saunders Co.

Comroe, J. H., Jr.: Physiology of respiration, Chicago, 1965, Year Book Medical Publishers, Inc.

Dejours, P.: Respiration. Translated by L. E. Farhi, New York, 1966, Oxford University Press, Inc.

de Rueck, A. V. S., and O'Connor, M., editors: Pulmonary structure and function, a CIBA Foundation Symposium, Boston, 1962, Little, Brown & Co.

Fenn, W. O., and Rahn, H., editors: Handbook of physiology, section 3, Respiration, vol. 1, Baltimore, 1964, The Williams & Wilkins Co.

Fenn, W. O., and Rahn, H., editors: Handbook of physiology, section 3, Respiration, vol. 2, Baltimore, 1965, The Williams & Wilkins Co.

Gordon, B. L., editor: Clinical cardiopulmonary physiology, ed. 3, New York, 1969, Grune & Stratton, Inc.

Grover, R. F., editor: Progress in research in emphysema and chronic bronchitis, vol. 1, Normal and abnormal pulmonary circulation, Basel, 1963, S. Karger AG.

Mitchell, R. S., editor: Progress in research in emphysema and chronic bronchitis, vol. 2, The pathogenesis of the chronic obstructive bronchopulmonary disease, Basel, 1965, S. Karger AG.

Negus, Sir V.: The biology of respiration, Baltimore, 1965, The Williams & Wilkins Co.

Peters, J. P., and Van Slyke, D. D.: Quantitative clinical chemistry, vol. 1, Interpretations, ed. 2, Baltimore, 1946, The Williams & Wilkins Co.

Rushmer, R. F., editor: Methods in medical research, vol. 11, Chicago, 1966, Year Book Medical Publishers, Inc.

SOURCES OF DATA

Altman, P. L., and Dittmer, D. S., editors: Biology data book, Washington, D. C., 1964, Federation of American Societies for Experimental Biology.

Altman, P. L., and Dittmer, D. S., editors: Environmental biology, Bethesda, Md., 1966, Federation of American Societies for Experimental Biology.

Altman, P. L., and Dittmer, D. S., editors: Respiration and circulation, Bethesda, Md., 1971, Federation of American Societies for Experimental Biology.

Carpenter, T. M.: Tables, factors, and formulas for computing respiratory exchange and biological transformations of energy, ed. 4, Washington, D. C., 1964, Carnegie Institution of Washington Publication 303C.

Cassels, D. E., and Morse, M.: Cardiopulmonary data for children and young adults, Springfield, Ill., 1962, Charles C Thomas, Publisher.

Cherniack, R. M.: Ventilatory function in normal children, Canad. Med. Ass. J. 87:80, 1962.

Dittmer, D. S., editor: Blood and other body fluids, Washington, D. C., 1961, Federation of American Societies for Experimental Biology.

Dittmer, D. S., and Grebe, R. M., editors: Handbook of respiration, Philadelphia, 1958, W. B. Saunders Co.

The Matheson Company, Inc.: Matheson gas data book, ed. 4, East Rutherford, N. J., 1966.

Slonim, N. B.: Cardiopulmonary physiological data for healthy Denver-acclimatized man, proceedings of a symposium, Denver, Colo., 1965, Cardiopulmonary Research Club of Colorado.

CHAPTER 1. RESPIRATION AND METABOLISM

Daggs, R. G.: Energy metabolism and metabolic reference standards. In Steele, J. M., editor: Methods in medical research, vol 6, Chicago, 1954, The Year Book Publishers, Inc., pp. 74-84.

Daggs, R. G.: Respiratory exchange. In Steele, J. M., editor: Methods in medical research, vol. 6, Chicago, 1954, The Year Book Publishers, Inc., pp. 60-73.

Wolf, W., editor: Rhythmic functions in the living system, Ann. N. Y. Acad. Sci. **98**:753, 1962.

CHAPTER 2. LAWS DESCRIBING THE BEHAVIOR OF GASES

Crank, J.: The mathematics of diffusion, London, 1964, Oxford University Press.

CHAPTER 4. LUNG VOLUME AND ITS SUBDIVISIONS

de Reuck, A. V. S., and Porter, R., editors: Development of the lung, a CIBA Foundation Symposium, Boston, 1967, Little, Brown & Co.

Weibel, E. R.: Morphometry of the human lung, New York, 1963, Academic Press, Inc.

CHAPTER 6. PULMONARY CIRCULATION

de Reuck, A. V. S., and O'Connor, M., editors: Problems of pulmonary circulation, CIBA Foundation Study Group No. 8, London, 1961, J. & A. Churchill, Ltd.

Gorlin, R., and Warren, J. V.: Hemodynamic methods—heart and lungs. In Warren, J. V., editor: Methods in medical research, vol. 7, Chicago, 1958, The Year Book Publishers, Inc., pp. 60-127.

CHAPTER 7. BLOOD-GAS TRANSPORT

Henderson, L. J.: Blood, a study in general physiology, New Haven, 1928, Yale University Press.

CHAPTER 9. DISTRIBUTION OF INSPIRED GAS, DISTRIBUTION OF PULMONARY BLOOD FLOW, AND VENTILATION-PERFUSION RATIO

Rahn, H., and Fenn, W. O.: A graphical analysis of the respiratory gas exchange; the O_2-CO_2 diagram, Washington, D. C., 1955, American Physiological Society.

West, J. B.: Ventilation/blood flow and gas exchange, Oxford, 1965, Blackwell Scientific Publications.

CHAPTER 10. pH HOMEOSTASIS

Davenport, H. W.: The ABC of acid-base chemistry, ed. 4, Chicago, 1958, The University of Chicago Press.

Peters, J. P., and Van Slyke, D. D.: Hemoglobin and oxygen, carbonic acid and acid-base balance, Baltimore, 1931, The Williams & Wilkins Co.

Slonim, N. B., and Estridge, N. K.: The acid-base surface: a three-dimensional visual model for analysis of acid-base information, J. Med. Educ. **45**:826, 1970.

Woolmer, R. F., editor: A symposium on pH and blood gas measurement, methods and interpretation, London, 1959, J. & A. Churchill, Ltd.

CHAPTER 12. REGULATION OF PULMONARY VENTILATION

Brooks, C. M., Kao, F. F., and Lloyd, B. B., editors: Cerebrospinal fluid and the regulation of ventilation, Philadelphia, 1965, F. A. Davis Co.

Cunningham, D. J. C., and Lloyd, B. B., editors: The regulation of human respiration, proceedings of the J. S. Haldane Centenary Symposium, Philadelphia, 1963, F. A. Davis Co.

Howell, J. B. L., and Campbell, E. J. M.: Breathlessness, Philadelphia, 1966, F. A. Davis Co.

CHAPTER 14. RESPIRATORY RESPONSES TO UNUSUAL ENVIRONMENTS AND SPECIAL ATMOSPHERES

Slonim, N. B., and Estridge, N. K.: Carbon dioxide—environmental health aspects, J. Environ. Health **33**:171, 1970.

Slonim, N. B., and Estridge, N. K.: Ozone—an underestimated environmental hazard, J. Environ. Health **31**:577, 1969.

United States Department of Health, Education, and Welfare: Smoking and health, report of the Advisory Committee to the Surgeon General of the Public Health Service, Public Health Service Publication No. 1103, Washington, D. C., 1964, Government Printing Office.

CHAPTER 15. CLINICAL EVALUATION OF PULMONARY FUNCTION

Comroe, J. H., Jr.: Pulmonary function tests. In Comroe, J. H., Jr., editor: Methods in medical research, vol. 2, Chicago, 1950, The Year Book Publishers, Inc., pp. 74-244.

Comroe, J. H., Jr., Forster, R. E., II, Dubois, A. B., Briscoe, W. A., and Carlsen, E.: The lung, ed. 2, Chicago, 1962, Year Book Medical Publishers, Inc.

Darling, R. C., Cournand, A., and Richards, D. W., Jr.: Studies on the intrapulmonary mixture of gases. III. An open circuit method for measuring residual air, J. Clin. Invest. **19**:609, 1940.

Knowles, J. H.: Respiratory physiology and its clinical application, Cambridge, Mass., 1959, Harvard University Press.

Leuallen, E. C., and Fowler, W. S.: Maximal midexpiratory flow, Am. Rev. Tuberc. **72**:783, 1955.

Rossier, P. H., Buhlmann, A. A., and Wiesinger, K.: Respiration; physiologic principles and their clinical applications, edited and translated by C. Luchsinger and K. M. Moser, St. Louis, 1960, The C. V. Mosby Co.

Slonim, N. B., Bell, B. P., and Christensen, S. E.: Cardiopulmonary laboratory basic methods and calculations, a manual of cardiopulmonary technology, Springfield, Ill., 1967, Charles C Thomas, Publisher.

Index